# Coronary Artery Disease and Related Conditions Management

## Clinical Pathways, Guidelines, and Patient Education

### Health & Administration Development Group

**Jo Gulledge**
Executive Director

**Shawn Beard**
Research Editor

AN ASPEN PUBLICATION®
Aspen Publishers, Inc.
Gaithersburg, Maryland
1999

ASPEN CHRONIC DISEASE MANAGEMENT SERIES

Library of Congress Cataloging-in-Publication Data

Coronary artery disease and related conditions management:
clinical pathways, guidelines, and patient
education / Health & Administration Development Group;
Jo Gulledge, executive director; Shawn Beard, research editor.
p. cm. — (Aspen chronic disease management series)
Includes index.
ISBN: 0-8342-1704-X
1. Coronary heart disease Handbooks, manuals, etc.
I. Gulledge, Jo. II. Beard, Shawn. III. Health and
Administration Development Group (Aspen Publishers) IV. Series.

RC685.C6  C63134  1999
616.1'23—dc21      99-31850
CIP

Editorial Services: Marsha Davies

Copyright © 1999 by Aspen Publishers, Inc.

Orders: (800) 638-8437
Customer Service: (800) 234-1660

**About Aspen Publishers** • For more than 35 years, Aspen has been a leading professional publisher in a variety of disciplines. Aspen's vast information resources are available in both print and electronic formats. We are committed to providing the highest quality information available in the most appropriate format for our customers. Visit Aspen's Internet site for more information resources, directories, articles, and a searchable version of Aspen's full catalog, including the most recent publications: **http://www.aspenpublishers.com**
**Aspen Publishers, Inc.** • The hallmark  of quality in publishing
Member of the worldwide Wolters Kluwer group

Library of Congress Catalog Card Number: 99-31850
ISBN: 0-8342-1704-X

*Printed in the United States of America*

1 2 3 4 5

# Table of Contents

# Editorial Board

**Claire B. Rossé, RN, BS, MBA**
Founder and CEO
FutureHealth Corporation
Timonium, Maryland

**Rachel Stipe, RN, BS, CPHQ**
Quality Improvement/Reimbursement Specialist
Spectracare, Inc.
Louisville, Kentucky

**Maura J. Sughrue, MD**
Medical Director
Fairfax Family Practice Centers
Fairfax, Virginia

**Warren E. Todd, MBA**
Vice President, Business Development
Hastings Healthcare Group
Pennington, New Jersey

**Marcus D. Wilson, PharmD**
President
Health Core, Inc.
Newark, Delaware

# Introduction

Disease management is based on the understanding that a small proportion of the population—individuals with chronic conditions—consumes the vast majority of health care resources. Focusing on chronic illnesses, disease management programs strive to reduce costly hospitalizations through continual, rather than episodic, care. The logic is straightforward: providing a continuum of care dramatically reduces the incidence of acute episodes requiring inpatient treatment.

Because of disease management's emphasis on continual care, effective education of patients, families, and other informal caregivers is a vital component. Providers form partnerships with patients and families, teaching them to take daily responsibility for managing disease.

Coronary artery disease, and its related conditions, is one of several chronic disease states affecting millions of Americans. In fact, coronary heart disease is the leading cause of death for men and women in the United States. Because of its prevalence and gravity, it is imperative to create a disease-management program that aids clinicians in diagnosing and effectively treating the disease.

*Coronary Artery Disease and Related Conditions Management* provides comprehensive, detailed guidelines on all aspects of managing heart disease from the initial diagnosis in the clinical examination to the treatment strategy, which may include drug therapy, lifestyle modification, and nutrition intervention. *Coronary Artery Disease and Related Conditions Management* couples these clinical guidelines with patient education handouts, which teach patients to comply with interventions, while also learning the principles of demand management: recognizing and prioritizing their health care needs. Through education, patients know when professional interventions are required, and use resources accordingly.

To ensure quick access to the information clinicians need most, *Coronary Artery Disease and Related Conditions Management* is divided into two parts.

Part I, "Managing Coronary Artery Disease and Related Conditions: Clinical Pathways and Guidelines," addresses the essentials of administering heart disease management programs, with information on developing and implementing clinical guidelines/pathways, measuring and managing outcomes, and monitoring and improving patient satisfaction. While the guidelines originate from nationally recognized sources, their purpose is to serve as a starting point for providers and payers pursuing disease management. They are meant to be adapted to meet the needs of specific populations and to be further refined for individual patients.

Part II, "Self-Management of Coronary Artery Disease and Related Conditions: Patient Education," recognizes the patient education component of disease management. Consisting entirely of large-print patient handouts, including Spanish-language patient information sheets, this section is designed for clinicians across the care continuum to distribute freely to patients. The educational materials encourage patients and their families to become active partners in managing chronic conditions.

*Coronary Artery Disease and Related Conditions Management* is not intended to add new information to the abundant literature relevant to disease management, but rather to extract from hundreds of publications the most sound and useful information available. The goal is to provide this information in such a man-ner that is concise, practical, and pertinent. To that end, *Coronary Artery Disease and Related Conditions Management* distills the traditional narrative text and presents it in a quick-read format.

*Shawn K. Beard*
Research Editor
Health & Administration Development Group

ix

# Acknowledgments

Creating a reference volume such as *Coronary Artery Disease and Related Conditions Management* demands tremendous effort during the development period—shaping the manual's focus, collecting and evaluating materials, and ensuring that the format is practical and easy to use.

Foremost among the people who help us fulfill these responsibilities are the editorial board members. By answering queries, providing contacts, and reviewing materials, they play an instrumental role in the development of a high quality resource.

I am grateful to all the health care facilities, organizations, individual professionals, and others who generously shared their clinical guidelines, pathways, and patient education materials with us—special thanks to Lillian Gray, MS, Vice President of Medical Administration, Spaulding Rehabilitation Hospital, Boston, Massachusetts and Lynette Bennett, RN, Northwest Health Systems, Springdale, Arkansas.

In addition, this project never could have progressed from a bare-bones idea to a comprehensive resource without the untiring support of Rosemarie Cooper, Administrative Assistant; the skill of Marsha Davies, Editorial Services, and the guidance of Jo Gulledge, Executive Director, Health & Administration Development Group.

*Shawn Beard*
Research Editor
Health & Administration Development Group

# Tracking Form

## POLICY

Patient education documentation

## PURPOSE

To provide interdisciplinary documentation of patient/family education

## PROCEDURE

1. On admission, stamp the Tracking Form with patient's Addressograph plate and place in front of chart.
2. Within first three days of admission, have licensed nursing/therapy staff identify patient/family educational needs.
3. Read and follow directions 1–3 on the Tracking Form.
4. Fill out specific sections of the Tracking Form.

- **Document:** List of materials from manual by chapter.
- **Initial/Date Given:** As material is given, initial and date in the space provided.
- **Primary Caregiver:** Indicate who is receiving education information (the caregiver or the patient).
- **Comments:** Write comments regarding when material was reviewed (provide date/initials), with whom, and any required special needs.
- **Demonstrates Understanding of Activity:** Initial and date when primary caregiver has demonstrated understanding of activity (must be completed before discharge).
- **Other Classes Attended:** List other education opportunities (classes attended and additional handouts) not already listed.

5. Sign full name, with initials and title, on back of form.

### Place Facility Logo Here

A D D R E S S O G R A P H

## Coronary Artery Disease and Related Conditions Management

DIRECTIONS:
1. Highlight APPROPRIATE patient education materials.
2. Initial and date when material was given/reviewed/completed.
3. Use comments column for:
   a. Charting dates reviewed.
   b. Special patient/family needs.
   c. Receiver of education.

| DOCUMENT | Init/Date Given | Primary Caregiver | COMMENTS Init/Dates Material Reviewed • Special Needs • Who Received Education | Init/Date States &/or Demonstrates Understanding of Activity |
|---|---|---|---|---|
| **5. Overview of Coronary Artery Disease** | | | | |
| Facts about Coronary Heart Disease | | | | |
| Women and Coronary Heart Disease | | | | |
| **6. Unstable Angina and Myocardial Infarction** | | | | |
| Unstable Angina | | | | |
| La angina de pecho inestable | | | | |
| Heart Attack | | | | |
| Nitroglycerin | | | | |
| **7. Heart Failure** | | | | |
| What Is Heart Failure? | | | | |
| Managing Heart Failure | | | | |
| Medicines for Heart Failure | | | | |
| Medication Information for the Patient Who Has Heart Failure | | | | |
| Weekly Medicine Record | | | | |
| Diet and Heart Failure | | | | |
| Lifestyle and Heart Failure | | | | |
| Chest Pain and Heart Failure | | | | |
| Chest Pain Chart | | | | |
| Surgery for Heart Failure | | | | |
| Post Coronary Artery Bypass Graft (CABG) | | | | |
| La insuficiencia cardíaca | | | | |
| Pulmonary Edema | | | | |
| **8. Thrombophlebitis and Pulmonary Embolism** | | | | |
| Thrombophlebitis | | | | |
| Pulmonary Embolism | | | | |

| DOCUMENT | Init/Date Given | Primary Caregiver | COMMENTS Init/Dates Material Reviewed • Special Needs • Who Received Education | Init/Date States &/or Demonstrates Understanding of Activity | |
|---|---|---|---|---|---|
| **9. Cardiac Rehabilitation** | | | | | |
| Recovering from Heart Problems through Cardiac Rehabilitation | | | | | |
| How To Take Your Pulse— Determining Heart Rate | | | | | |
| Target Zone Heart Rate | | | | | |
| Walking for Heart Health | | | | | |
| Calories Burned during Physical Activities | | | | | |
| **10. Cholesterol and Heart** | | | | | |
| What Makes Blood Cholesterol High or Low | | | | | |
| Cholesterol and Your Risk of Heart Disease | | | | | |
| What Your Blood Cholesterol Levels Mean If You **Do Not** Have Heart Disease | | | | | |
| What Your Blood Cholesterol Levels Mean If You **Do** Have Heart Disease | | | | | |
| Questions You May Have about Your High Blood Cholesterol | | | | | |
| Three Steps To Reducing Your High Blood Cholesterol Levels | | | | | |
| Proteja su corazón—Baje su colesterol | | | | | |
| Ask Your Health Professionals about High Blood Cholesterol | | | | | |
| High Blood Cholesterol Glossary | | | | | |
| Know Your Cholesterol Level | | | | | |
| Conozca su nivel de colesterol | | | | | |
| Medicine for High Blood Cholesterol | | | | | |
| **11. Nutrition for Heart Disease** | | | | | |
| Heart-Healthy Eating: the Step I and Step II Diets | | | | | |
| Sample Menus—Traditional American-Style Foods | | | | | |
| Sample Menus—Southern-Style Foods | | | | | |
| Sample Menus—Mexican American-Style Foods | | | | | |
| The Heart-Healthy Eating Plan | | | | | |
| Your Diet after Coronary Artery Bypass Graft | | | | | |
| Congestive Heart Failure and Your Diet | | | | | |

| DOCUMENT | Init/Date Given | Primary Caregiver | COMMENTS Init/Dates Material Reviewed • Special Needs • Who Received Education | Init/Date States &/or Demonstrates Understanding of Activity |
|---|---|---|---|---|
| Myocardial Infarction and Your Diet | | | | |
| Shop to Your Heart's Content | | | | |
| Serving Sizes for Meat and Cheese | | | | |
| Reduzca la grasa—No el sabor | | | | |
| Cooking the Heart-Healthy Way | | | | |
| New Ways To Use Favorite Recipes | | | | |
| Eat Right When Eating Out | | | | |
| Saturated Fat, Total Fat, Cholesterol, Calories, and Sodium in Basic Foods | | | | |

| OTHER CLASSES ATTENDED/HANDOUTS GIVEN | INIT | SIGNATURE |
|---|---|---|
| | | |
| | | |
| | | |
| | | |
| | | |

# PART I

# Managing Coronary Artery Disease and Related Conditions: Clinical Pathways and Guidelines

# 1. Coronary Artery Disease and Disease Management

## IMPORTANCE*

Mortality from coronary artery disease (CAD) has been declining in the United States over the past two decades, but CAD and related diagnoses are a major cause of morbidity and mortality among adults. In 1990, almost 500,000 deaths were attributable to CAD. From 1973 through 1987, cardiovascular mortality decreased 42% in the age group under 54 years and decreased 33% in the age group 55–84 years. Annually, about 1.5 million people are newly diagnosed with CAD and the direct and indirect health care costs are estimated to be $47 billion.

## EFFICACY OR EFFECTIVENESS OF INTERVENTIONS*

There are a number of risk factors that, if modified, can prevent development of CAD, including elevated serum cholesterol, low levels of high-density lipoprotein cholesterol, uncontrolled hypertension, cigarette smoking, obesity, and physical inactivity.

An analysis of 19 randomized trials that evaluated the effect of cholesterol reduction on total mortality and the incidence of CAD found that reducing cholesterol was effective in lowering the incidence of CAD but reductions had to be at least 8% to 9% to effectively reduce total mortality. For every 1% reduction in cholesterol, an estimated 2.5% reduction in disease incidence was found. The trials showed greater effect from cholesterol-lowering drugs than from dietary modifications. The US Preventive Services Task Force (USPSTF) has recommended that all adults have their blood cholesterol and serum cholesterol checked every five years.

Hypertension is a risk factor for CAD as well as for stroke and cerebrovascular disease. If the average diastolic blood pressure for the entire population was reduced by 6–8 mm Hg, the incidence of CAD would be reduced by 25%. Although there is general agreement that high blood pressure control should contribute to reductions in the incidence of and mortality from CAD, hypertension intervention trials involving diuretics and beta-blockers have not demonstrated significant reductions in CAD. This may be because multiple risk factors for heart disease (eg, serum cholesterol and smoking) tend to cluster together and multifactorial treat-

ment may be required. The Public Health Service (PHS) recommends that blood pressure be measured regularly to screen for hypertension in all individuals who are three years of age or older and that the measurements be made every two years if the last blood pressure readings were in the normal range (140 mm Hg systolic and 85 mm Hg diastolic) and annually if the last diastolic blood pressure was 85–89 mm Hg. Once hypertension is confirmed, the patient should receive counseling about exercise, weight reduction, dietary sodium intake, and alcohol consumption. The *Healthy People 2000* objectives for the nation call for 50% of persons with hypertension to have their blood pressure under control and for 90% to be taking actions to bring their blood pressure under control.

Smoking is responsible for over 115,000 deaths annually from CAD. About 27% of American adults smoke. Smoking cessation can contribute to reductions in deaths from CAD; the benefits become evident as soon as two years after quitting. Clinical trials of smoking cessation techniques have concluded that effectiveness depends on several factors, including: use of multiple modes, frequent contact with the patient, longer-length intervention, the use of face-to-face techniques, and both physician and nonphysician staff. Nicotine gum can increase long-term smoking cessation rates by about one third. Patient factors are also important (eg, level of dependence, motivation to quit). A meta-analysis of 38 clinical trials found differences in cessation rates of unselected patients to be 8% after six months and 6% after one year.

Obesity is a risk factor for CAD; about 10% of women and 20% of men in the Framingham study were obese. It is difficult to assess the independent effect of weight reduction on cardiovascular risk because of the close association between obesity and other risk factors (eg, hypercholesterolemia). Many weight reduction interventions that have been studied demonstrate short-term efficacy but the results are not maintained in the long term. The best results have been achieved in conservative programs that involve behavior therapy, nutrition education, and exercise programs and that are typically targeted at persons with mild to moderate obesity. The USPSTF recommends that persons who are 20% or more above their desired weight (as determined by standard life insurance tables) be referred to appropriate nutritional and exercise counseling.

The relationship between cardiovascular fitness and exercise is strongly positive, but the clinical and public health implications of this finding are less clear. Efficacy studies limited to secondary prevention trials report a 66% compliance rate and a 15% reduction in total mortality. Two recent studies have found that regular exercise provides a protective effect against triggering sudden onset of a myocardial infarction during strenuous exercise. The risk of heart attack among sedentary people during vigorous exercise was 7 times greater in one study and 100 times greater in the other

---

*Source: Elizabeth A. McGlynn, "Choosing Chronic Disease Measures for HEDIS: Conceptual Framework and Review of Seven Clinical Areas," *Managed Care Quarterly*, Vol. 4:3, Aspen Publishers, Inc., © 1996.

study than during lighter activity or no activity. In both studies, among people who exercise regularly, there was no increase in the risk of heart attack. There is some suggestion that regular, heavy exertion exercise may prevent the development and progression of heart disease.

The other preventive strategy that has been recommended (by the USPSTF) for men is low doses of aspirin on alternate days to prevent a first myocardial infarction. A review of three female cohort studies did not support a general recommendation that asymptomatic women take aspirin as a preventive measure; there was some evidence of benefit among high-risk women.

Thus, a number of primary prevention strategies have been suggested as important for reducing the likelihood of developing CAD. The risk profile of the population enrolled in a health plan may provide some measure of the potential for preventing the development of heart disease. In the short run, the success of programs designed to modify these risk factors might be examined.

There are a number of secondary and tertiary prevention interventions available for the treatment of heart disease. Lowering plasma cholesterol can slow the progression of established coronary artery disease. Effective medications are available for the treatment of chronic angina and unstable angina. Improved prehospital care for acute myocardial infarction has been shown to reduce mortality. Major advances have been made in the acute and postacute treatment of myocardial infarction. Some deaths among patients hospitalized for acute myocardial infarction may be preventable. Thrombolytic therapy after acute myocardial infarction may reduce mortality among those hospitalized by an average of 24% with the largest benefit accruing to those receiving therapy within six hours of the onset of symptoms. The benefits of thrombolytic therapy are even greater among the elderly; 2.1 nonelderly lives versus 4.2 elderly lives per 100 admissions for heart attack would be saved with this therapy. Similarly, the use of beta-blockers after myocardial infarction proportionally reduces the risk of death by about 22%.

Three leading cardiac procedures are used in the diagnosis and treatment of persons with heart disease: coronary angiography, coronary artery bypass graft surgery (CABG), and percutaneous transluminal coronary angioplasty (PTCA). Previous studies of angiography and CABG have found significant numbers of these interventions performed for inappropriate clinical indications. Although more recent studies have reported considerably lower rates of inappropriate procedure use, these studies were done in New York State, which has an active program to monitor outcomes of cardiac procedures. It is likely that other regions of the country would not produce the impressive results found in New York State.

## POTENTIAL FOR IMPROVING QUALITY*

Considerable potential exists for improving the quality of care for persons at risk for developing or who have already developed CAD, including primary, secondary, and tertiary interventions.

About 10% of adults have serum cholesterol levels that are associated with a fourfold increase in the risk of coronary death. The recent HEDIS pilot study found that among persons continuously enrolled for five years in any one of the 21 participating health plans, 67% had a cholesterol screen in the previous five years; the range by individual health plan was from 34% to 87%. Reducing cholesterol levels by 10% among half of the high-risk population has been estimated to result in a 3.5% reduction in coronary mortality. Thus, continued efforts to identify persons with high cholesterol and to reduce cholesterol levels will contribute to reduced incidence of heart disease and coronary deaths.

The second National Health and Nutrition Examination Survey (NHANES II) found that 54% of adults with hypertension were aware they had high blood pressure, but only 11% had their blood pressure under control. Another study found that 66% of hypertensives knew they had high blood pressure but only 24% had their blood pressure under control. A recent study of unionized New York City health care workers found that 71% of hypertensives were aware of their condition but only 12% had their blood pressure controlled. The findings of this study are particularly important for quality improvement because the study subjects had fairly high levels of physician visits (9.6 annually in the uncontrolled group versus 19.4 in the controlled group).

The USPSTF has estimated that if every primary care provider offered the brief smoking cessation counseling intervention that has been shown to be effective to all of their patients who currently smoke, an additional 1 million Americans would quit smoking annually; currently 1.3 million quit annually. One study found that more than one third of smokers seen in university internal medicine practices reported that a physician had never suggested that they stop smoking.

Increasing the use of thrombolytic therapy for persons with a recent myocardial infarction from 40% to about 75% of eligible patients has been estimated to reduce mortality by 9.3%. On average, only about 18% of all patients with a heart attack currently receive thrombolytic therapy. Similarly, increasing the use of beta-blockade after myocardial infarc-

*Source: Elizabeth A. McGlynn, "Choosing Chronic Disease Measures for HEDIS: Conceptual Framework and Review of Seven Clinical Areas," *Managed Care Quarterly*, Vol. 4:3, Aspen Publishers, Inc., © 1996.

tion from 40% to 75% of eligibles could reduce coronary mortality by 8.4%.

Because coronary angiography is the most common cardiac procedure and provides a pathway to both CABG surgery and PTCA, examining the appropriateness of use of this procedure may be an excellent quality indicator. In addition to examining appropriateness, examining the volume of procedures performed by hospitals providing care for managed care enrollees might provide additional indirect evidence of quality.

## COST-EFFECTIVENESS OF INTERVENTIONS*

An Australian study investigated the cost-effectiveness of three alternative strategies for reducing blood cholesterol levels: a high-risk strategy (identifying and treating men with cholesterol levels greater than 6.5 mmol/L with diet and drug), a moderate/high-risk strategy (diet counseling for those with 5.5 to 6.5 mmol/L cholesterol levels plus the same strategy for high-risk persons), and a population strategy (dietary change for the entire population regardless of cholesterol levels). The cost-effectiveness ratios (costs per heart disease events saved) in Australian dollars were $482,224 (high-risk), $369,098 (moderate/high-risk), and $46,667 (population-based). The authors suggest further research on strategies to alter the eating habits of the entire population. A US study comparing targeted versus populationwide interventions for lowering serum cholesterol also concluded that populationwide strategies were indicated.

Another study compared the cost-effectiveness of treatment alternatives for elevated serum cholesterol, hypertension, and symptomatic CAD in reducing the risk of CAD. The author concluded that the recommendations from the National Cholesterol Education program went beyond the scientific evidence and did not adequately account for problems with adherence to diet and drug regimens as well as the costs of widespread implementation. The cost-effectiveness of drug treatment for both high cholesterol and hypertension depends on the target population.

Evaluations of thrombolytic therapy and beta-blockage have demonstrated the cost-effectiveness of these therapeutic interventions.

An analysis of the cost-effectiveness of CABG surgery as compared to medical therapy found that surgery was an excellent value for persons with three-vessel or left main disease and a reasonable value for persons with two-vessel disease who had severe angina that was uncontrollable by medication. The results of cost-effectiveness comparisons of CABG and PTCA are dependent on the time frame evaluated because of the high rate of PTCA failure; five-year costs are $39,656 for CABG and $32,838 for PTCA.

## HEALTH PLAN ROLE IN PROVIDING INTERVENTIONS*

The role of health plans in providing secondary and tertiary interventions for the treatment of CAD is noncontroversial. The considerable expense and potential for negative outcomes associated with mismanaging these patients suggests careful attention to best practices is warranted. More controversial may be the role of the health plan in risk factor modification. For many of these activities, the health plan itself may not reap the benefits of the intervention (ie, if the person does not remain with the health plan for life). The surveillance and intervention programs are not inexpensive and health plans may argue that public health interventions for certain aspects of risk factor modification (eg, smoking cessation, dietary changes) may be more appropriate. The presence of quality indicators in these areas, however, would send a strong signal that health plans should be responsible for offering these interventions.

Areas for quality measurement development are:

1. rates of cholesterol screening within the past five years by age and gender
2. adequacy of follow-up for elevated cholesterol levels (eg, dietary counseling, drug therapy)
3. proportion of persons in the plan with coronary artery disease who have elevated cholesterol levels
4. proportion of persons in the plan with hypertension whose blood pressure is outside the normal range
5. proportion of persons in the plan who smoke who have not received a smoking cessation intervention in the past two years
6. proportion of persons with myocardial infarctions who appropriately receive thrombolytic therapy

*Source: Elizabeth A. McGlynn, "Choosing Chronic Disease Measures for HEDIS: Conceptual Framework and Review of Seven Clinical Areas," *Managed Care Quarterly*, Vol. 4:3, Aspen Publishers, Inc., © 1996.

*Source: Elizabeth A. McGlynn, "Choosing Chronic Disease Measures for HEDIS: Conceptual Framework and Review of Seven Clinical Areas," *Managed Care Quarterly*, Vol. 4:3, Aspen Publishers, Inc., © 1996.

# 2. Assessment

**EMERGENCY DEPARTMENT (ED) ALGORITHM/PROTOCOL FOR PATIENTS WITH SYMPTOMS AND SIGNS OF AMI**

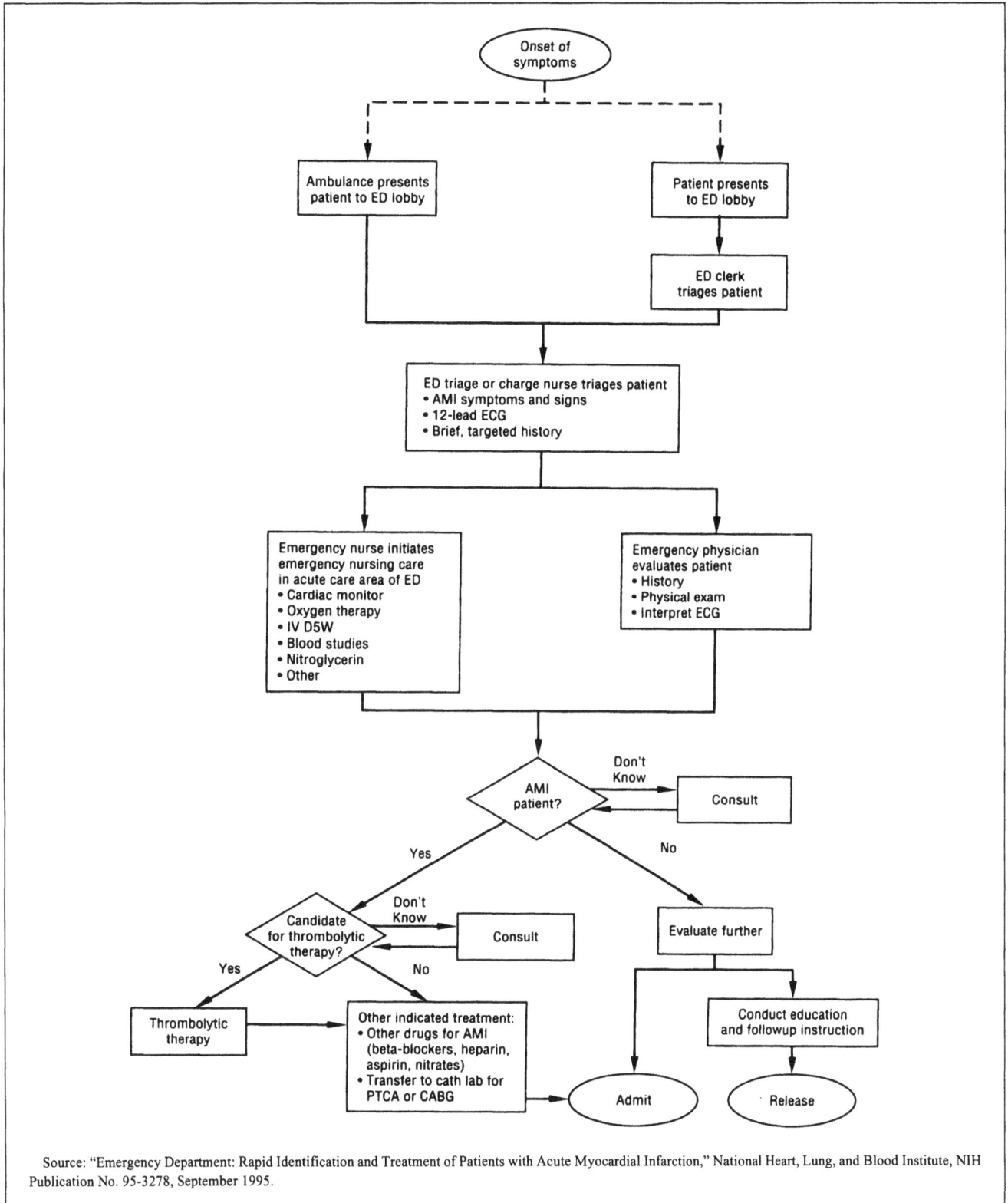

Source: "Emergency Department: Rapid Identification and Treatment of Patients with Acute Myocardial Infarction," National Heart, Lung, and Blood Institute, NIH Publication No. 95-3278, September 1995.

7

## TIME AS CRITICAL TO OPTIMAL OUTCOME FOR AMI*

Time is critical to an optimal outcome for patients with acute myocardial infarction (AMI). Major trials of thrombolytic therapy—the definitive therapy for AMI in 1993—have documented maximum treatment benefit during the first one to two hours following symptom onset. Additionally, one half of AMI deaths occur suddenly, within one hour of the onset of symptoms.

An ultimate goal of the National Heart Attack Alert Program (NHAAP) is to reduce the interval between the onset of symptoms (Time 0) and definitive treatment in the emergency department (ED Time 4). The following exhibits examine the emergency department's contribution to overall delay and recommend measures that will shorten the time that lapses between the patient's arrival at the emergency department and the administration of thrombolytic therapy (the "door-to-drug" or "door-to-needle" time, or ED Time 1 to ED Time 4).

*Source: "Emergency Department: Rapid Identification and Treatment of Patients with Acute Myocardial Infarction," National Heart, Lung, and Blood Institute, NIH Publication No. 95-3278, September 1995.

The AHA has recommended that thrombolytic treatment of eligible AMI patients occur within 30 to 60 minutes of their arrival in the emergency department. Emergency departments should strive to achieve the minimum 30-minute, door-to-drug time goal recommended by the AHA for patients with a clear diagnosis of AMI. Published reports and analyses of AMI diagnosis and treatment have demonstrated that a door-to-drug time of 30 minutes for the clearly defined AMI patient is feasible and reasonable. Emergency departments can move toward this goal by assessing the time they spend on each critical interval and instituting policies and protocols to evaluate and expedite the care processes for patients with symptoms and signs of AMI. Recommendations for changes in care should be based on an analysis of the data coupled with an understanding of the operational characteristics unique to that emergency department. Changes should be made while continuing to monitor time-interval data and other aspects of patient care. Continued refinements should be based on ongoing data analysis.

It is hoped this will facilitate the treatment of AMI patients by emergency departments with the same sense of urgency as victims of trauma. Other educational efforts will need to be undertaken to bring these patients to the emergency department door early after symptom onset so they can receive maximum benefit from the state-of-the-art, emergency department AMI care.

## AMI TIME-TO-TREATMENT FLOWSHEET

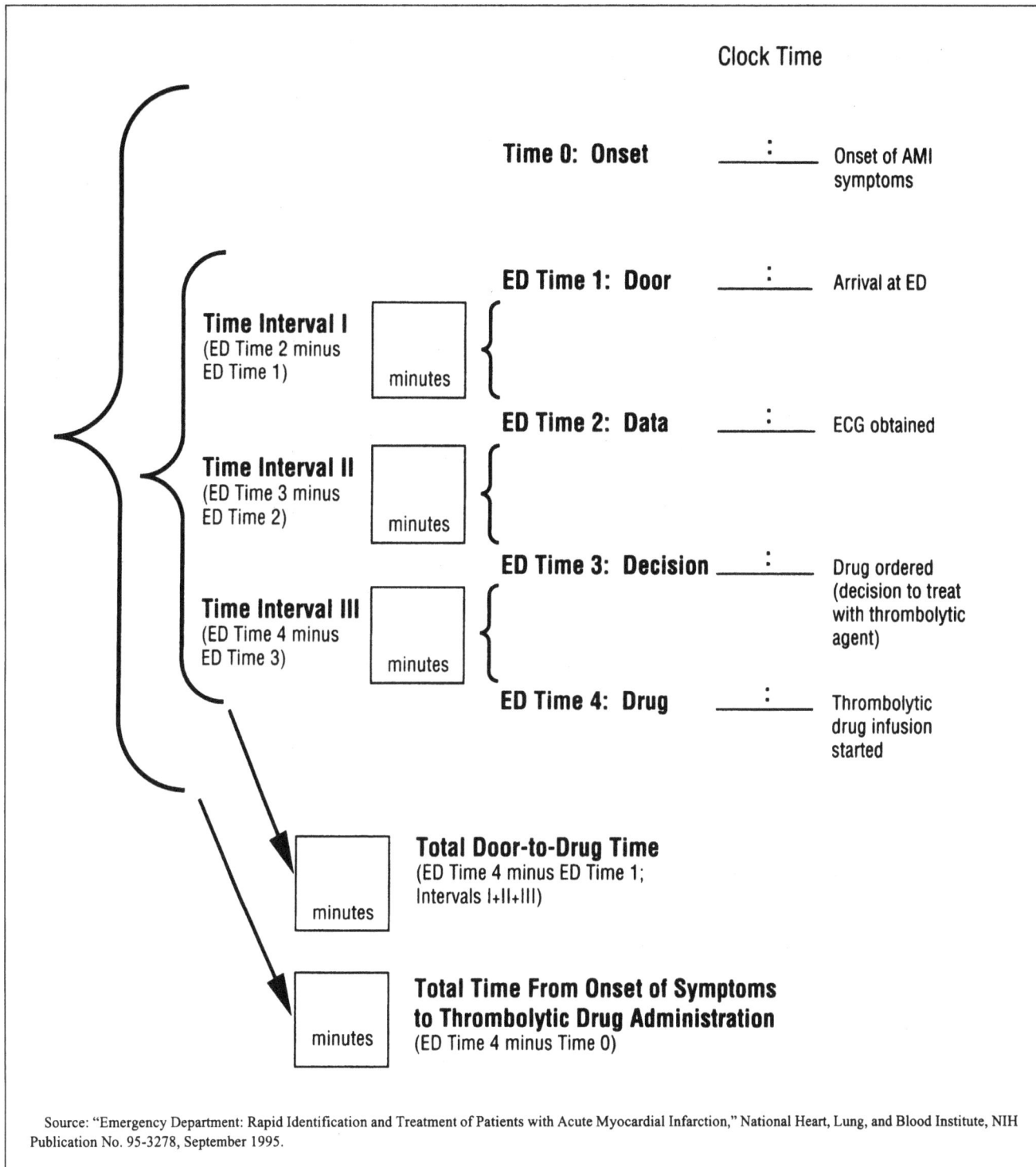

Clock Time

**Time 0: Onset** _____:_____ Onset of AMI symptoms

**Time Interval I**
(ED Time 2 minus
ED Time 1)

| minutes |

**ED Time 1: Door** _____:_____ Arrival at ED

**ED Time 2: Data** _____:_____ ECG obtained

**Time Interval II**
(ED Time 3 minus
ED Time 2)

| minutes |

**ED Time 3: Decision** _____:_____ Drug ordered (decision to treat with thrombolytic agent)

**Time Interval III**
(ED Time 4 minus
ED Time 3)

| minutes |

**ED Time 4: Drug** _____:_____ Thrombolytic drug infusion started

| minutes |

**Total Door-to-Drug Time**
(ED Time 4 minus ED Time 1;
Intervals I+II+III)

| minutes |

**Total Time From Onset of Symptoms
to Thrombolytic Drug Administration**
(ED Time 4 minus Time 0)

Source: "Emergency Department: Rapid Identification and Treatment of Patients with Acute Myocardial Infarction," National Heart, Lung, and Blood Institute, NIH Publication No. 95-3278, September 1995.

## EMERGENCY DEPARTMENT IDENTIFICATION AND TREATMENT OF AMI—TIMEPOINTS FOR CQI

The following questions about each of the four timepoints of care may help an emergency department examine and refine its care of AMI patients:

**Door**

- Is there appropriate prehospital communication with rescue units?
- How does a patient who arrives ambulatory with symptoms suggesting AMI move into a clinical treatment area?
- How does a patient whom the prehospital care provider or triage nurse suspects may be having an AMI come to the attention of the treating physician?

**Data**

- Who has the authority to order an ECG on an emergency department patient, and what criteria are used to determine whether it is needed?
- How rapidly is an ECG obtained once it is ordered?
- What is the process and how swift is the process for getting the ECG and/or its interpretation to the treating physician?

**Decision**

- Who has the authority to order thrombolytic therapy for an emergency department patient having an ST-segment-elevation AMI?
- What is the mechanism for obtaining appropriate consultation when the emergency physician is uncertain of what to do?

**Drug**

- Is thrombolytic therapy routinely administered in the emergency department or deferred to the coronary care unit?
- What is the process by which the thrombolytic drug is prepared for infusion once the decision to use it has been made?
- Are aspirin, heparin, nitrates, and beta-blockers appropriately administered to AMI patients in the emergency department without delaying initiation of thrombolytic therapy?
- Is the information needed to obtain the patient's informed consent presented clearly and efficiently?

Source: "Emergency Department: Rapid Identification and Treatment of Patients with Acute Myocardial Infarction," National Heart, Lung, and Blood Institute, NIH Publication No. 95-3278, September 1995.

# GUIDELINES FOR EMERGENCY DEPARTMENT REGISTRATION CLERK'S AND/OR TRIAGE NURSE'S IDENTIFICATION OF AMI PATIENTS

## REGISTRATION/CLERICAL STAFF

Patients over 30 years of age with the following chief complaints require immediate assessment by the triage nurse and should be referred for further evaluation:

### Chief Complaint

- Chest pain, pressure, tightness, or heaviness. Radiating pain in neck, jaw, shoulders, back, or one or both arms
- Indigestion or "heartburn"/nausea and/or vomiting
- Persistent shortness of breath
- Weakness/dizziness/light-headedness/loss of consciousness

## TRIAGE NURSE

Patients with the following symptoms and signs require immediate assessment by the triage nurse for initiating the AMI protocol:

### Chief Complaint

- Chest pain. Patients over 30 years of age with chest pain or severe epigastric pain, nontraumatic in origin, having components typical of myocardial ischemia or infarction:
  - central/substernal compression or crushing chest pain
  - pressure, tightness, heaviness, cramping, burning, aching sensation
  - unexplained indigestion/belching
  - radiating pain in neck, jaw, shoulders, back, or one or both arms
- Associated dyspnea
- Associated nausea/vomiting
- Associated diaphoresis

If these symptoms are present, obtain stat ECG.

### Medical History

The triage nurse should do a brief, targeted, initial history assessing for current or past history of:

- coronary artery bypass grafting, angioplasty, coronary artery disease, or AMI
- nitroglycerin use to relieve pain
- risk factors including smoking, hyperlipidemia, hypertension, diabetes mellitus, family history, cocaine use

This brief history **must not** delay entry into the AMI protocol.

### Special Considerations

- Questions have been raised as to whether women may present more frequently with atypical chest pain and symptoms.
- Diabetic patients may have atypical presentations due to autonomic dysfunction.
- Elderly patients may have stroke, syncope, or change in mental status.

Source: "Emergency Department: Rapid Identification and Treatment of Patients with Acute Myocardial Infarction," National Heart, Lung, and Blood Institute, NIH Publication No. 95-3278, September 1995.

## GENERALLY ACCEPTED ELIGIBILITY/EXCLUSION CRITERIA: THROMBOLYTIC THERAPY FOR AMI

### 1. ELIGIBILITY CRITERIA

**Clinical**

Chest pain or chest-pain-equivalent syndrome consistent with AMI $\leq$12 hours from symptom onset with:

**ECG**

- $\geq$1 mm ST elevation in $\geq$2 contiguous limb leads
- $\geq$2 mm ST elevation in $\geq$2 contiguous precordial leads
- New bundle branch block

**Cardiogenic Shock**

Emergency catheterization and revascularization if possible; consider thrombolysis if catheterization not immediately available.

### 2. CONTRAINDICATIONS

**Absolute Contraindications**

Require consideration of other reperfusion strategy, such as PTCA or CABG

- altered consciousness
- active internal bleeding
- known spinal cord or cerebral arteriovenous malformation or tumor
- recent head trauma
- known previous hemorrhagic cerebrovascular accident
- intracranial or intraspinal surgery within 2 months
- trauma or surgery within 2 weeks, which could result in bleeding into a closed space
- persistent blood pressure >200/120 mm Hg
- known bleeding disorder
- pregnancy
- suspected aortic dissection
- previous allergy to a streptokinase product (but not a contraindication to use of other thrombolytic agents)

**Relative Contraindications**

- active peptic ulcer disease
- history of ischemic or embolic cerebrovascular accident (CVA)
- current use of oral anticoagulants
- major trauma or surgery >2 weeks, <2 months
- history of chronic, uncontrolled hypertension (diastolic >100 mm Hg), treated or untreated
- subclavian or internal jugular venous cannulation

Source: "Emergency Department: Rapid Identification and Treatment of Patients with Acute Myocardial Infarction," National Heart, Lung, and Blood Institute, NIH Publication No. 95-3278, September 1995.

# 3. Guidelines for Managing CAD and Related Conditions

## GUIDELINES FOR DETECTING AND MANAGING HIGH BLOOD CHOLESTEROL*

### Background

An increased blood cholesterol level, specifically high LDL-cholesterol, increases risk for coronary heart disease (CHD). Conversely, lowering total cholesterol and LDL-cholesterol levels reduces CHD risk. Two approaches can be taken to lower blood cholesterol levels in the American population. One is a clinical approach that identifies individuals at high risk who need intensive intervention efforts. The second is a public health (population) approach that aims to shift the distribution of cholesterol levels in the entire population to a lower range through dietary change. The two approaches are complementary and together represent a coordinated strategy for reducing coronary risk.

The first Adult Treatment Panel (ATP) report published in 1988 outlined a systematic clinical approach to treatment of high blood cholesterol in adults. It was followed in 1990 by the report of the Laboratory Standardization Panel, which made recommendations for improving the accuracy of cholesterol measurement, and by the report of the Population Panel, which set forth a public health approach, and in 1991 by the Children's Panel report. Together these four reports provide the basis for the National Cholesterol Education Program's (NCEP) strategy for control of high blood cholesterol in Americans.

Since the first ATP report was published in 1988, several issues have emerged and will be summarized briefly here.

### CHD Risk Status as a Guide to Intensity of Therapy

The intensity of treatment of the individual patient depends on the patient's risk status. Those at higher risk for CHD should receive more aggressive intervention than patients at lower risk. There is a spectrum of risk from very high to low, and patients should be categorized into three general risk categories when a decision is made about the appropriate cholesterol-lowering therapy; these include (1) those at highest risk for future CHD events because of prior CHD or other atherosclerotic disease (eg, peripheral arterial disease or symptomatic carotid artery disease); (2) patients without evident CHD who are at high risk because of high blood cholesterol together with multiple other CHD risk factors; and (3) patients with high blood cholesterol but who are at low risk otherwise. The latter group especially includes young adult men (<35 years) or premenopausal women.

### Cholesterol Management in Patients with CHD and Other Atherosclerotic Diseases

Clinical trials demonstrate conclusively that serum cholesterol lowering will reduce morbidity and mortality from CHD in patients with established CHD. In addition, pooling of data from available clinical trials reveals a definite trend toward decreased total mortality in these patients. Treatment of elevated LDL-cholesterol in patients with prior CHD and/or other atherosclerotic disease is called "secondary prevention," whereas clinical management of patients without CHD is called "primary prevention." This distinction is somewhat arbitrary, since atherosclerosis is a long-term process and the risk status of high-risk individuals is not fundamentally different on the day before their myocardial infarction than on the day after it. Secondary prevention nonetheless receives increased emphasis in this report, since a substantial proportion of new CHD events occurs in patients with established CHD, and it appears that many CHD patients are not getting the aggressive cholesterol-lowering therapy that is warranted.

### The Total Mortality Issue in Primary Prevention of CHD

Clinical trials demonstrate that serum cholesterol lowering will reduce new CHD events and CHD mortality in primary prevention, ie, in patients without established CHD. An important question is whether cholesterol lowering will also reduce total mortality in primary prevention. Individual clinical trials have not had the size or power to evaluate the issue of total mortality and have not provided a conclusive answer to this question. Neither individual clinical trials nor meta-analyses of pooled data reveal a reduction in total mortality. Some analyses of drug trials raise the possibility of increases in non-CHD mortality resulting from drug therapy that offset the benefit of reduction in CHD mortality. However, the causes of non-CHD mortality are different in different trials, and it is not known whether these reported increases in non-CHD mortality are due to drug therapy or to chance. Dietary therapy has not been found to be associated with increased non-CHD mortality. Therefore, evidence that cholesterol lowering will reduce CHD morbidity and mortality supports efforts to use dietary therapy in primary prevention for patients with high cholesterol levels and to reserve

*Source: Second Report of the Expert Panel on Detection, Evaluation, and Treatment of High Blood Cholesterol in Adults, National Cholesterol Education Program, National Heart, Lung, and Blood Institute, NIH Publication No. 93-3096, September 1993.

drug treatment for high-risk patients in whom the benefits outweigh the potential side effects. The possibility of adverse effects from drug treatment as well as considerations of cost warrants the recommendation to be cautious about drug therapy in primary prevention for patients not at high risk from multiple risk factors or very high LDL-cholesterol levels. Cholesterol lowering through dietary means and physical activity is safer, and these should be the major form of therapy for primary prevention. Therefore, it is recommended that drug treatment be used sparingly in young adult men and premenopausal women.

## Low HDL-Cholesterol

There is growing evidence that a low HDL-cholesterol level imparts increased risk for CHD. Therefore, a low HDL-cholesterol (<35 mg/dL) is classified as a major risk factor for CHD, and HDL-cholesterol should be measured in initial risk assessment when accurate testing is available. A high HDL-cholesterol also appears to be protective against CHD, and levels $\geq$60 mg/dL can be called a "negative" risk factor. LDL-cholesterol is the primary target of cholesterol-lowering therapy because direct clinical trial evidence for the benefit of lowering LDL is strong, and similar evidence for raising HDL is less conclusive. However, therapeutic decisions should take into account HDL-cholesterol levels. For low HDL levels, hygienic therapies are the first line of treatment: physical activity, smoking cessation, and weight loss in the overweight. If drug therapy is needed to lower LDL levels in a patient with a high LDL who also has a low HDL, agents that raise HDL levels should be considered.

## Young Adults

In young men (<35 years) and premenopausal women, elevated total and LDL-cholesterol levels increase the long-term risk of CHD. Nevertheless, young men and premenopausal women with moderately high LDL-cholesterol levels (160 to 220 mg/dL) are at relatively low risk for CHD in the near future unless they have multiple other risk factors, particularly diabetes mellitus or a family history of premature CHD. For these patients who are otherwise at low risk, cholesterol lowering through dietary means and increased physical activity is warranted, but drug therapy should be delayed. For most young adult men and premenopausal women, drug therapy should be considered when LDL-cholesterol levels are very high ($\geq$220 mg/dL) or multiple other risk factors are also present.

## High Blood Cholesterol in Women

Elevated blood cholesterol levels increase the risk of CHD in women, although after age 65 the relationship is somewhat less consistent than before that age. In general, women are at lower risk for CHD than are men of the same age. As indicated above, premenopausal women in particular are at low risk. Although CHD risk in women lags behind that of men by about 10 years, risk increases progressively after the menopause. Therefore, dietary therapy, combined with weight reduction in the obese, and increased physical activity are indicated in women with high cholesterol levels, but a more cautious approach in use of drugs is warranted for women compared to men of the same age. In premenopausal women, drug therapy for high cholesterol levels should generally be delayed. If postmenopausal women have unusually high LDL-cholesterol levels or multiple other risk factors, they can be considered for drug therapy; however, in many women with high LDL-cholesterol levels, use of estrogen replacement therapy may obviate the need for drug treatment.

## Age

CHD rates are much higher in elderly patients than in younger groups. As a result, despite the fact that the relative risk of CHD conferred by an elevated cholesterol is weaker in the elderly than in young or middle-aged adults, a high cholesterol level leads to more events in the elderly. A high proportion of all CHD events occurs in the elderly. While there are limited clinical trial data available in the elderly population, extrapolation of data from trials showing reduction in CHD risk in middle-aged patients seems reasonable. Angiographic studies show that even advanced coronary atherosclerosis responds to cholesterol-lowering treatment. These considerations suggest that substantial benefit in CHD risk reduction for the elderly may be achieved by cholesterol lowering. In spite of these generalizations, many elderly patients will not be suitable candidates for aggressive cholesterol lowering. These include patients of advanced physiologic or chronologic age or those with severe competing illnesses (eg, chronic congestive heart failure, dementia, advanced cerebrovascular disease, or active malignancy). On the other hand, elderly patients who are otherwise in good health and who can expect a reasonably long life in the absence of CHD should not be excluded from cholesterol-lowering therapy. The level of aggressiveness in cholesterol lowering depends on the assessment of CHD risk. Patients with established CHD or with multiple risk factors may warrant drug therapy, in addition to dietary therapy, whereas those at lower risk should be treated prudently with diet and exercise.

Consideration of all the above issues led the panel to make two changes in the guidelines. (1) The presence of CHD now places a patient in a separate category in which the goal for LDL-cholesterol lowering is set lower than before. (2) As in the first ATP report, determination of the risk status in patients without CHD depends not only on LDL-cholesterol levels but on other CHD risk factors as well. However, ATP

II identifies and defines the risk factors that modify the target goal for LDL-cholesterol (see the exhibit, "Risk Status Based on Presence of CHD Risk Factors Other Than LDL-Cholesterol") somewhat differently from ATP I. These now include age (≥45 years in men and ≥55 years in women), a family history of premature CHD, cigarette smoking, hypertension, low levels of HDL-cholesterol (<35 mg dL), and diabetes mellitus. A high level of HDL-cholesterol (≥60 mg/dL) is called a "negative" risk factor. In addition to these listed risk factors, obesity and physical inactivity are important CHD risk factors which physicians should treat as targets of intervention.

## Clinical Management of High Blood Cholesterol

Serum total cholesterol should be measured in all adults 20 years of age and over at least once every five years; HDL-cholesterol should be measured at the same time if accurate results are available. These measurements may be made in the nonfasting state. In individuals free of CHD, total cholesterol levels below 200 mg/dL are classified as "desirable blood cholesterol," those 200 to 239 mg/dL as "borderline-high blood cholesterol," and those 240 mg/dL and above as "high blood cholesterol." The cutpoint that defines high blood cholesterol (240 mg/dL) is a value above which risk for CHD rises more steeply and corresponds approximately to the 80th percentile of the adult US population (NHANES III). An HDL-cholesterol level below 35 mg/dL is defined as "low," and a low HDL-cholesterol level constitutes a CHD risk factor. The exhibit, "Initial Classification Based on Total Cholesterol and HDL-Cholesterol," summarizes these categories.

For primary prevention in adults without evidence of CHD, initial classification based on total cholesterol and HDL-cholesterol is outlined in the exhibit, "Primary Prevention in Adults without Evidence of CHD: Initial Classification Based on Total Cholesterol and HDL Cholesterol." For individuals with desirable blood cholesterol (<200 mg/dL), the level of HDL-cholesterol determines the appropriate follow-up. Those with HDL-cholesterol of ≥35 mg/dL are given general educational materials about dietary modification, physical activity, and other risk-reduction activities and advised to have repeat total cholesterol and HDL-cholesterol analysis in five years. Those with HDL-cholesterol levels less than 35 mg/dL should proceed to lipoprotein analysis. For individuals with total cholesterol levels of 200 to 239 mg/dL, the level of HDL-cholesterol and the presence or absence of multiple other CHD risk factors determine the follow-up. Those with an HDL-cholesterol of 35 mg/dL or greater and fewer than two other risk factors are given instruction in dietary modification, physical activity, and other risk-reduction activities and are advised to repeat total cholesterol

and HDL-cholesterol analysis in one to two years. Patients with total cholesterol levels of 200 to 239 mg/dL who have an HDL-cholesterol less than 35 mg/dL or two or more other risk factors should have a lipoprotein analysis. Lipoprotein analysis is also required for those whose total cholesterol is 240 mg/dL or greater. Lipoprotein analysis includes measurement of fasting levels of total cholesterol, total triglyceride, and HDL-cholesterol. From these values, LDL-cholesterol is calculated as follows:

$$\text{LDL-cholesterol} = \text{Total cholesterol} - \text{HDL-cholesterol} - (\text{triglyceride}/5)$$

Levels of LDL-cholesterol of 160 mg/dL or greater are classified as "high-risk LDL-cholesterol," those 130–159 mg/dL as "borderline-high-risk LDL-cholesterol," and those <130 mg/dL as "desirable LDL-cholesterol."

The clinical evaluation should include a complete history, physical examination, and basic laboratory tests. The aim is to determine whether a high LDL-cholesterol level is secondary to another disease or a drug, and whether a familial lipoprotein disorder is present. The patient's total coronary risk and clinical status, including age and sex, should be considered in developing a cholesterol-lowering program.

For primary prevention, subsequent classification based on LDL-cholesterol is shown in the exhibit, "Primary Prevention in Adults without Evidence of CHD: Subsequent Classification Based on LDL-Cholesterol." Individuals with desirable LDL-cholesterol levels (<130 mg/dL) do not need further evaluation and active medical therapy; they should be given information on diet and exercise designed for the general population and be reevaluated at five years. Those with borderline-high-risk LDL-cholesterol levels (130–159 mg/dL) who have fewer than two other CHD risk factors should be given instruction in dietary modification and physical activity and be reevaluated in one year. Patients with high-risk LDL-cholesterol levels (160 mg/dL) and those with borderline-high-risk LDL-cholesterol (130–159 mg/dL) who have two or more risk factors should be evaluated clinically and begin active cholesterol-lowering dietary therapy. Assignment of patients to these last two categories should be done on the basis of the average of two LDL-cholesterol determinations (see footnote to the following exhibit) to account for biologic variation.

For secondary prevention in adults with evidence of CHD or other clinical atherosclerotic disease, lipoprotein analysis is required in all patients and classification is based on LDL-cholesterol (see exhibit, "Secondary Prevention in Adults with Evidence of CHD: Classification Based on LDL-Cholesterol"). For these patients, the optimal LDL-cholesterol is 100 mg/dL or lower. When a patient has an optimal LDL-cholesterol level, instruction on diet and physical activity should be individualized and lipoprotein analysis repeated annually. When the LDL-cholesterol level is above

## RISK STATUS BASED ON PRESENCE OF CHD RISK FACTORS OTHER THAN LDL-CHOLESTEROL

Positive Risk Factors

- Age
  - Male: ≥45 years
  - Female: ≥55 years, or premature menopause without estrogen replacement therapy
- Family history of premature CHD (definite myocardial infarction or sudden death before 55 years of age in father or other male first-degree relative, or before 65 years of age in mother or other female first-degree relative)
- Current cigarette smoking
- Hypertension (≥140/90 mm Hg,* or on antihypertensive medication)
- Low HDL-cholesterol (<35 mg/dL*)
- Diabetes mellitus

Negative Risk Factor**

- High HDL-cholesterol (≥60 mg/dL)

High risk, defined as a net of two or more CHD risk factors, leads to more vigorous intervention. Age (defined differently for men and for women) is treated as a risk factor because rates of CHD are higher in the elderly than in the young, and in men than in women of the same age. Obesity is not listed as a risk factor because it operates through other risk factors that are included (hypertension, hyperlipidemia, decreased HDL-cholesterol, and diabetes mellitus), but it should be considered a target for intervention. Physical inactivity is similarly not listed as a risk factor, but it too should be considered a target for intervention, and physical activity is recommended as desirable for everyone.

*Confirmed by measurements on several occasions.
**If the HDL-cholesterol level is ≥60 mg/dL, subtract one risk factor (because high HDL-cholesterol levels decrease CHD risk).

Source: Second Report of the Expert Panel on Detection, Evaluation, and Treatment of High Blood Cholesterol in Adults, National Cholesterol Education Program, National Heart, Lung, and Blood Institute, NIH Publication No. 93-3096, September 1993.

## INITIAL CLASSIFICATION BASED ON TOTAL CHOLESTEROL AND HDL-CHOLESTEROL

Total Cholesterol

| | |
|---|---|
| <200 mg/dL | Desirable Blood Cholesterol |
| 200–239 mg/dL | Borderline-High Blood Cholesterol |
| ≥240 mg/dL | High Blood Cholesterol |

HDL-Cholesterol

| | |
|---|---|
| <35 mg/dL | Low HDL-Cholesterol |

Source: Second Report of the Expert Panel on Detection, Evaluation, and Treatment of High Blood Cholesterol in Adults, National Cholesterol Education Program, National Heart, Lung, and Blood Institute, NIH Publication No. 93-3096, September 1993.

without CHD or other atherosclerotic disease, the LDL-cholesterol levels for initiation of dietary therapy are: (a) ≥160 mg/dL in patients with fewer than two other CHD risk factors or (b)≥130 mg/dL in patients with two (or more) CHD risk factors. The goals of therapy are to lower LDL-cholesterol to levels below the cutpoints for initiating therapy: (a) to below 160 mg/dL if fewer than two other risk factors are present or (b) to below 130 mg/dL if two (or more) CHD risk factors are present. Patients whose LDL-cholesterol exceeds these levels are candidates for dietary therapy and increased physical activity. However, if an elevated LDL-cholesterol persists after an appropriate trial of dietary therapy, drug therapy may be considered. Candidates for drug therapy include patients with multiple CHD risk factors or severe forms of hypercholesterolemia. A limited number of patients with less severe elevations of LDL-cholesterol and fewer than two other CHD risk factors also may be candidates for drug therapy; examples are patients with diabetes mellitus or a family history of premature CHD. The LDL-cholesterol levels at which drug therapy may be considered after an adequate trial of dietary therapy are: (a) ≥190 mg/dL in patients with fewer than two other CHD risk factors, or (b) ≥160 mg/dL in patients with two (or more) CHD risk factors. Often drug therapy can be delayed in young adult men (<35 yrs) and premenopausal women who have LDL-cholesterol levels below 220 mg/dL and who are not otherwise at high risk.

In patients with CHD, therapy should be initiated if the LDL-cholesterol level is >100 mg/dL. The goal of therapy is to reduce LDL-cholesterol to 100 mg/dL or below. Maximal dietary therapy should be employed in patients in this category. If the LDL-cholesterol level remains ≥130 mg/dL with dietary therapy, drug treatment should be considered. However, if the LDL-cholesterol level is 100 to 129 mg/dL

optimal (>100 mg/dL), appropriate clinical evaluation should be carried out (see exhibit, "Secondary Prevention in Adults with Evidence of CHD: Classification Based on LDL-Cholesterol") and cholesterol-lowering therapy should be initiated.

The exhibit, "Treatment Decisions Based on LDL-Cholesterol," summarizes the levels for initiating dietary therapy and considering drug treatment in patients with and without CHD, and the LDL goals in these patients. For patients

**PRIMARY PREVENTION IN ADULTS WITHOUT EVIDENCE OF CHD: INITIAL CLASSIFICATION BASED ON TOTAL CHOLESTEROL AND HDL-CHOLESTEROL**

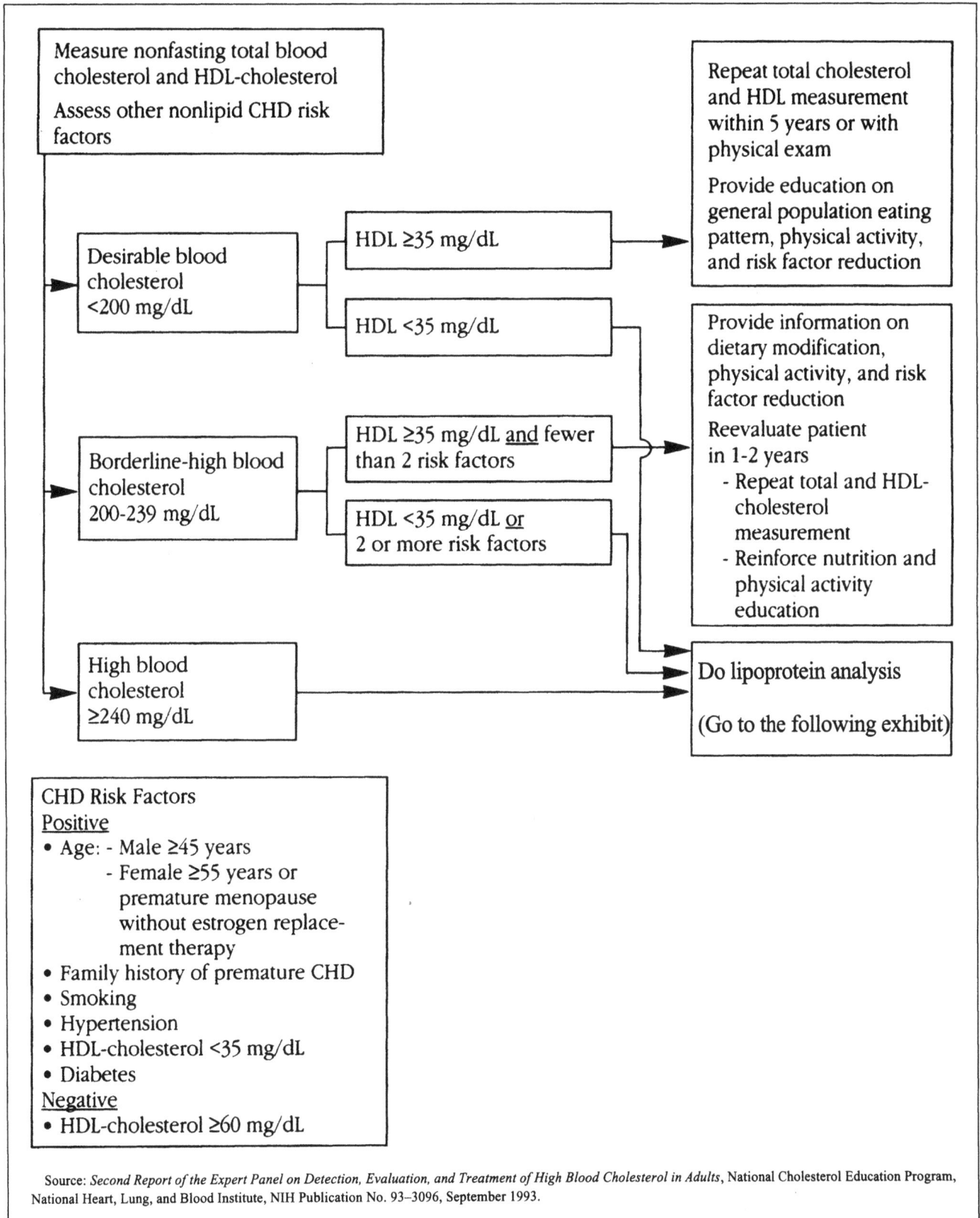

Measure nonfasting total blood cholesterol and HDL-cholesterol

Assess other nonlipid CHD risk factors

Repeat total cholesterol and HDL measurement within 5 years or with physical exam

Provide education on general population eating pattern, physical activity, and risk factor reduction

Desirable blood cholesterol <200 mg/dL

HDL ≥35 mg/dL

HDL <35 mg/dL

Borderline-high blood cholesterol 200-239 mg/dL

HDL ≥35 mg/dL <u>and</u> fewer than 2 risk factors

HDL <35 mg/dL <u>or</u> 2 or more risk factors

Provide information on dietary modification, physical activity, and risk factor reduction

Reevaluate patient in 1-2 years
 - Repeat total and HDL-cholesterol measurement
 - Reinforce nutrition and physical activity education

High blood cholesterol ≥240 mg/dL

Do lipoprotein analysis

(Go to the following exhibit)

CHD Risk Factors
<u>Positive</u>
• Age: - Male ≥45 years
        - Female ≥55 years or premature menopause without estrogen replace-ment therapy
• Family history of premature CHD
• Smoking
• Hypertension
• HDL-cholesterol <35 mg/dL
• Diabetes
<u>Negative</u>
• HDL-cholesterol ≥60 mg/dL

Source: *Second Report of the Expert Panel on Detection, Evaluation, and Treatment of High Blood Cholesterol in Adults*, National Cholesterol Education Program, National Heart, Lung, and Blood Institute, NIH Publication No. 93–3096, September 1993.

**PRIMARY PREVENTION IN ADULTS WITHOUT EVIDENCE OF CHD: SUBSEQUENT CLASSIFICATION BASED ON LDL-CHOLESTEROL**

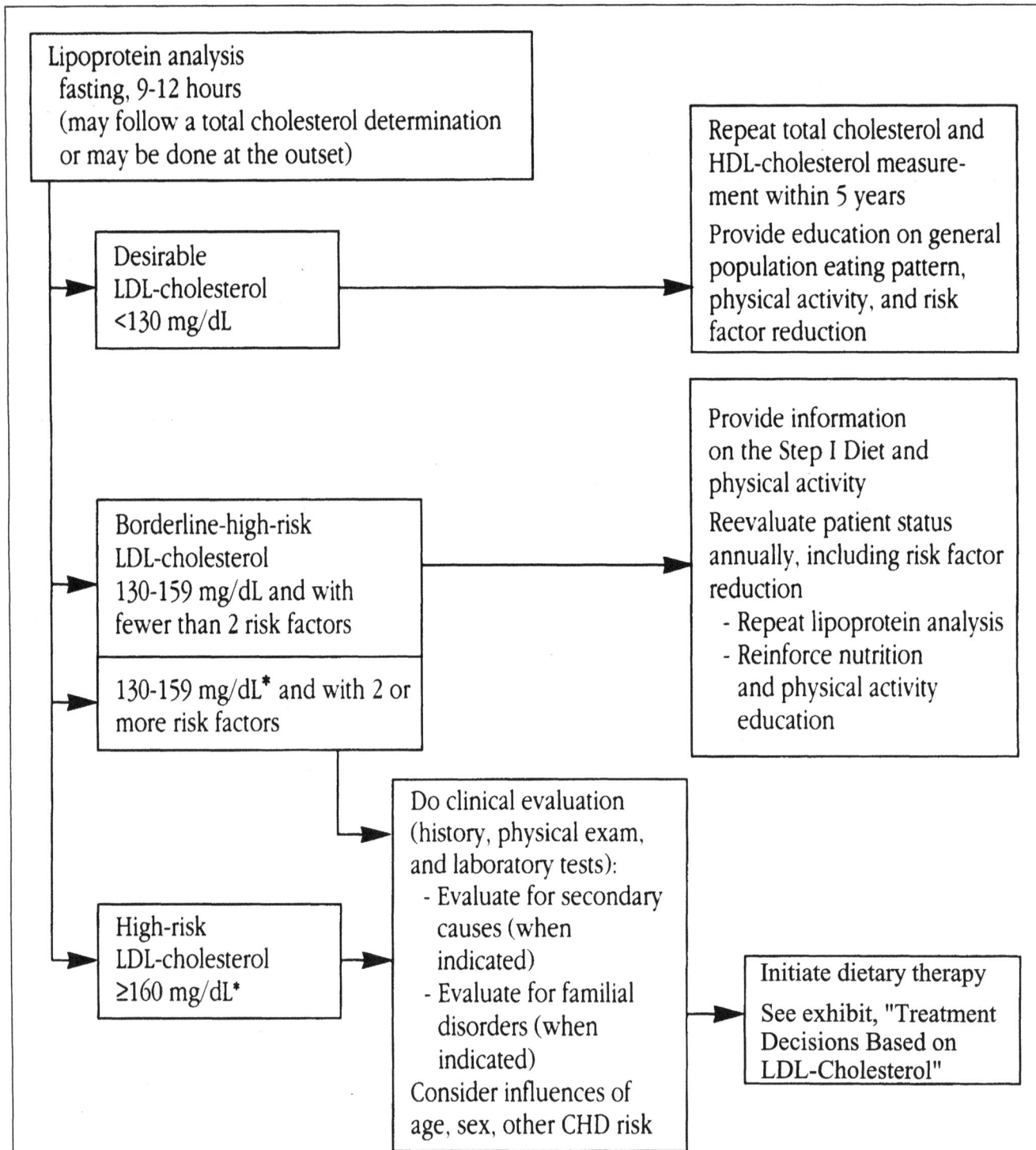

Lipoprotein analysis
fasting, 9-12 hours
(may follow a total cholesterol determination
or may be done at the outset)

Desirable
LDL-cholesterol
<130 mg/dL

→ Repeat total cholesterol and HDL-cholesterol measurement within 5 years

Provide education on general population eating pattern, physical activity, and risk factor reduction

Borderline-high-risk
LDL-cholesterol
130-159 mg/dL and with
fewer than 2 risk factors

130-159 mg/dL* and with 2 or
more risk factors

→ Provide information on the Step I Diet and physical activity

Reevaluate patient status annually, including risk factor reduction
- Repeat lipoprotein analysis
- Reinforce nutrition and physical activity education

Do clinical evaluation
(history, physical exam,
and laboratory tests):
- Evaluate for secondary
  causes (when
  indicated)
- Evaluate for familial
  disorders (when
  indicated)
Consider influences of
age, sex, other CHD risk

High-risk
LDL-cholesterol
≥160 mg/dL*

Initiate dietary therapy

See exhibit, "Treatment
Decisions Based on
LDL-Cholesterol"

*On the basis of the average of two determinations. If the first two LDL-cholesterol tests differ by more than 30 mg/dL, a third test should be obtained within one to eight weeks and the average value of the three tests used.

Source: *Second Report of the Expert Panel on Detection, Evaluation, and Treatment of High Blood Cholesterol in Adults*, National Cholesterol Education Program, National Heart, Lung, and Blood Institute, NIH Publication No. 93–3096, September 1993.

**SECONDARY PREVENTION IN ADULTS WITH EVIDENCE OF CHD:**
**CLASSIFICATION BASED ON LDL-CHOLESTEROL**

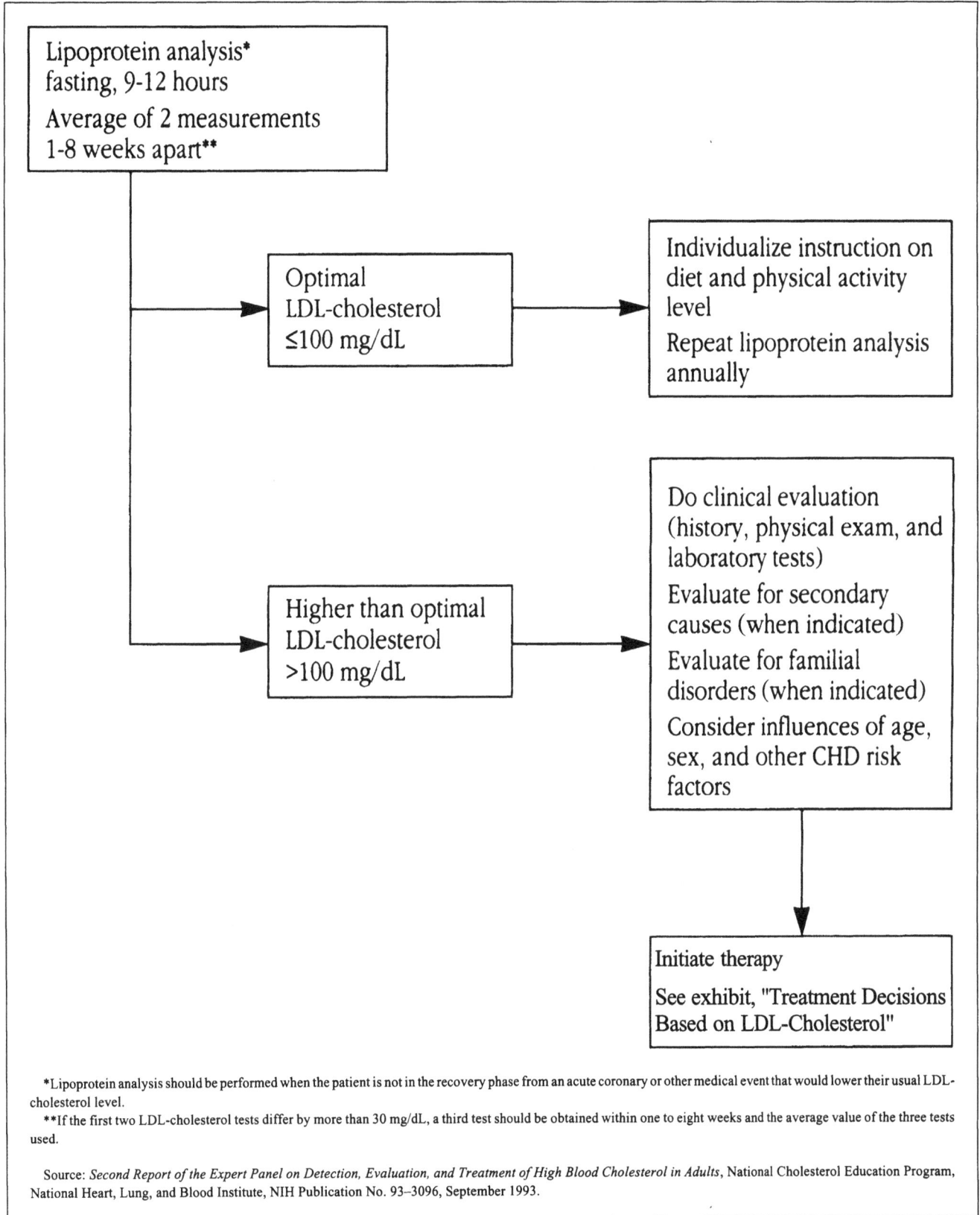

Lipoprotein analysis*
fasting, 9-12 hours
Average of 2 measurements
1-8 weeks apart**

Optimal
LDL-cholesterol
≤100 mg/dL

Individualize instruction on diet and physical activity level

Repeat lipoprotein analysis annually

Higher than optimal
LDL-cholesterol
>100 mg/dL

Do clinical evaluation (history, physical exam, and laboratory tests)

Evaluate for secondary causes (when indicated)

Evaluate for familial disorders (when indicated)

Consider influences of age, sex, and other CHD risk factors

Initiate therapy

See exhibit, "Treatment Decisions Based on LDL-Cholesterol"

*Lipoprotein analysis should be performed when the patient is not in the recovery phase from an acute coronary or other medical event that would lower their usual LDL-cholesterol level.

**If the first two LDL-cholesterol tests differ by more than 30 mg/dL, a third test should be obtained within one to eight weeks and the average value of the three tests used.

Source: *Second Report of the Expert Panel on Detection, Evaluation, and Treatment of High Blood Cholesterol in Adults*, National Cholesterol Education Program, National Heart, Lung, and Blood Institute, NIH Publication No. 93–3096, September 1993.

## TREATMENT DECISIONS BASED ON LDL-CHOLESTEROL

### Dietary Therapy

|  | Initiation Level | LDL Goal |
|---|---|---|
| Without CHD and with fewer than 2 risk factors | ≥160 mg/dL | <160 mg/dL |
| Without CHD and with 2 or more risk factors | ≥130 mg/dL | <130 mg/dL |
| With CHD | >100 mg/dL | ≤100 mg/dL |

### Drug Treatment

|  | Consideration Level | LDL Goal |
|---|---|---|
| Without CHD and with fewer than 2 risk factors | ≥190 mg/dL* | <160 mg/dL |
| Without CHD and with 2 or more risk factors | ≥160 mg/dL | <130 mg/dL |
| With CHD | ≥130 mg/dL** | ≤100 mg/dL |

*In men under 35 years of age and premenopausal women with LDL-cholesterol levels 190–219 mg/dL, drug therapy should be delayed except in high-risk patients such as those with diabetes.

**In CHD patients with LDL-cholesterol levels 100–129 mg/dL, the physician should exercise clinical judgment in deciding whether to initiate drug treatment.

Source: *Second Report of the Expert Panel on Detection, Evaluation, and Treatment of High Blood Cholesterol in Adults*, National Cholesterol Education Program, National Heart, Lung, and Blood Institute, NIH Publication No. 93–3096, September 1993.

with maximal dietary therapy, clinical judgment must be used as to whether to use cholesterol-lowering drugs. Likewise, if one drug brings the LDL-cholesterol level to this range, clinical judgment is required as to whether to add a second drug.

## Dietary Therapy and Physical Activity

The general aim of dietary therapy is to reduce elevated serum cholesterol while maintaining a nutritionally adequate eating pattern. Dietary therapy should occur in two steps, the Step I and Step II Diets; these are designed to progressively reduce intakes of saturated fatty acids (saturated fat) and cholesterol and to promote weight loss in patients who are overweight by eliminating excess total calories and increasing physical activity. The appropriate use of physical activity is considered an essential element in the nonpharmacologic therapy of elevated serum cholesterol.

The NCEP's eating pattern recommendation for the general public is similar in nutrient intake to the Step I Diet. Consequently, at time of detection of high blood cholesterol, many patients may already be adhering to the recommended diet. Therefore, an assessment of the patient's current dietary habits is necessary before prescribing a therapeutic diet. If the patient has not adopted the Step I Diet, this should be the first step of dietary therapy. The Step I Diet should be prescribed and explained by the physician and other involved health professionals. This diet involves an intake of saturated fat of 8% to 10% of total calories, 30% or less of calories from total fat, and cholesterol less than 300 mg/day. If the patient is already adhering to the Step I Diet at the time of detection, or if this diet proves inadequate to achieve the goals of dietary therapy, the patient should proceed to the Step II Diet. This diet calls for further reduction in saturated fat intake to less than 7% of calories and in cholesterol to less than 200 mg/day. The Step I Diet calls for the reduction of the major and obvious sources of saturated fat and cholesterol in the diet; for many patients this can be achieved without a radical alteration in dietary habits. The Step II Diet requires careful attention to the whole diet so as to reduce intake of saturated fat and cholesterol to a minimal level while maintaining an acceptable and nutritious diet. Involvement of a registered dietitian or other qualified nutrition professional is very useful, particularly for intensive dietary therapy such as the Step II Diet.

Weight reduction in overweight patients and increased physical activity are extremely important elements of therapy for high blood cholesterol. Weight reduction enhances the LDL-cholesterol lowering that can be achieved by reducing intakes of saturated fats and cholesterol. Both weight reduction and exercise not only promote reduction of cholesterol levels but have other benefits, ie, reducing triglycerides, raising HDL-cholesterol, reducing blood pressure, and decreasing the risk for diabetes mellitus. Thus they reduce risk for CHD in several ways beyond lowering LDL-cholesterol levels.

Patients with established CHD or other atherosclerotic disease should begin immediately on the Step II Diet. If the goals of therapy are achieved, as outlined above for secondary prevention, the patient will remain on this therapy. Assistance from a dietitian can facilitate maintenance of the Step II Diet in CHD patients. If the goals of therapy are not met, consideration can be given to using drugs. Dietary therapy is particularly important in these patients at high risk of recurrent CHD events, but the period for observing the results of the diet before initiating drug therapy can be relatively short.

In patients without CHD, after starting the therapeutic diet, the serum total cholesterol level should be measured and adherence to the diet assessed at four to six weeks and at three months. Although the goal of therapy is to lower LDL-cholesterol, most patients can be managed during dietary therapy on the basis of their total cholesterol levels. This has the advantage of avoiding the additional cost and the inconvenience of obtaining a fasting blood sample required to estimate LDL-cholesterol levels. For most patients, serum total cholesterol levels of 240 and 200 mg/dL correspond roughly to LDL-cholesterol levels of 160 and 130 mg/dL, respectively. Thus, the monitoring goals during dietary therapy are to lower serum total cholesterol to below 240 mg/dL for patients with an LDL-cholesterol goal of less than 160 mg/dL, or to below 200 mg/dL for patients with an LDL-cholesterol goal of less than 130 mg/dL. If the total cholesterol monitoring goal is met, then the LDL-cholesterol level should be measured to confirm that the LDL goal has been achieved. If this is the case, the patient enters a long-term monitoring program, and is seen quarterly for the first year and twice yearly thereafter. At these visits total cholesterol levels should be measured, and dietary and physical activity recommendations reinforced.

If the cholesterol goal has not been achieved with the Step I Diet, the patient generally should be referred to a dietitian. With the aid of the dietitian, the patient should progress to the Step II Diet, or to another trial on the Step I Diet (with progression to the Step II Diet if the response is still not satisfactory). On the Step II Diet, total cholesterol levels again should be measured and adherence to the diet assessed after four to six weeks and at three months of therapy. If the desired goal for total cholesterol (and for LDL-cholesterol) lowering has been attained, long-term monitoring can begin. If not, there is the option for the patient to further reduce saturated fat, and total fat if additional weight loss is needed. If the LDL-cholesterol level remains substantially above the target goal after dietary therapy, drug therapy should be considered. A minimum of six months of intensive dietary therapy and counseling generally should be carried out in primary prevention before initiating drug therapy; shorter periods can be considered in patients with severe elevations

of LDL-cholesterol (≥220 mg/dL). Drug therapy should be added to dietary therapy and not substituted for it.

## Drug Treatment

For primary prevention, drug treatment can be considered for an adult patient who despite dietary therapy has an LDL-cholesterol level of (a) 190 mg/dL or higher without two other risk factors, or (b) 160 mg/dL with two other risk factors. The goals of drug therapy are the same as those of dietary therapy: to lower LDL-cholesterol to below 160 mg/dL, or to below 130 mg/dL if two other risk factors are present. These are minimal goals; if possible, lowering levels of LDL-cholesterol even more is desirable. Drug therapy should be delayed in young adult men (<35 yrs) and premenopausal women without other risk factors whose LDL-cholesterol levels are in the range of 190 to 220 mg/dL.

Particularly in primary prevention, individualized clinical judgment is needed for patients who do not meet the criteria for drug therapy, but have not attained their minimal goals on dietary therapy and physical activity. These patients include those without two other risk factors whose LDL-cholesterol remains in the range of 160–190 mg/dL (or young adults in the range of 190–220 mg/dL) and patients with two other risk factors in the range of 130–160 mg/dL, on adequate dietary therapy. In general, maximal efforts should be made in this group to achieve lower cholesterol levels and lower CHD risk by means of nonpharmacologic approaches (diet, physical activity, and reduction of other CHD risk factors). Consideration may also be given to use of low doses of bile acid sequestrants in patients in these categories, especially in men.

For secondary prevention, the goal of therapy is an LDL-cholesterol of 100 mg/dL or lower. Drug therapy generally is indicated in patients with established CHD or other atherosclerotic disease if LDL-cholesterol levels are 130 mg/dL or greater after maximal dietary therapy. If the level is in the range of 100 to 129 mg/dL, clinical judgment that weighs potential benefit, possible side effects, and costs must be used in the decision for drug therapy.

In this report, drugs are classified into major drugs (bile acid sequestrants, nicotinic acid, and HMG CoA reductase inhibitors [statins]) and other drugs (fibric acids and probucol). Estrogen replacement in postmenopausal women is listed as a possible alternative or adjunct to drug therapy in those with elevated LDL-cholesterol levels.

Bile acid sequestrants (cholestyramine and colestipol) have a strong efficacy and safety record. They are especially valuable in patients with moderately elevated LDL-cholesterol, in primary prevention, and when drug therapy is necessary in young adult men and premenopausal women.

They also have utility in severe forms of hypercholesterolemia in combination with other drugs (eg, statins). Low doses of bile acid sequestrants can be effective in many patients whose LDL-cholesterol is not markedly elevated above the goal of therapy.

Nicotinic acid is effective in lowering total cholesterol and triglycerides and raising HDL-cholesterol levels. There is evidence that it reduces total mortality in secondary prevention trials. However, nicotinic acid has several side effects that limit its use in some patients; these include flushing and itching of the skin, gastrointestinal distress, liver toxicity, hyperglycemia, and hyperuricemia. Nicotinic acid is valuable in treating high blood cholesterol in patients with low HDL-cholesterol levels or when combined hyperlipidemia (elevated cholesterol and triglyceride) is present.

Statins (lovastatin, pravastatin, and simvastatin) are highly effective in lowering LDL-cholesterol. They appear to be relatively safe but long-term safety remains to be demonstrated. Therefore, they should be used with particular caution in young adult men and premenopausal women. The statins have not been proven to reduce risk for CHD when used alone, but in view of their efficacy for lowering LDL-cholesterol, they are attractive for treatment of severe forms of hypercholesterolemia and for maximal lowering of LDL levels in secondary prevention.

Fibric acids (eg, gemfibrozil) are effective triglyceride-lowering drugs. In some patients, they modestly lower LDL-cholesterol and raise HDL-cholesterol levels. They are not listed as major drugs because they do not usually produce substantial reductions in LDL-cholesterol levels. Thus they are not appropriate for maximal lowering of LDL levels in secondary prevention. However, these agents are valuable for treatment of very high triglyceride levels and for patients with familial dysbetalipoproteinemia (type 3 hyperlipoproteinemia). They also may have therapeutic utility for combined hyperlipidemia, as suggested by a controlled clinical trial, and for diabetic patients with elevated triglycerides.

Probucol is approved for treatment of high cholesterol levels. However, it has only a modest LDL-lowering effect and it has not been proven to reduce CHD rates in a clinical trial. It is therefore not listed as a major cholesterol-lowering drug.

For postmenopausal women with high serum cholesterol, consideration can be given to estrogen replacement therapy. Estrogens lower LDL-cholesterol levels and raise HDL-cholesterol levels. Epidemiologic studies suggest that their use reduces the risk for CHD, but there have been no large-scale controlled clinical trials to confirm this effect. In addition to CHD risk reduction, there is evidence for a retardation of osteoporosis. However, unopposed estrogen use is associated with side effects including increased risk for uterine cancer. Estrogen replacement therapy can be employed in postmenopausal women with elevated LDL-cholesterol, although confirmation of benefit in CHD risk reduction from clinical trials is still needed for certainty. Epidemiologic evidence for benefit of estrogen therapy is especially strong for secondary prevention in women with prior CHD.

After starting drug therapy, the LDL-cholesterol level should be measured at four to six weeks, and then again at three months. If the response to drug therapy is adequate (ie, the LDL-cholesterol goal has been achieved), the patient should be seen every four months, or more frequently when drugs requiring closer follow-up are used, to monitor the cholesterol response and possible side effects of therapy. For long-term monitoring, serum total cholesterol alone can be measured at most follow-up visits, with lipoprotein analysis (and LDL-cholesterol estimation) carried out once a year.

If the response to initial drug therapy is not adequate, the patient should be switched to another drug, or to a combination of two drugs. The combination of a bile acid sequestrant with either nicotinic acid or a statin has the potential of lowering LDL-cholesterol levels by 40% to 50% or more. For most patients, the judicious use of one or two drugs should provide an adequate LDL-cholesterol–lowering effect. Combined drug therapy is particularly indicated in those with severe forms of hypercholesterolemia and combined hyperlipidemia. Most cholesterol-lowering drugs can be used in combination, but a statin plus fibric acid (and possibly a statin plus nicotinic acid) carries an increased risk of myopathy.

Drug therapy is likely to continue for many years or a lifetime. Hence, the decision to add drug therapy to the regimen should be made only after vigorous efforts at dietary therapy have not proven sufficient. The patient must be well informed about the goals and side effects of medication and the need for long-term commitment. Consultation with a lipid specialist generally is needed only for patients with unusually severe, complex, or refractory lipid disorders, and the primary care provider can oversee the management of high blood cholesterol in most patients.

## Other Issues

### Hypertriglyceridemia

Elevated serum triglycerides are positively correlated with risk for CHD in univariate analysis, but they lose some or most of their ability to predict CHD in multivariate analysis, ie, when other lipid risk factors are added to the model. The link between triglycerides and CHD appears to be complex, and it may be explained by the association between high triglycerides, low HDL levels, and unusually atherogenic forms of LDL. In addition, elevated triglycerides often reflect an increase in triglyceride-rich, remnant lipoproteins that have atherogenic potential. In this document, triglyceride levels are classified as normal (<200 mg/dL), borderline-high (200–400 mg/dL), high (400–1000 mg/dL), and very high (>1000 mg/dL). Patients with borderline-high and high triglycerides may have accompanying dyslipidemias that increase risk for CHD (eg, familial combined hyperlipidemia and diabetic dyslipidemia). Those with triglyceride levels in excess of 1000 mg/dL are at increased risk for acute pancreatitis. Nonpharmacologic therapy (weight reduction in overweight patients, alcohol restriction, and increased physical activity) is recommended for all patients with elevated triglycerides. When triglycerides are elevated in association with "atherogenic" dyslipidemias (eg, familial combined hyperlipidemia), drug therapy may be indicated; the choice of drug preferably is one that effectively lowers triglycerides (eg, nicotinic acid). Drug therapy (fibric acids or nicotinic acid) generally is indicated in patients with very high triglycerides to prevent acute pancreatitis.

## Secondary Dyslipidemias

Common causes of secondary dyslipidemia include diabetes mellitus, the nephrotic syndrome, chronic renal failure, and hypothyroidism. Noninsulin-dependent diabetes mellitus (NIDDM) is frequently accompanied by elevated triglycerides and low HDL-cholesterol; in addition, LDL-cholesterol levels commonly are in the borderline-high-risk range. Because of the high risk for CHD resulting from NIDDM, aggressive lowering of LDL-cholesterol levels, similar to that recommended for established CHD, can be applied to diabetic patients. This is true for women diabetic patients as well as men because the protection against CHD normally afforded to women appears to be abolished in the presence of diabetes. Although nicotinic acid produces a favorable modification of the lipoprotein profile in NIDDM patients, it tends to worsen glucose tolerance, which limits the drug's utility. When high cholesterol levels predominate in diabetic patients, bile acid sequestrants or statin drugs appear to be preferable, whereas fibric acids may be preferred when elevated triglycerides predominate.

The dyslipidemia of the nephrotic syndrome should first be addressed with treatment of the underlying renal disease. Hypercholesterolemia is the major lipid abnormality in the chronic nephrotic syndrome, and it is responsive to the statins. Nicotinic acid (or fibric acids) can be used when the predominant abnormality is hypertriglyceridemia. The major lipid abnormality with chronic renal failure is hypertriglyceridemia, and because of potential side effects of lipid-lowering drugs the preferred therapy is nonphar-macologic, ie, weight control and minimizing use of drugs that raise triglyceride levels.

## Severe Forms of Hypercholesterolemia

Most severe forms of hypercholesterolemia in the absence of obvious disorders that might produce a secondary eleva-

tion of cholesterol levels are the result of genetic disorders of lipoprotein metabolism. Three such disorders are the most readily identified in clinical practice. Familial hypercholesterolemia occurs in 1 in 500 people and is characterized by severe elevations of LDL-cholesterol (often over 260 mg/dL), tendon xanthomas, and frequently premature CHD. Severe polygenic hypercholesterolemia manifests as LDL-cholesterol levels exceeding 220 mg/dL, and it occurs in about 1% of the adult population; premature CHD is common. Familial combined hyperlipidemia is characterized by elevations of total cholesterol, triglycerides, or both in different members of the same family; it also occurs in about 1% of the population, and affected patients are prone to premature CHD. Patients presenting with severe forms of hypercholesterolemia should undergo family screening to detect other candidates for therapy.

## High Blood Cholesterol and Concomitant Hypertension

Both high blood cholesterol and high blood pressure are common and frequently coexist in US adults. Both should be identified and treated appropriately. Diet, exercise, and other nonpharmacologic therapies are the essential first step for elevations of both blood pressure and cholesterol. Emphasis should be on weight reduction in overweight patients, but decreases in intakes of saturated fat, total fat, cholesterol, and alcohol consumption also are indicated. If drug therapy is required for blood pressure lowering, preference should be given to drugs that do not adversely affect plasma lipids; however, even though thiazides and beta-blockers may adversely affect lipids in some patients, they still may have utility in many patients because of efficacy, safety, and cost considerations. In some instances, drugs affecting lipid metabolism may interact adversely with antihypertensive agents, and awareness of possible interaction is needed in drug selection.

## Cost-Effectiveness Issues

The aggregate cost of CHD in the United States is enormous, costing the nation between $50 billion and $100 billion per year for medical treatment and lost wages. Prevention of CHD therefore could greatly reduce this economic toll. The least expensive way to reduce CHD is through the public health approach. This approach targets the whole population in an effort to reduce the major risk factors for CHD—especially smoking, hypertension, and high blood cholesterol—by public education, governmental policy, and private sector and industry commitment. The clinical strategy, which aims to identify and treat individuals at greatest risk for CHD, complements the public health approach. The clinical strategy, although necessary for risk reduction in high-risk patients, nonetheless carries costs for detection, therapy, and long-term monitoring in patients at risk from high blood cholesterol.

Cost-effectiveness analyses have been carried out for drug treatment of high blood cholesterol. According to these analyses, the cost to produce health benefits (increased longevity and improved quality of life) will be lowest in groups with the highest near-term risk for CHD. Three categories of patients have been identified for whom the cost-effectiveness of cholesterol-lowering drug treatment differs. Those at highest near-term risk for future CHD events and mortality are patients with established CHD, and the cost to produce health benefits is lowest for these patients. Next are patients with multiple risk factors or severely high choles-terol levels who also have a high risk for developing CHD in the near future. Costs are highest in those who have only moderate elevations of blood cholesterol and absence of other risk factors. These concepts parallel those for benefit/risk ratios: the greatest benefit relative to risk from choles-terol-lowering drug therapy is seen in patients at high risk for CHD. These parallel findings support the concept that drug therapy should be reserved primarily for high-risk patients, whereas those with high blood cholesterol who are otherwise at lower risk should be treated with dietary therapy and physical activity, which are safer and less expensive. None-theless these general principles may not always pertain to individual patients, and clinical judgment is required for shaping the best therapy for individuals.

## FOLLOW-UP TO CHOLESTEROL SCREENING

### Initial Classification Based on Total Cholesterol and HDL-Cholesterol

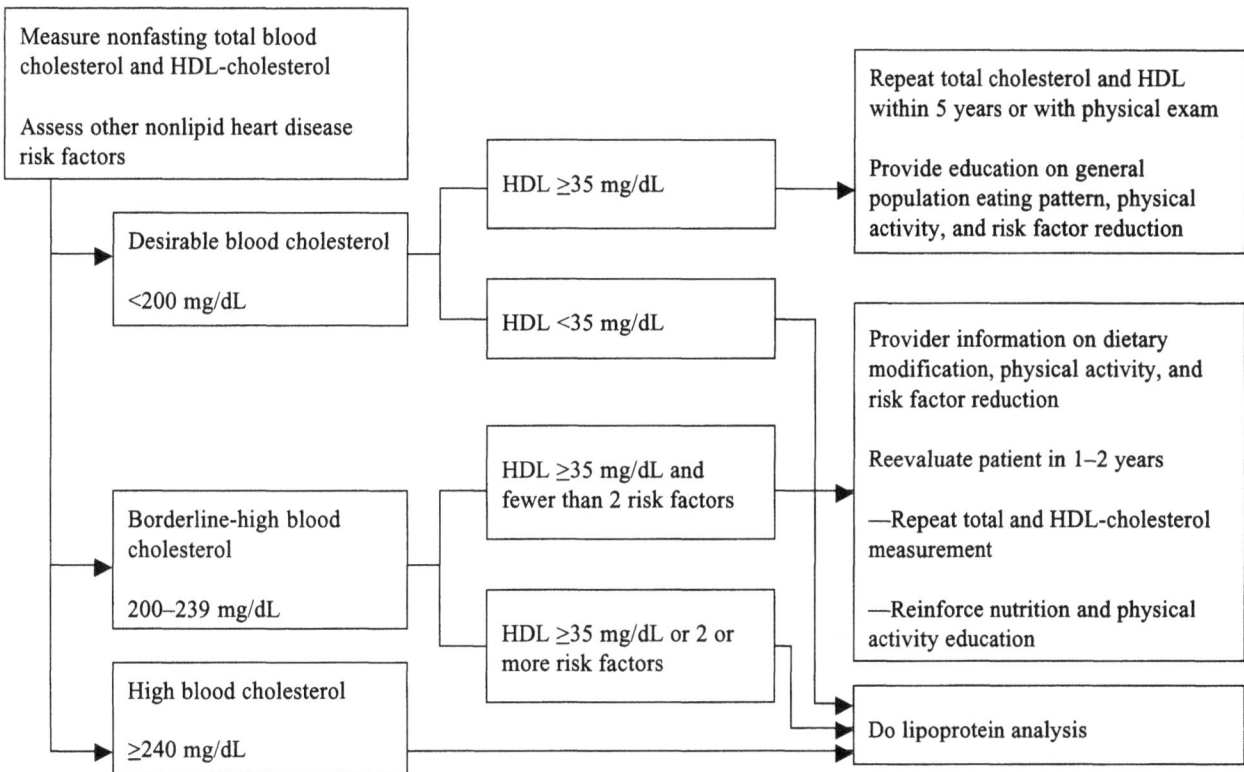

*Total Cholesterol*

| | |
|---|---|
| <200 mg/dL | Desirable blood cholesterol |
| 200–239 mg/dL | Borderline-high blood cholesterol |
| ≥240 mg/dL | High blood cholesterol |

*HDL-Cholesterol*

| | |
|---|---|
| <35 mg/dL | Low HDL-cholesterol |

### Primary Prevention in Adults without Evidence of Heart Disease
### Initial Classification Based on Total Cholesterol and HDL-Cholesterol

Measure nonfasting total blood cholesterol and HDL-cholesterol

Assess other nonlipid heart disease risk factors

Desirable blood cholesterol

<200 mg/dL

→ HDL ≥35 mg/dL → Repeat total cholesterol and HDL within 5 years or with physical exam

Provide education on general population eating pattern, physical activity, and risk factor reduction

→ HDL <35 mg/dL →

Provider information on dietary modification, physical activity, and risk factor reduction

Reevaluate patient in 1–2 years

—Repeat total and HDL-cholesterol measurement

—Reinforce nutrition and physical activity education

Borderline-high blood cholesterol

200–239 mg/dL

→ HDL ≥35 mg/dL and fewer than 2 risk factors →

→ HDL ≥35 mg/dL or 2 or more risk factors →

High blood cholesterol

≥240 mg/dL →

Do lipoprotein analysis

### Heart Disease Risk Factors

*Positive:*

- Age:  Male ≥45 years
        Female ≥55 years or premature menopause without estrogen replacement therapy
- Family history of premature heart disease
- Smoking
- Hypertension
- HDL-cholesterol <35 mg/dL
- Diabetes

*Negative*

- HDL-cholesterol ≥60 mg/dL

Source: National Cholesterol Education Program, *Second Report of the Expert Panel on Detection, Evaluation, and Treatment of High Blood Cholesterol in Adults.* National Heart, Lung, and Blood Institute, NIH Publication No. 93-3095, September 1993.

## HIGHLIGHTS OF AHCPR CLINICAL PRACTICE GUIDELINE—DIAGNOSING AND MANAGING UNSTABLE ANGINA*

### Purpose and Scope

Unstable angina is a transitory syndrome that causes significant disability and death in the United States. In 1991 alone, 570,000 hospitalizations for this principal diagnosis resulted in 3.1 million hospital days. Unstable angina most often results from disruption of an atherosclerotic plaque and the subsequent cascade of pathologic processes that critically decrease coronary blood flow. In most but not all patients presenting with angina, symptoms will be caused by significant coronary artery disease (CAD).

The following highlights include recommendations and supporting evidence for all aspects of the diagnosis and treatment of unstable angina in both the inpatient and outpatient settings. The management of patients with acute myocardial infarction or stable angina is addressed only when these related conditions border indistinguishably with unstable angina.

Unstable angina is defined as a clinical syndrome falling between stable angina and myocardial infarction in the spectrum of patients with CAD.

### Abstract

This guide contains recommendations on the care of patients with unstable angina based on a combination of evidence obtained through extensive literature reviews and consensus among members of a private-sector, expert panel. Principal conclusions include:

- Many patients suspected of having unstable angina can be discharged home after adequate initial evaluation.
- Further outpatient evaluation may be scheduled for up to 72 hours after initial presentation for patients with clinical symptoms of unstable angina judged at initial evaluation to be at low risk for complications.
- Patients with acute ischemic heart disease judged to be at intermediate or high risk of complications should be hospitalized for careful monitoring of their clinical course.
- Intravenous thrombolytic therapy should not be administered to patients without evidence of acute myocardial infarction.

*Source: Braunwald E, Mark DB, Jones RH et al. Diagnosing and Managing Unstable Angina. Quick Reference Guide for Clinicians. Number 10. AHCPR Publication No. 94-0603. Rockville, MD. U.S. Department of Health and Human Services, Public Health Service, Agency for Health Care Policy and Research and National Heart, Lung, and Blood Institute. March 1994.

- Assessment of prognosis by noninvasive testing often aids selection of appropriate therapy.
- Coronary angiography is appropriate for patients judged to be at high risk for cardiac complications or death based on their clinical course or results of noninvasive testing.
- Coronary artery bypass surgery should be recommended for almost all patients with left main disease and many patients with three-vessel disease, especially those with left ventricular dysfunction.
- The discharge care plan should include continued monitoring of symptoms; appropriate drug therapy, including aspirin; risk-factor modification; and counseling.

### Initial Evaluation and Treatment

#### Initial Evaluation

Diagnosis of unstable angina depends on a careful clinical history, physical examination, and examination of a resting 12-lead electrocardiogram (ECG). Therefore, the initial evaluation of patients with symptoms consistent with ischemic pain usually should take place in a medical facility and not by telephone.

- The ECG provides crucial information in the diagnosis of unstable angina, and recordings taken both during periods of pain and after pain relief are useful.
- In patients with symptoms suggesting unstable angina, there are two complementary and equally important components to the initial assessment: (1) assessment of the likelihood of CAD (see exhibit "Likelihood of Significant CAD in Patients with Symptoms Suggesting Unstable Angina") and (2) assessment of the risk of adverse outcomes (see exhibit, "Short-Term Risk of Death or Nonfatal Myocardial Infarction in Patients with Symptoms Suggesting Unstable Angina").

At the conclusion of this initial evaluation, the patient can be assigned to one of four diagnostic categories: not coronary artery disease, stable angina, acute myocardial infarction (MI), or unstable angina (see exhibit, "Diagnosis and Risk Stratification").

#### Initial Medical Treatment

The certainty of diagnosis, severity of symptoms, hemodynamic state, and medication history will determine the choice and timing of drugs used in individual patients. Drugs to be considered for use at the time of initial evaluation and treatment of patients with unstable angina include aspirin, heparin, nitrates, and beta-blockers (See exhibit, "Drugs Commonly Used in Intensive Medical Management of Patients with Unstable Angina").

## UNSTABLE ANGINA PRESENTATIONS

- Rest angina within one week of presentation
- New onset angina of Canadian Cardiovascular Society Classification (CCSC) class III or IV within two months of presentation
- Angina increasing in CCSC class to at least CCSC III or IV
- Variant angina
- Non–Q-wave myocardial infarction
- Postmyocardial infarction angina (>24 hours)

Source: Braunwald E, Mark DB, Jones RH et al. Diagnosing and Managing Unstable Angina. Quick Reference Guide for Clinicians. Number 10. AHCPR Publication No. 94-0603. Rockville, MD, U.S. Department of Health and Human Services, Public Health Service, Agency for Health Care Policy and Research and National Heart, Lung, and Blood Institute, March 1994.

- Begin treatment with an indicated drug in the emergency department; pharmacologic treatment should not be delayed until hospital admission. The aggressiveness of drug dosage will depend on the severity of symptoms and, for many drugs, will require modification throughout the subsequent hospital course.
- Institute anti-ischemic therapy in the emergency department as soon as the working diagnosis of unstable angina is made.
- Give supplemental oxygen to patients with cyanosis, respiratory distress, or high-risk features. Monitor for adequate arterial oxygenation with finger pulse oximetry or blood gas determinations.
- Place patients with intermediate- or high-risk unstable angina on continuous ECG monitoring for ischemia and arrhythmia detection.
- Intravenous thrombolytic therapy is not indicated in patients who do not have evidence of acute ST-segment elevation or left bundle branch block on their 12-lead ECG.

## LIKELIHOOD OF SIGNIFICANT CAD IN PATIENTS WITH SYMPTOMS SUGGESTING UNSTABLE ANGINA

| High Likelihood | Intermediate Likelihood | Low Likelihood |
|---|---|---|
| Any of the following features: | Absence of high-likelihood features and any of the following: | Absence of high- or intermediate-likelihood features but may have: |
| Known history of CAD | Definite angina: males <60 or females <70 | Chest pain, probably not angina |
| Definite angina: males ≥60 or females ≥70 | Probable angina: males >60 or females >70 | One risk factor but not diabetes |
| Hemodynamic changes or ECG changes with pain | Probably not angina in diabetics or in nondiabetics with ≥ two other risk factors* | T wave flat or inverted <1 mm in leads with dominant R waves |
| Variant angina | Extracardiac vascular disease | Normal ECG |
| ST increase or decrease ≥1 mm | ST depression .05 to 1 mm | |
| Marked symmetrical T-wave inversion in multiple precordial leads | T-wave inversion ≥1 mm in leads with dominant R waves | |

*CAD risk factors include diabetes, smoking, hypertension, and elevated cholesterol.

Source: Braunwald E, Mark DB, Jones RH et al. Diagnosing and Managing Unstable Angina, Quick Reference Guide for Clinicians, Number 10. AHCPR Publication No. 94–0603. Rockville, MD. U.S. Department of Health and Human Services, Public Health Service, Agency for Health Care Policy and Research and National Heart, Lung, and Blood Institute, March 1994.

**SHORT-TERM RISK OF DEATH OR NONFATAL MYOCARDIAL INFARCTION IN PATIENTS WITH SYMPTOMS SUGGESTING UNSTABLE ANGINA**

| High Risk | Intermediate Risk | Low Risk |
|---|---|---|
| At least one of the following features must be present: | No high-risk feature but must have any of the following: | No high- or intermediate-risk feature but may have any of the following: |
| Prolonged ongoing (>20 mins) rest pain | Rest angina now resolved but not low likelihood of CAD | Increased angina frequency, severity, or duration |
| Pulmonary edema | Rest angina (>20 mins or relieved with rest or nitroglycerin) | Angina provoked at a lower threshold |
| Angina with new or worsening mitral regurgitation murmurs | Angina with dynamic T-wave changes | New onset angina within 2 weeks to 2 months |
| Rest angina with dynamic ST changes ≥1 mm | Nocturnal angina | Normal or unchanged ECG |
| Angina with S3 or rales | New onset CCSC III or IV angina in past 2 weeks but not low likelihood of CAD | |
| Angina with hypotension | Q waves or ST depression ≥1 mm in multiple leads<br>Age >65 years | |

Source: Braunwald E, Mark DB, Jones RH et al. Diagnosing and Managing Unstable Angina. Quick Reference Guide for Clinicians. Number 10, AHCPR Publication No. 94–0603. Rockville, MD. U.S. Department of Health and Human Services, Public Health Service, Agency for Health Care Policy and Research and National Heart, Lung, and Blood Institute. March 1994.

## Outpatient Care

Patients with unstable angina who are judged in the initial evaluation and treatment phase to be at low risk for adverse outcomes can, in many cases, be safely evaluated further as outpatients. Typically, these are patients who have experienced new onset or worsening symptoms that may be due to ischemia, but they have not had severe, prolonged, or rest episodes in the preceding two weeks.

- Schedule a follow-up evaluation as soon as possible, generally within 72 hours after the initial presentation.
- Conduct a systematic search for precipitating noncardiac causes that might explain the new development of unstable angina symptoms or the conversion from a stable to an unstable course. Thus, at the follow-up evaluation, each patient should have: a second ECG to look for asymptomatic ischemia or arrhythmias; measurement of body temperature and blood pressure; a hemoglobin or hematocrit determination; and a physical examination for evidence of other cardiac diseases (particularly aortic valve disease and hypertrophic cardiomyopathy) or hyperthyroidism.

- Review the patient's history to determine additional potential exacerbating factors, such as a recent increase in physical activity level (especially in combination with environmental temperature extremes), noncompliance with medical therapy, or a recent increase in psychological stress levels.
- Advise patients diagnosed with unstable angina to take aspirin, 80 to 324 mg per day, unless contraindications are present. For patients unable to take aspirin because of a history of true hypersensitivity or recent significant gastrointestinal bleeding, ticlopidine, 250 mg twice a day, may be used as a substitute.
- Begin therapy for newly diagnosed patients, generally with sublingual nitroglycerin as needed, followed by oral beta-blockers and/or long-acting topical or oral nitrates. Review the medical regimen of patients with established coronary artery disease already on medical therapy, and increase dosages as appropriate for symptom management and as tolerated.

**DIAGNOSIS AND RISK STRATIFICATION**

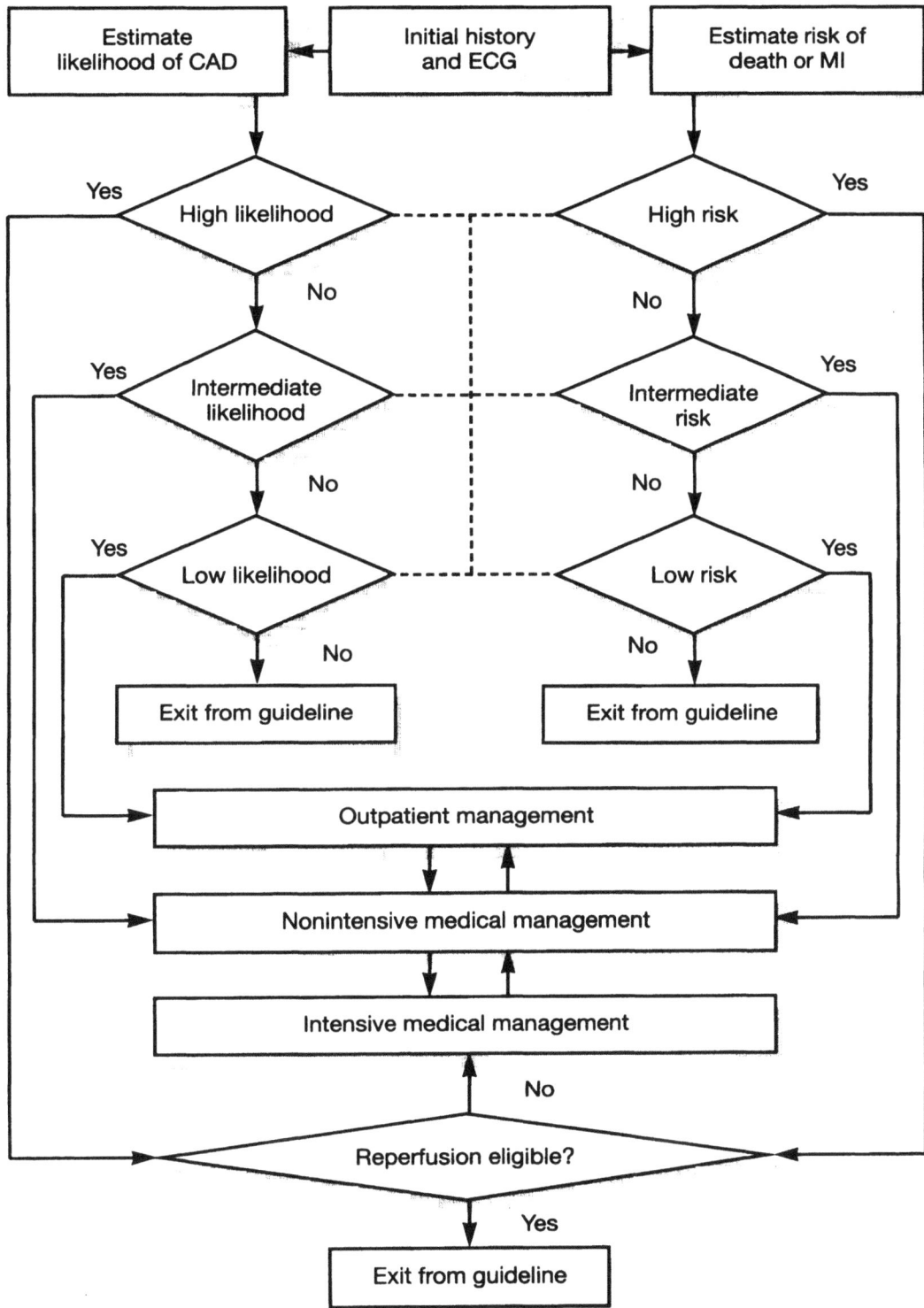

Source: Braunwald E, Mark DB, Jones RH et al. Diagnosing and Managing Unstable Angina. Quick Reference Guide for Clinicians, Number 10. AHCPR Publication No. 94–0603. Rockville, MD. U.S. Department of Health and Human Services, Public Health Service, Agency for Health Care Policy and Research and National Heart, Lung, and Blood Institute, March 1994.

## DRUGS COMMONLY USED IN INTENSIVE MEDICAL MANAGEMENT OF PATIENTS WITH UNSTABLE ANGINA

| Drug Category | Clinical Condition | When To Avoid[1] | Dose |
|---|---|---|---|
| Aspirin[2] | Unstable angina | • Hypersensitivity<br>• Active bleeding<br>• Severe bleeding risk | • 324 mg (160–324) daily |
| Heparin | Unstable angina in high-risk category | • Active bleeding<br>• History of heparin-induced thrombocytopenia<br>• Severe bleeding risk<br>• Recent stroke | • 80 units/kg intravenous (IV) bolus<br>• Constant intravenous infusion at 18 units/kg/hr<br>• Titrated to maintain aPTT between 1.5 to 2.5 times control |
| Nitrates | Symptoms are not fully relieved with three sublingual nitroglycerin tablets and initiation of beta-blocker therapy | • Hypotension | • 5 to 10 mcg/min by continuous infusion<br>• Titrated up to 75 to 100 mcg/min until relief of symptoms or limiting side effects (headache or hypotension with a systolic blood pressure <90 mm Hg or more than 30% below starting mean arterial pressure levels if significant hypertension is present)<br>• Topical, oral, or buccal nitrates are acceptable alternatives for patients without ongoing or refractory symptoms |
| Beta-blockers[3] | Unstable angina | • PR ECG segment >0.24 second<br>• 2° or 3° atrioventricular (AV) block<br>• Heart rate <60<br>• Blood pressure <90 mm Hg<br>• Shock<br>• Left ventricular failure with congestive heart failure<br>• Severe reactive airway disease | **Metoprolol**<br>• 5-mg increments by slow (over 1 to 2 minutes) intravenous administration<br>• Repeated every 5 minutes for a total initial dose of 15 mg<br>• Followed in 1 to 2 hours by 25 to 50 mg by mouth every 6 hours<br>• If a very conservative regimen is desired, initial doses can be reduced to 1 to 2 mg<br>**Propranolol**<br>• 0.5- to 1.0-mg intravenous dose<br>• Followed in 1 to 2 hours by 40 to 80 mg by mouth every 6 to 8 hours<br>**Esmolol**<br>• Starting maintenance dose of 0.1 mg/kg/min intravenously<br>• Titration in increments of 0.05 mg/kg/min every 10 to 15 minutes as tolerated by blood pressure until the desired therapeutic response has been obtained, limited symptoms develop, or a dose of 0.20 mg/kg/min is reached<br>• Optional loading dose of 0.5 mg/kg may be given by slow intravenous administration (2 to 5 minutes) for more rapid onset of action<br>**Atenolol**<br>• 5-mg intravenous dose<br>• Followed 5 minutes later by a second 5-mg intravenous dose and then 50 to 100 mg orally every day initiated 1 to 2 hours after the intravenous dose |

*continues*

**Drugs Commonly Used in Intensive Medical Management of Patients with Unstable Angina** continued

| Drug Category | Clinical Condition | When To Avoid[1] | Dose |
|---|---|---|---|
| Calcium channel blockers | Patients already on adequate doses of nitrates and beta-blockers or in patients unable to tolerate adequate doses of one or both of these agents or in patients with variant angina. | • Pulmonary edema<br>• Evidence of left ventricular dysfunction | • Dependent on specific agent |
| Morphine sulfate | Patients whose symptoms are not relieved after three serial sublingual nitroglycerin tablets or whose symptoms recur with adequate anti-ischemic therapy | • Hypotension<br>• Respiratory depression<br>• Confusion<br>• Obtundation | • 2- to 5-mg intravenous dose<br>• May be repeated every 5 to 30 minutes as needed to relieve symptoms and maintain patient comfort |

[1]Allergy or prior intolerance contraindication for all categories of drugs listed in this chart.

[2]Patients unable to take aspirin because of a history of hypersensitivity or major gastrointestinal intolerance should be started on ticlopidine 250 mg twice a day, as a substitute.

[3]Choice of the specific agent is not as important as ensuring that appropriate candidates receive this therapy. If there are concerns about patient intolerance due to existing pulmonary disease, especially asthma, left ventricular dysfunction, or risk of hypotension or severe bradycardia, initial selection should favor a short-acting agent, such as propranolol or metoprolol or the ultra short-acting agent, esmolol. Mild wheezing or a history of chronic obstructive pulmonary disease should prompt a trial of a short-acting agent at a reduced dose (eg, 2.5 mg intravenous metoprolol, 12.5 mg oral metoprolol, or 25 mcg/kg/min esmolol as initial doses) rather than complete avoidance of beta-blocker therapy.

*Note:* Some of the recommendations in this guide suggest the use of agents for purposes or in doses other than those specified by the Food and Drug Administration (FDA). Such recommendations are made after consideration of concerns regarding nonapproved indications. Where made, such recommendations are based on more recent clinical trials or expert consensus.

Source: Braunwald E, Mark DB, Jones RH et al. Diagnosing and Managing Unstable Angina. Quick Reference Guide for Clinicians. Number 10. AHCPR Publication No. 94-0603. Rockville, MD. U.S. Department of Health and Human Services, Public Health Service Agency for Health Care Policy and Research and National Heart, Lung, and Blood Institute, March 1994.

• Consider prescribing long-acting forms of antianginal drugs for enhanced patient compliance.

## Intensive Medical Management

Intensive medical treatment should begin immediately in the emergency department in patients at high or intermediate risk of death or nonfatal MI. For high-risk patients, such as those with ongoing angina at rest and/or those who appear unstable, simultaneous evaluation and treatment assume an urgency greater than for intermediate-risk patients, such as those with prior discomfort who are asymptomatic during the initial evaluation.

• Establish intravenous access while simultaneously obtaining a brief cardiovascular history, physical examination, and ECG.
• Institute daily aspirin and intravenous heparin plus nitrates and beta-blockers (see exhibit, "Drugs Commonly Used in Intensive Medical Management of Patients with Unstable Angina").
• Consider adding calcium channel blockers in the subset of patients who have significant hypertension (systolic blood pressure ≥150 mm Hg), in patients who have refractory ischemia on beta-blockers, and in those with variant angina.

Recurrent symptoms after the initial hemodynamic goals of therapy have been achieved may be regarded as a failure of medical therapy and should prompt consideration of urgent cardiac catheterization. Although it is theoretically desirable to have the maximal medical regimen in place for ≥24 hours before declaring any patient a failure of medical therapy, to do so in all cases may be inappropriate or even dangerous.

• Assign patients who have one or more recurrent severe, prolonged (>20 minutes) ischemic episodes, particularly when accompanied by pulmonary edema, a new or worsening mitral regurgitation murmur, hypotension, or new ST or T-wave changes, to the high-risk category regardless of the level of medical therapy and triage them to early cardiac catheterization.

- Assign patients with shorter, less severe ischemic episodes without accompanying hemodynamic or ECG changes to a substantially lower-risk category and continue medical therapy.

## Monitoring Medical Therapy

During the period of intensive medical therapy, appropriate monitoring includes:

## Heparin

- Obtain an aPTT (activated partial thromboplastin time) six hours after initial therapy is started or any dosage change occurs and every six hours thereafter until a therapeutic level of 1.5 to 2.5 times control is obtained on two consecutive aPTTs.
- Obtain an aPTT every 24 hours, once a therapeutic range is achieved.
- Obtain an immediate aPTT if the patient's clinical condition changes significantly (eg, recurrent definite ischemia, bleeding, hypotension). Obtain an immediate hemoglobin/hematocrit and platelet determination if any of the following occur: clinically significant bleeding, recurrent symptoms, or hemodynamic instability. A drop in platelets necessitates close monitoring for heparin-induced thrombocytopenia.
- Monitor hemoglobin/hematocrit and platelets daily for the first three days of heparin therapy.

## Beta-Blockers

- Monitor heart rate and blood pressure (target heart rate for beta-blockade is 50 to 60 beats per minute).
- Monitor for congestive heart failure and bronchospasm.
- Utilize continuous ECG monitoring.

## Discontinuation of Intravenous Therapy

- Discontinue heparin after three to five days.
- Convert to an oral regimen of beta-blockers after the initial intravenous load in patients without limiting side effects. Selection of the oral agent should be based on the clinician's familiarity with the agent as well as the risk of adverse effects.
- Change to oral or topical nitrate therapy when the patient has been symptom-free for 24 hours. Tolerance to nitrates is dose- and duration-dependent and typically becomes significant after only 24 hours of continuous

therapy. Responsiveness can be enhanced by increasing the dose; switching the patient to a topical, oral, or buccal form of therapy; and using a nitrate-free interval of six to eight hours.

## Reassessing Persistent Symptoms

Most patients stabilize and have improvement in their chest pain after 30 minutes of aggressive medical management and can be admitted to an intensive care unit or intermediate care unit. Failure to respond to initial therapy should prompt reconsideration of other possible catastrophic causes of chest pain including:

- ongoing acute myocardial infarction
- aortic dissection
- pulmonary embolism
- pneumothorax
- esophageal rupture
- rupture or ischemia of intra-abdominal organs

## Treatment of Severe Ischemia Refractory to Aggressive Initial Therapy

Patients considered to have unstable angina after further evaluation and who fail to respond within 30 minutes to initial treatment are at increased risk for myocardial infarction or cardiac death. The major ischemic complications seen in unstable angina are recurrent unstable angina, acute ischemic pulmonary edema, new or worsening mitral regurgitation, cadiogenic shock, malignant ventricular arrhythmias, and advanced atrioventricular block. For these patients, in addition to maximizing the medical regimen described in the previous section and instituting appropriate adjunctive therapy (eg, pulmonary artery pressure monitoring and inotropic therapy for shock, antiarrhythmic therapy for malignant ventricular arrhythmias, pacemaker for symptomatic high-grade atrioventricular block), the clinician should consider insertion of an intra-aortic balloon pump and cardiac catheterization.

If emergency cardiac catheterization is not possible, an intra-aortic balloon pump should be placed in unstable angina patients who have symptoms refractory to medical management and those who have symptoms in conjunction with hemodynamic instability. An intra-aortic balloon pump can also serve as a bridge to stabilize the patient on the way to the catheterization laboratory or operating room. Exceptions to this recommendation include patients with severe peripheral vascular disease, significant aortic insufficiency, or known severe aortoiliac disease, including aortic aneurysm.

- Refer for urgent diagnostic catheterization patients who have received an intra-aortic balloon pump for stabilization.
- Transfer patients who have received an intra-aortic balloon pump for stabilization to a facility capable of providing diagnostic catheterization and revascularization.
- Reevaluate patients who have not stabilized after placement of the pump to reaffirm the diagnosis of acute ischemic heart disease and then consider for emergency catheterization.

## Selection of Further Therapy in Stabilized Patients

For patients who stabilize after initial treatment, two alternative strategies for definitive treatment of unstable angina are proposed, termed "early invasive" and "early conservative."

Patients who prefer continued intensive medical management and patients who are not candidates for revascularization will continue to receive care at a level and duration dictated by the level of their disease activity. (See exhibit, "Cardiac Catheterization and Myocardial Revascularization.")

## Progression to Nonintensive Medical Therapy

Most patients with unstable angina stabilize and become pain-free with appropriate intensive medical management. Transfer from intensive to nonintensive medical management occurs when:

1. The patient is hemodynamically stable (including no uncompensated congestive heart failure) for ≥24 hours.
2. Ischemia has been successfully suppressed for ≥24 hours.

Once these criteria are reached:

- Convert parenteral to nonparenteral medications.
- Reassess heparin use. Discontinue in selected patients (for example, those found to have a secondary cause for ischemia such as anemia). Continue for two to five days in others.
- Continue aspirin at 80 to 324 mg/day.
- Ensure that appropriate enzyme levels are obtained: Total CK (creatinine kinase) and CK-MB (cardiac muscle) every 6 to 8 hours for the first 24 hours after admission. Lactate dehydrogenase levels may be useful in detecting cardiac damage in patients presenting between 24 and 72 hours after symptom onset.

---

### Early invasive strategy

All hospitalized patients with unstable angina and without contraindications receive cardiac catheterization within 48 hours of presentation.

### Early conservative strategy

Unless contraindicated, hospitalized patients with unstable angina receive a cardiac catheterization if they have one or more of the following high-risk indicators: prior revascularization; associated congestive heart failure or depressed left ventricular function (ejection fraction <.50) by noninvasive study; malignant ventricular arrhythmia; persistent or recurrent pain/ischemia; and/or a functional study indicating high risk. All other patients receive medical management and undergo cardiac catheterization only when medical management fails.

---

- Obtain a follow-up 12-lead ECG 24 hours after admission or whenever the patient has recurrent symptoms or a change in clinical status.
- Obtain a chest X-ray within 48 hours of admission in all stable patients. In hemodynamically unstable patients, obtain a chest X-ray initially and repeat as necessary.
- Measure resting left ventricular function in patients who do not have early cardiac catheterization but who have had previous infarct or who have cardiomegaly by physical examination or chest radiograph. Either a radionuclide ventriculogram or a two-dimensional echocardiogram may be used.

## Nonintensive Medical Management

Patients with unstable angina judged to be at moderate risk may be admitted initially to a monitored intermediate care unit until the diagnosis of myocardial infarction can be excluded and it is clear that the patient's symptoms are adequately controlled on medical therapy. These patients then enter the nonintensive phase of management.

Other moderate-risk and some low-risk patients may be admitted directly to a regular hospital bed with telemetry capabilities, thereby proceeding directly to the nonintensive phase. High-risk unstable angina patients will be moved to the nonintensive phase after one or more days of intensive management and stabilization.

Once patients reach the nonintensive phase of management, reasons for continued hospitalization include optimization of medical therapy, evaluation of the propensity for recurrent ischemia or ischemic complications, and risk stratification to determine the need for catheterization and revascularization.

- Discontinue continuous monitoring of the ECG in this phase for most patients.
- Instruct all patients to notify nursing personnel immediately if chest discomfort recurs.
- Recurrent ischemic episodes should prompt a brief nursing assessment and an ECG and should be brought to the attention of a physician.
- Reevaluate the patient's medical regimen and adjust doses of anti-ischemic agents as tolerated.
- Encourage the patient to progress gradually to a level of activity, under the observation of the health care team, commensurate with that required to perform activities of daily living.
- Advise the patient and his or her family regarding risk-factor modification and have them work with the health care team to set appropriate goals.

Many patients reaching this phase will be referred within one to two days for either noninvasive functional testing or cardiac catheterization.

### Recurrence of Pain and Return to Intensive Management

- Transfer patients who have pain or ECG evidence of ischemia increasing in severity >20 minutes and are unresponsive to nitroglycerin back to the intensive medical management phase protocol.
- Patients who respond to sublingual nitroglycerin generally do not need to return to intensive medical management. However, a second recurrence of chest pain of at least 20 minutes' duration in the setting of appropriate medical therapy should prompt return of the patient to a monitored environment and the management steps outlined in the intensive management phase.

## Noninvasive Testing

The goals of noninvasive testing in a recently stabilized patient with unstable angina are to estimate the subsequent prognosis, especially for the next three to six months, decide which additional tests and adjustments in therapy are required based on this prognosis, and provide the patient with the information and reassurances necessary to return to a lifestyle as full and productive as possible (see exhibit, "Noninvasive Testing").

- Conduct exercise or pharmacologic stress testing of low-risk patients with unstable angina who are to be managed as outpatients, unless contraindicated.
- Perform noninvasive testing within 72 hours of presentation (in most cases) in low-risk patients who are to be managed as outpatients.
- Perform noninvasive exercise or pharmacologic stress testing in low- or intermediate-risk patients hospitalized with unstable angina who have been stabilized and free of angina and congestive heart failure for a minimum of 48 hours, unless cardiac catheterization is indicated.

### Choice of Test

- Base the choice of the stress testing modality on an evaluation of the patient's resting ECG, ability to perform exercise, and the local expertise and technologies available.
- Employ the exercise treadmill test as the standard mode of stress testing in patients with a normal ECG who are not taking digoxin. Test patients with widespread resting ST depression (≥1 mm), ST changes secondary to digoxin, left ventricular hypertrophy, left bundle branch block/significant intraventricular conduction deficit, or pre-excitation using an imaging modality.
- Use pharmacologic stress testing in combination with an imaging modality for patients unable to exercise due to physical limitations (eg, arthritis, amputation, severe peripheral vascular disease, general debility).

An exercise treadmill is the most commonly used stress test and has the largest reported experience for use in patients with unstable angina. A nomogram useful to convert results from this test into an assessment of risk has been derived on a large sample of patients with coronary artery disease exclusively (not in patients presenting with unstable angina) (see the *Clinical Practice Guideline, Unstable Angina: Diagnosis and Management*). Use of this nomogram to quantitate risk from results of treadmill examinations provides more clinically useful information than a simple normal/abnormal reading.

### Interpreting Noninvasive Test Results

Implications and appropriate follow-up for the exercise treadmill tests are outlined in the exhibit, "Implications of Stress Test Results."

**CARDIAC CATHETERIZATION AND MYOCARDIAL REVASCULARIZATION**

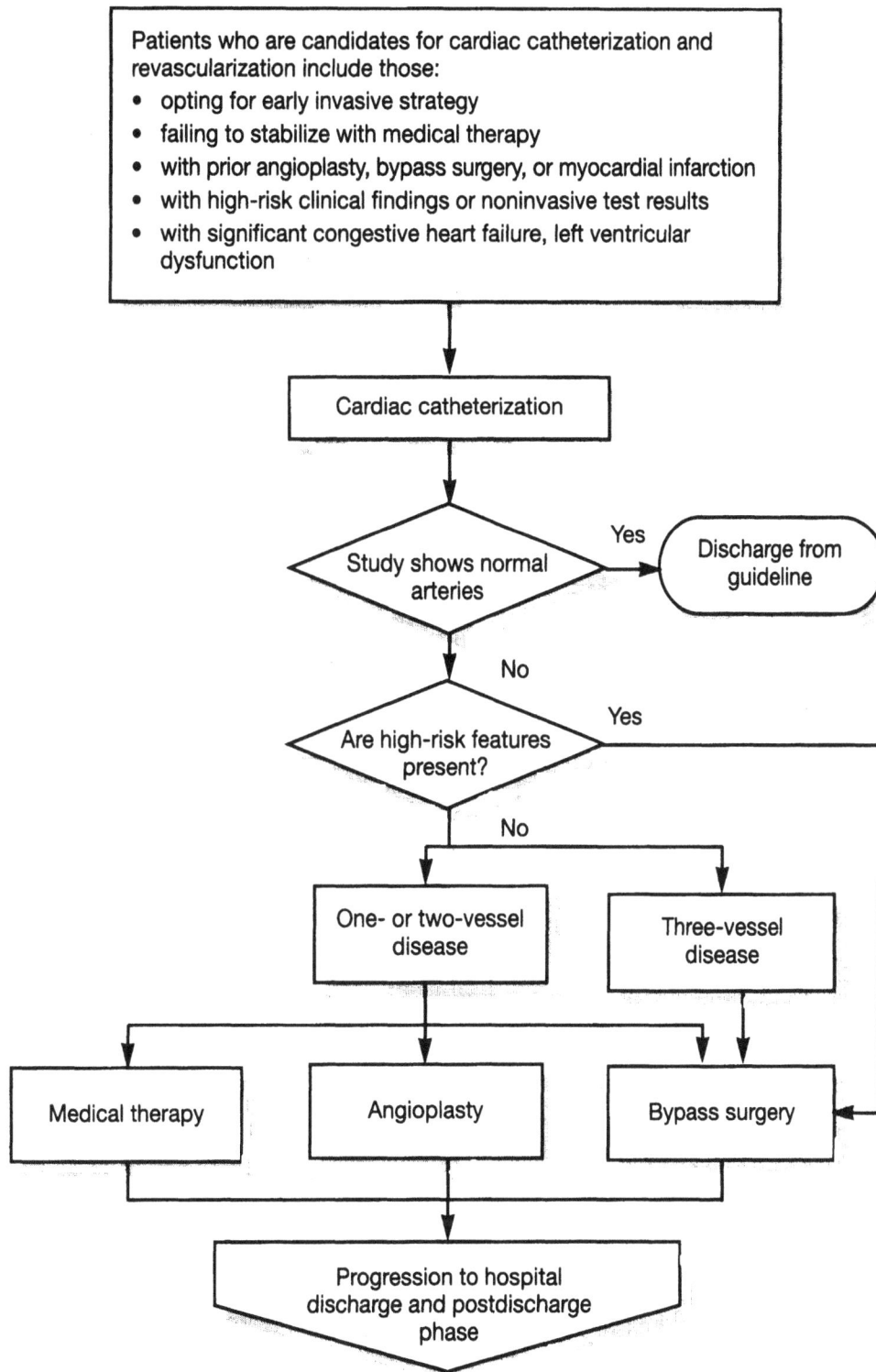

Patients who are candidates for cardiac catheterization and revascularization include those:
- opting for early invasive strategy
- failing to stabilize with medical therapy
- with prior angioplasty, bypass surgery, or myocardial infarction
- with high-risk clinical findings or noninvasive test results
- with significant congestive heart failure, left ventricular dysfunction

↓

Cardiac catheterization

↓

Study shows normal arteries — **Yes** → Discharge from guideline

**No**
↓

Are high-risk features present? — **Yes** →

**No**
↓

One- or two-vessel disease          Three-vessel disease

Medical therapy          Angioplasty          Bypass surgery

↓

Progression to hospital discharge and postdischarge phase

Source: Braunwald E, Mark DB, Jones RH et al. Diagnosing and Managing Unstable Angina. Quick Reference Guide for Clinicians. Number 10. AHCPR Publication No. 94-0603. Rockville, MD. U.S. Department of Health and Human Services, Public Health Service, Agency for Health Care Policy and Research and National Heart, Lung, and Blood Institute. March 1994.

**NONINVASIVE TESTING**

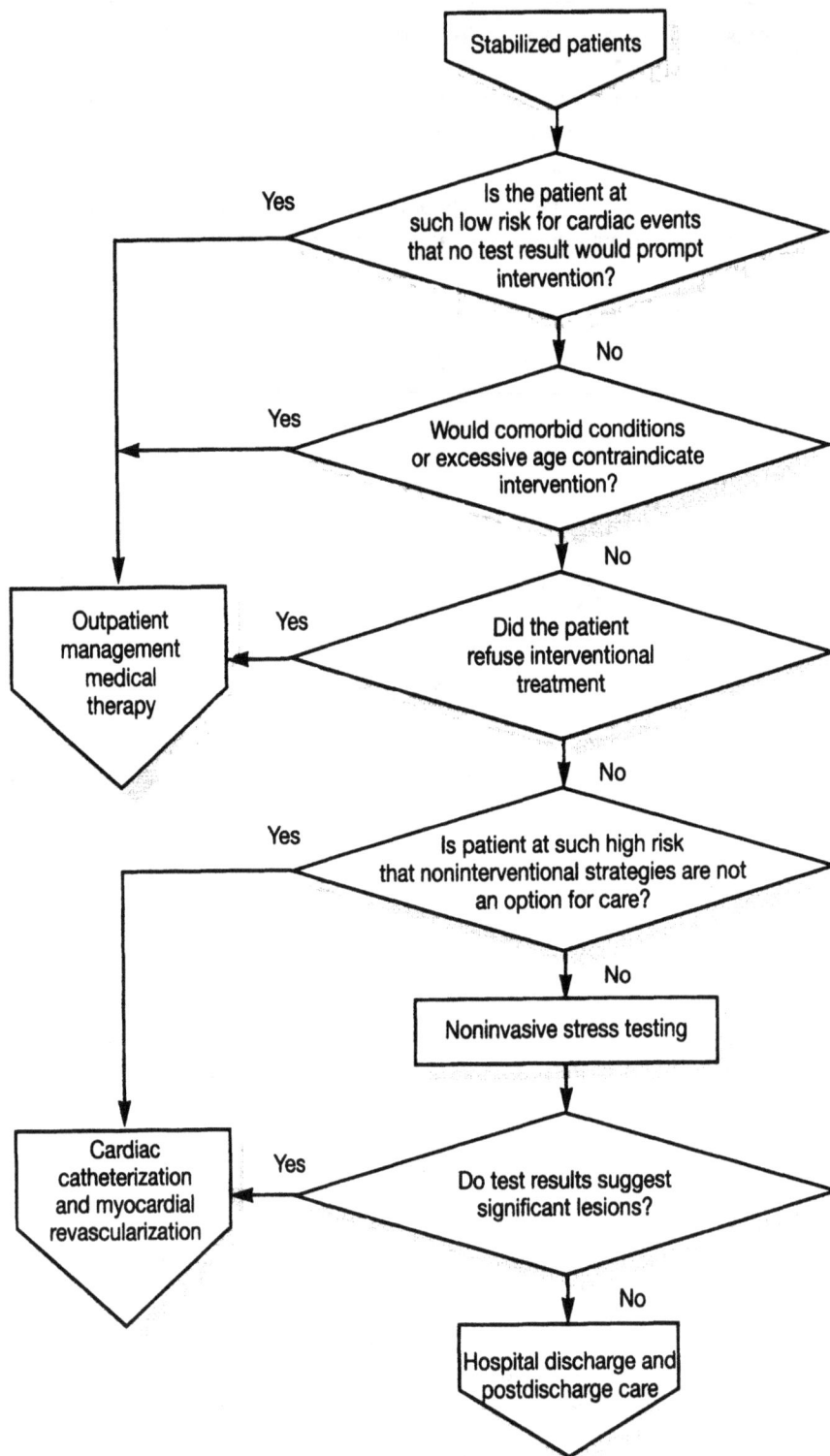

```
                        ┌─────────────────┐
                        │ Stabilized patients │
                        └─────────────────┘
                                 │
                                 ▼
      Yes            ◇ Is the patient at
     ◄───────────────  such low risk for cardiac events
                        that no test result would prompt
                        intervention? ◇
                                 │ No
                                 ▼
      Yes            ◇ Would comorbid conditions
     ◄───────────────  or excessive age contraindicate
                        intervention? ◇
                                 │ No
                                 ▼
   Outpatient   Yes   ◇ Did the patient
   management  ◄───────  refuse interventional
   medical               treatment ◇
   therapy                        │ No
                                 ▼
      Yes            ◇ Is patient at such high risk
     ◄───────────────  that noninterventional strategies are not
                        an option for care? ◇
                                 │ No
                                 ▼
                        ┌─────────────────┐
                        │ Noninvasive stress testing │
                        └─────────────────┘
                                 │
                                 ▼
   Cardiac      Yes   ◇ Do test results suggest
   catheterization ◄──  significant lesions? ◇
   and myocardial                │ No
   revascularization             ▼
                        ┌─────────────────────┐
                        │ Hospital discharge and │
                        │ postdischarge care     │
                        └─────────────────────┘
```

Source: Braunwald E, Mark DB, Jones RH et al. Diagnosing and Managing Unstable Angina. Quick Reference Guide for Clinicians. Number 10. AHCPR Publication No. 94–0603. Rockville, MD. U.S. Department of Health and Human Services, Public Health Service, Agency for Health Care Policy and Research and National Heart, Lung, and Blood Institute. March 1994.

**IMPLICATIONS OF STRESS TEST RESULTS**

| Prognosis[1] | Implications | Treatment |
|---|---|---|
| Predicted average annual cardiac mortality <1%/year | Low risk | Manage medically, no need for referral to cardiac catheterization |
| Predicted average annual cardiac mortality 2% to 3%/year | Intermediate risk[2] | Refer for additional testing, either cardiac catheterization or an alternate exercise imaging study |
| Predicted average annual cardiac mortality ≥4%/year | High risk | Refer for prompt cardiac catheterization |

[1]Predicted average annual cardiac mortality based on test results interpreted using exercise testing nomogram in Mark DB, Shaw L, Harrell FE et al., Prognostic value of a treadmill exercise score in outpatients with suspected coronary artery disease. N Engl J Med 1991 Sep;325:849–53.

[2]A stress test result of intermediate risk combined with evidence of left ventricular dysfunction should prompt referral to cardiac catheterization.

Source: Braunwald E, Mark DB, Jones RH et al. Diagnosing and Managing Unstable Angina. Quick Reference Guide for Clinicians. Number 10. AHCPR Publication No. 94-0603. Rockville, MD. U.S. Department of Health and Human Services, Public Health Service, Agency for Health Care Policy and Research and National Heart, Lung, and Blood Institute. March 1994.

## Cardiac Catheterization and Myocardial Revascularization

### Indications for Cardiac Catheterization

The goal of cardiac catheterization in patients with unstable angina is to provide detailed structural information necessary to assess prognosis and select an appropriate long-term management strategy. The procedure is usually helpful in choosing between medical therapy, percutaneous transluminal coronary angioplasty, and coronary artery bypass graft surgery in patients at significant risk for future cardiac events (see exhibit "Cardiac Catheterization and Myocardial Revascularization.")

Patients undergoing cardiac catheterization include those managed under either the "early invasive" or "early conservative" strategies mentioned in the section on intensive medical management, patients undergoing emergency catheterization directly from the emergency room, and those who experienced recurrent ischemic episodes while being managed as outpatients.

- Patients with contraindications to revascularization because of extensive comorbidity and patients who do not wish to consider interventional therapy should not undergo diagnostic catheterization.

- Consider the possibility of noncoronary symptom etiologies in patients found at catheterization to have normal coronary arteries or insignificant lesions.

### Myocardial Revascularization

- Refer patients found at catheterization to have significant left main disease (≥50%) or significant (≥70%) three-vessel disease with depressed left ventricular function (ejection fraction <0.50) for coronary artery bypass graft surgery.
- Refer patients with two-vessel disease with proximal severe subtotal stenosis (≥95%) of the left anterior descending artery and depressed left ventricular function for revascularization.
- Consider for prompt revascularization (angioplasty or coronary artery bypass grafting) patients with significant coronary artery disease if they have any of the following: failure to stabilize with medical treatment; recurrent angina/ischemia at rest or with low-level activities; and/or ischemia accompanied by congestive heart failure symptoms, an $S_3$ gallop, new or worsening mitral regurgitation, or definite ECG changes.

For some patients without these high-risk features, revascularization may still be an option depending on recurrent symptoms, test results, and patient preferences.

The health care team should educate the patient, his or her family, and advocate about the expected risks and benefits of revascularization and determine individual patient preferences and fears that may affect the selection of therapy.

## Hospital Discharge and Postdischarge Care

The need for continued hospitalization of the patient with unstable angina is determined by whether the inpatient objectives of that hospital admission have been achieved. Patients who have undergone successful revascularization will usually have the remainder of their hospitalization defined by the standard protocol for the given procedure (eg, one to two days for angioplasty, five to seven days for coronary artery bypass graft surgery).

Patients opting for medical treatment after a cardiac catheterization or functional study include both a low-risk group that can be rapidly discharged (eg, one to two days after testing) and a high-risk group unsuitable for or unwilling to have coronary revascularization. These patients may require a prolonged hospitalization to ensure adequate (or as adequate as possible) symptom control.

The goal during the hospital discharge phase is to prepare the patient for normal activities to the extent possible.

### Patient Counseling

- Give specific instructions on smoking cessation, daily exercise, and diet.
- Consider referral, where possible and appropriate, to a smoking-cessation program or clinic and/or an outpatient cardiac rehabilitation program.
- Discuss resumption of sexual relations (eg, two weeks for low-risk patients to four weeks for postsurgery coronary artery bypass graft patients).
- Give specific instructions, beyond "daily exercise," on activities that are permissible and those that should be avoided (eg, heavy lifting, climbing stairs, yard work, household activities).
- Discuss resumption of driving and return to work.

### Discharge Medical Regimen

- Continue all patients on aspirin, 80 mg to 324 mg per day, indefinitely after discharge unless contraindications are present.
- Continue medications necessary to achieve adequate symptom control.
- Consider discontinuation of antianginal therapy in patients with successful revascularization without recurrent ischemia.
- If patients have unsuccessful revascularization or recurrent symptoms following revascularization, continue the antianginal regimen required in hospital to control their symptoms.
- Instruct patients who are continuing on antianginal therapy on the use of sublingual nitroglycerin.
- Continue antihypertensive and antihyperlipidemic workups and therapies started prior to admission or initiated in the hospital.
- Plan for follow-up medical care at the time of discharge whenever possible.

## Following and Monitoring Symptoms

- Schedule follow-up of low-risk patients and patients with successful coronary artery bypass grafting or angioplasty at two to six weeks and higher-risk patients at one to two weeks.
- Instruct the patient (and relevant family members or advocate) in the purpose, dose, and major side effects of each medicine prescribed, using language the patient can understand.
- Give specific instructions for the proper use of sublingual nitroglycerin, especially since response of chest pain to this medication is useful in assessing the nature of recurrent symptoms.
- Instruct the patient that recurrent symptoms lasting more than one to two minutes should prompt him or her to stop all activities, sit down, and place a nitroglycerin tablet under the tongue. This may be repeated twice at five-minute intervals for two additional tablets. If symptoms persist after three nitroglycerin tablets, the patient should promptly seek medical attention.
- Instruct the patient that if symptoms change in pattern (eg, asymptomatic to symptomatic, more frequent, or more severe symptoms), he or she should contact the primary care physician and discuss whether changes in the management plan are warranted.
- Instruct the patient to seek transportation to the nearest hospital emergency department, either by ambulance or the fastest available alternative, if he or she cannot reach a physician and chest pain persists for more than 20 minutes or despite three nitroglycerin tablets.

The natural history of unstable angina is typically characterized by either progression to nonfatal myocardial infarction or death, on the one hand, or resumption of the more quiescent clinical course of chronic stable angina/coronary artery disease, on the other. The acute phase of unstable angina is usually over within four to six weeks. The goal of postdischarge outpatient care is to make adjustments in the discharge regimen that appear most appropriate after an initial period away from direct patient care.

The long-term management of unstable angina ends as the patient reenters the stable phase of coronary artery disease.

**MEDICAL RECORD:**
**INFORMATION TO BE RECORDED IN THE MEDICAL RECORD SUMMARIZING**
**INITIAL EVALUATION AND MANAGEMENT FOR EACH PATIENT**

## AFTER INITIAL EVALUATION

- age and sex
- duration and nature of symptoms prior to presentation
- previous history of coronary artery disease; if yes, prior noninvasive test result, prior cardiac catheterization result, prior revascularization procedure (bypass or angioplasty)
- medication and drug use
- risk factors (diabetes, smoking, hypercholesterolemia, hypertension)
- systemic causes for precipitating or exacerbating ischemia
- electrocardiogram interpretation
- initial and final assignment of likelihood of coronary artery disease (high, intermediate, low) and basis
- initial and final risk assignment (high, intermediate, low) and basis
- summary of other pertinent positive and negative findings
- major or minor complications of diagnosis or treatment
- patient counseling, including assessment of patient response
- disposition for further care
- death classified as noncardiac or cardiac
- cardiac deaths classified as precipitated by arrhythmia, progressive ischemia, or progressive cardiac failure

## AFTER OUTPATIENT MANAGEMENT

- results of ancillary clinical studies
- final diagnosis
- final disposition
- effectiveness of antianginal medication used

## AFTER INTENSIVE MEDICAL MANAGEMENT

- intensity of pain (1–10) and duration (<20 minutes, <1 hour, >1 hour) of each episode of angina or equivalent ischemic symptoms
- duration of longest anginal episode during the phase
- summary of pharmacologic therapy used
- documentation of the status of patient teaching including evidence of what the patient appears to understand
- documentation of alternate treatment options discussed with the patient
- documented plan for further care as patient with stable CAD

## AFTER NONINTENSIVE MEDICAL MANAGEMENT

- medications at the beginning and conclusion of this phase
- number, severity, and duration of ischemic episodes

- complications during this phase
- evaluation of patient's understanding of recommended lifestyle changes and assessment of the patient's willingness to adhere to recommendations

## AFTER NONINVASIVE TESTING

- indications for test
- type of test performed
- summary of test results including electrocardiographic changes, symptoms, hemodynamic changes, reason for termination (exercise tests)
- test complications
- summary of posttest prognosis (low, intermediate, high risk, or probability of adverse event calculation)

## AFTER CARDIAC CATHETERIZATION AND MYOCARDIAL REVASCULARIZATION

- reasons for cardiac catheterization
- cardiac catheterization findings summarized by number of major coronary arteries with 70% or greater stenosis, presence or absence of a 50% or greater left main stenosis, left ventricular ejection fraction, presence and severity of valvular disease
- for patients undergoing interventional therapy, the primary reason for the procedure, indicated as enhanced survival, pain relief, both, or other
- complications occurring during one procedure that led to another, different procedure (angioplasty failure leading to coronary artery bypass graft surgery) including assessment of severity at the beginning of the second procedure

## AFTER HOSPITAL DISCHARGE

- discharge medical regimen
- major instructions about postdischarge activities and rehabilitation, and the patient's understanding and plan for adherence to the recommendations

## AT FINAL OUTPATIENT VISIT

- Summarize cardiac events.
- Document current symptoms.
- Note medication changes since hospital discharge or last outpatient visit.

Source: Braunwald E, Mark DB, Jones RH et al. Diagnosing and Managing Unstable Angina. Quick Reference Guide for Clinicians. Number 10. AHCPR Publication No. 94-0603. Rockville, MD. U.S. Department of Health and Human Services, Public Health Service, Agency for Health Care Policy and Research and National Heart, Lung, and Blood Institute. March 1994.

# HIGHLIGHTS OF AHCPR CLINICAL PRACTICE GUIDELINE—HEART FAILURE: MANAGEMENT OF PATIENTS WITH LEFT-VENTRICULAR SYSTOLIC DYSFUNCTION*

## Abstract

More than two million Americans have heart failure, and about 400,000 new cases are diagnosed each year. Mortality is high, with five-year mortality in the range of 50%. Many of the almost one million hospitalizations each year for heart failure might be prevented by improved evaluation and care.

The following recommendations are based on a combination of evidence obtained through extensive literature reviews and on expert judgment where evidence was lacking. Specific recommendations are made in the following areas:

- prevention of heart failure with asymptomatic left-ventricular systolic dysfunction
- approaches to diagnosis and initial evaluation of suspected heart failure
- hospital admission and discharge criteria
- pharmacological management
- patient counseling and education
- exercise and rehabilitation
- evaluation for myocardial revascularization
- patient monitoring and follow-up evaluation

*Source: Konstam M, Dracup K, Baker D, et al. *Heart Failure: Management of Patients with Left-Ventricular Systolic Dysfunction, Quick Reference Guide for Clinicians No. 11.* AHCPR Publication No. 94-0613. Rockville, MD: Agency for Health Care Policy and Research, Public Health Service, U.S. Department of Health and Human Services. June 1994.

## Purpose and Scope

Heart failure is a clinical syndrome or condition characterized by (1) signs and symptoms of intravascular and interstitial volume overload, including shortness of breath, rales, and edema, or (2) manifestations of inadequate tissue perfusion, such as fatigue or poor exercise tolerance.

Heart failure is a major public health problem. The National Heart, Lung, and Blood Institute estimates that over 2 million Americans have heart failure and that about 400,000 new cases of heart failure are diagnosed each year. Heart failure claims the lives of over 200,000 people in the United States every year. Almost one million hospitalizations occur each year for patients with this condition, at an estimated cost of over $7 billion. Total treatment costs for heart failure, including physician visits, drugs, and nursing home stays, were over $10 billion in 1990.

The following recommendations concern the outpatient evaluation and care of patients with heart failure due to left-ventricular systolic dysfunction, which is the most common cause of heart failure. They do not address the management of patients with heart failure occurring despite normal ventricular systolic performance or due to surgically correctable valvular disease.

These recommendations are intended for use by a broad range of health care practitioners, including family physicians, physician assistants, nurse practitioners, internists, cardiologists, cardiac surgeons, and clinical nurse specialists. Consultation is advised when patients remain symptomatic despite appropriate care or experience significant adverse effects, or when invasive management is contemplated.

The clinical algorithm is not intended as a rigid pathway that must be followed in all cases. The algorithm visually shows the conceptual organization, procedural flow, decision points, and preferred management pathways discussed in this guideline.

When applied to the individual patient, this algorithm should be adapted to accommodate patient preferences and overall patient goals. Numbers in the algorithm indicate the desired sequence of diagnostic, treatment, and management decisions and interventions.

**CLINICAL ALGORITHM FOR EVALUATION AND CARE OF PATIENTS WITH HEART FAILURE**

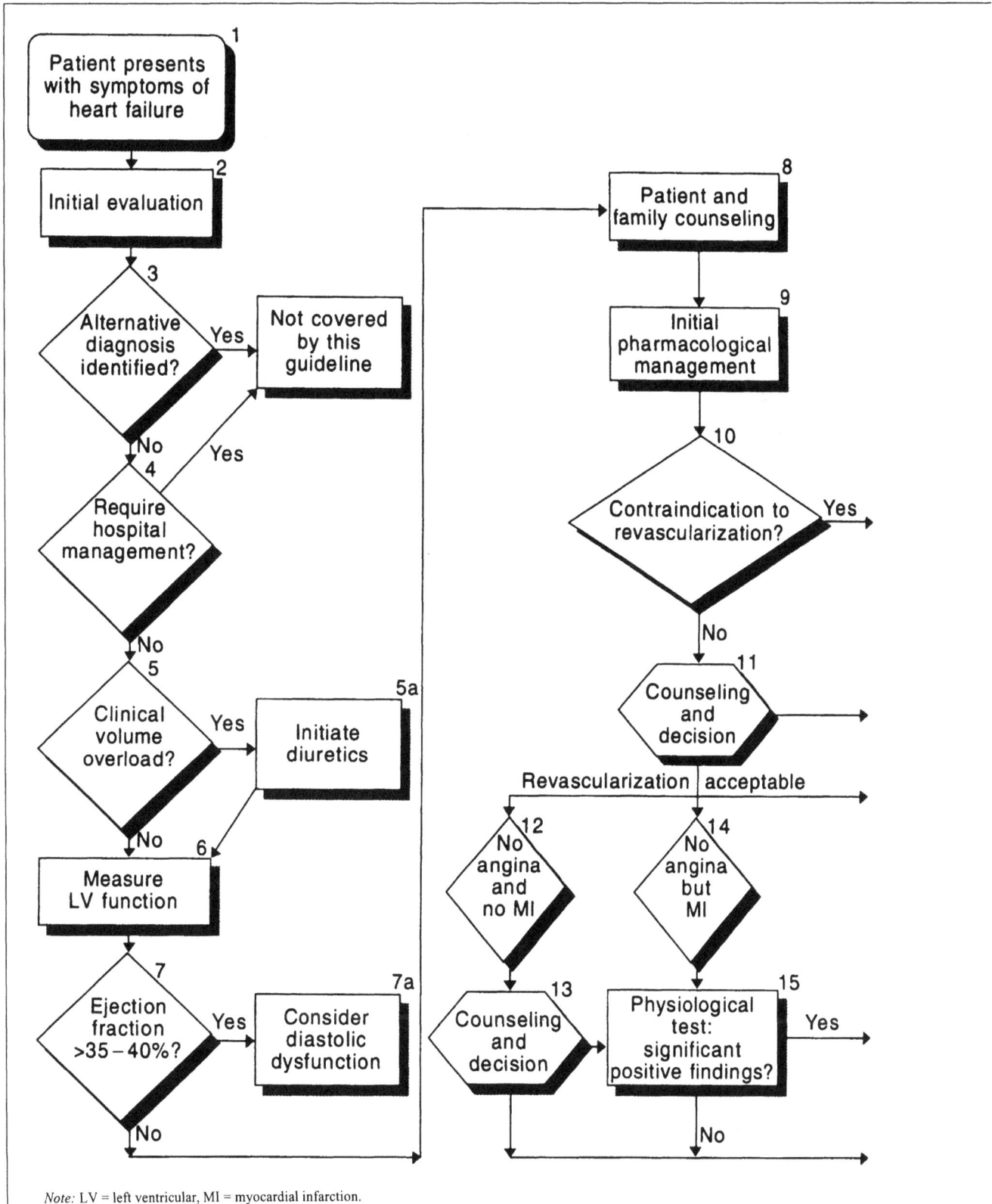

*Note:* LV = left ventricular, MI = myocardial infarction.

*continues*

**Clinical Algorithm for Evaluation and Care of Patients With Heart Failure** continued

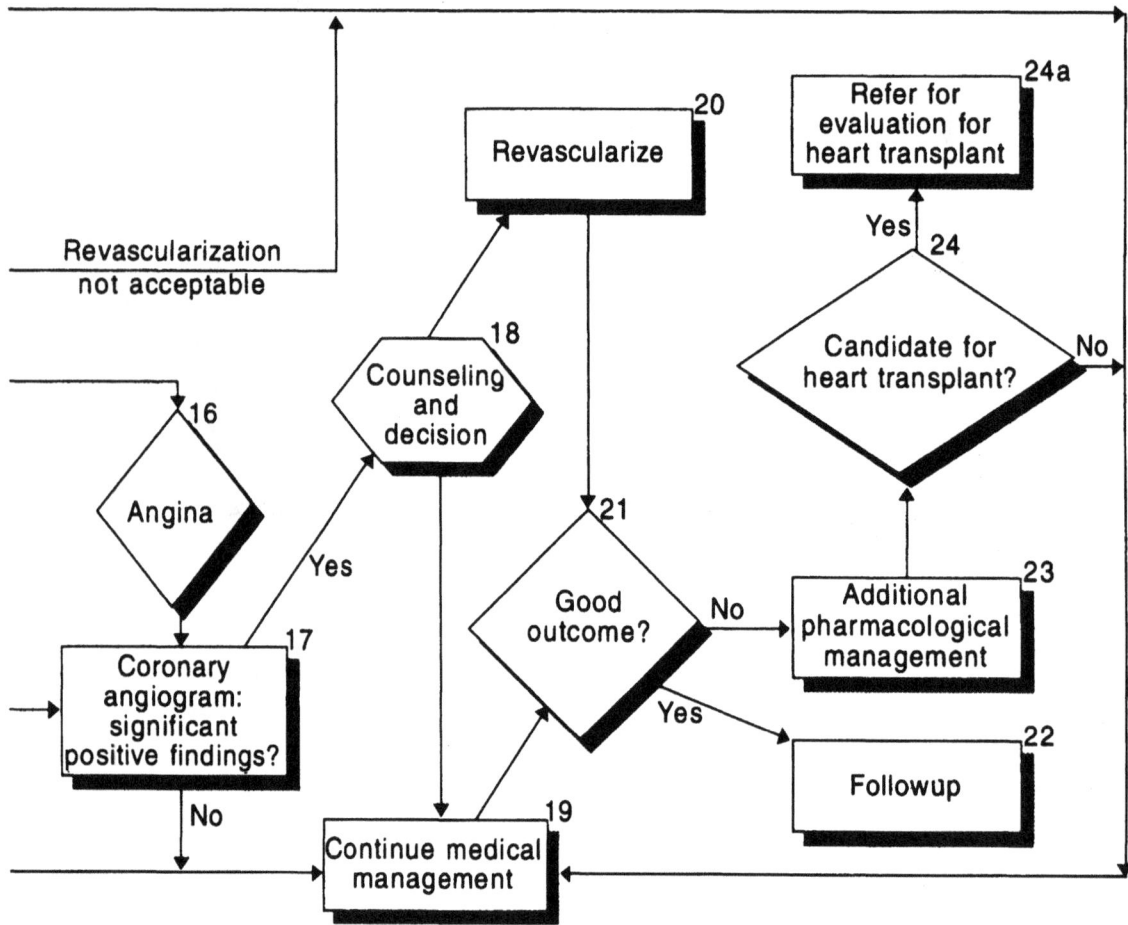

Source: Konstam M, Dracup K, Baker D, et al. *Heart Failure: Management of Patients with Left-Ventricular Systolic Dysfunction. Quick Reference Guide for Clinicians No. 11.* AHCPR Publication No. 94-0613. Rockville, MD: Agency for Health Care Policy and Research, Public Health Service, U.S. Department of Health and Human Services, June 1994.

## Highlights of Patient Management

### *Initial Evaluation*

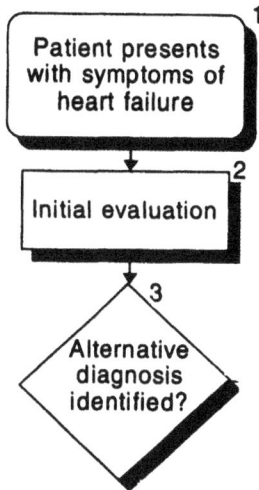

```
                    1
  ┌──────────────────┐
  │ Patient presents │
  │  with symptoms of│
  │   heart failure  │
  └──────────────────┘
           │
           ▼          2
  ┌──────────────────┐
  │ Initial evaluation│
  └──────────────────┘
           │
           ▼          3
        ◇ Alternative ◇
        ◇  diagnosis  ◇
        ◇ identified? ◇
```

All patients who complain of paraoxysmal nocturnal dyspnea, orthopnea, or new-onset dyspnea on exertion should undergo evaluation for heart failure unless history and physical examination clearly indicate a noncardiac cause for their symptoms, such as pulmonary disease.

Although the physical examination can provide important information about the etiology of patients' symptoms and about appropriate initial treatment, physical signs are not highly sensitive for detecting heart failure. Therefore, patients with symptoms highly suggestive of heart failure should undergo echocardiography or radionuclide ventriculography to measure left-ventricular ejection fraction (EF) even if physical signs of heart failure are absent. Patients with less specific symptoms (ie, fatigue, lower extremity edema) should undergo such testing only if there are physical or radiographic signs of heart failure.

Conversely, many physical findings of heart failure are not highly specific. Elevated jugular venous pressure and a third heart sound are the most specific findings and are virtually diagnostic in patients with compatible symptoms. Pulmonary rales or peripheral edema are relatively nonspecific findings, however. The presence of these signs does not require measurement of left-ventricular ejection fraction if other symptoms, signs, and radiographic findings of heart failure (eg, cardiomegaly and pulmonary vascular congestion) are absent or if they can be attributed to other causes.

The exhibit, "Recommended Tests for Patients with Signs or Symptoms of Heart Failure," summarizes the tests that should be performed to evaluate patients with new-onset signs or symptoms of heart failure for underlying causes.

A variety of conditions can mimic or provoke heart failure, including pulmonary disease, myocardial infarction (MI),

arrhythmias, anemia, renal failure, nephrotic syndrome, and thyroid disease. These conditions should be considered in every patient with suspected new-onset heart failure.

### *Hospital Management*

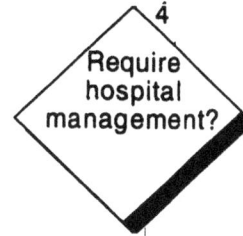

```
             4
         ◇ Require ◇
         ◇ hospital ◇
         ◇management?◇
```

The presence or suspicion of heart failure and any of the following findings usually indicate a need for hospitalization:

- clinical or electrocardiographic evidence of acute myocardial ischemia
- pulmonary edema or severe respiratory distress
- oxygen saturation below 90% (not due to pulmonary disease)
- severe complicating medical illness (eg, pneumonia)
- anasarca
- symptomatic hypotension or syncope
- heart failure refractory to outpatient therapy
- inadequate social support for safe outpatient management

Occasionally, patients with one of the above findings may be managed at home or in an assisted living or nursing home setting if the clinician believes it is safe to do so and adequate follow-up can be arranged. Heart failure is one of the most common causes for recurrent admission to hospitals, and many of these admissions may be avoidable. Readmission rates as high as 57% within 90 days have been reported in patients over the age of 70 years. Proper discharge planning is essential to prevent those unnecessary readmissions.

Patients with heart failure should be discharged from the hospital only when:

- Symptoms of heart failure have been adequately controlled.
- All reversible causes of morbidity have been treated or stabilized.
- Patients and caregivers have been educated about medications, diet, activity, and exercise recommendations, and symptoms of worsening heart failure.
- Adequate outpatient support and follow-up care have been arranged.

Patients who have been hospitalized for heart failure should be seen or contacted within one week of discharge to

**RECOMMENDED TESTS FOR PATIENTS WITH SIGNS OR SYMPTOMS OF HEART FAILURE**

| Test Recommendation | Finding | Suspected Diagnosis |
|---|---|---|
| Electrocardiogram | Acute ST-T wave changes | Myocardial ischemia |
| | Atrial fibrillation, other tachyarrhythmia | Thyroid disease or heart failure due to rapid ventricular rate |
| | Bradyarrhythmias | Heart failure due to low heart rate |
| | Previous MI (eg, Q waves) | Heart failure due to reduced left-ventricular performance |
| | Low voltage | Pericardial effusion |
| | Left-ventricular hypertrophy | Diastolic dysfunction |
| Complete blood count | Anemia | Heart failure due to or aggravated by decreased oxygen-carrying capacity |
| Urinalysis | Proteinuria | Nephrotic syndrome |
| | Red blood cells or cellular casts | Glomerulonephritis |
| Serum creatinine | Elevated | Volume overload due to renal failure |
| Serum albumin | Decreased | Increased extravascular volume due to hypoalbuminemia |
| T4 and TSH (obtain only if atrial fibrillation, evidence of thyroid disease, or patient age >65) | Abnormal T4 or TSH | Heart failure due to or aggravated by hypo/hyperthyroidism |

*Note:* TSH = Thyroid-stimulating hormone, MI = myocardial infarction.

Source: Konstam M, Dracup K, Baker D, et al., *Heart Failure: Management of Patients with Left-Ventricular Systolic Dysfunction. Quick Reference Guide for Clinicians No. 11.* AHCPR Publication No. 94-0613. Rockville, MD: Agency for Health Care Policy and Research, Public Health Service, U.S. Department of Health and Human Services. June 1994.

make sure that they are stable in the outpatient setting and to check their understanding of and compliance with the treatment plan.

## Clinical Volume Overload

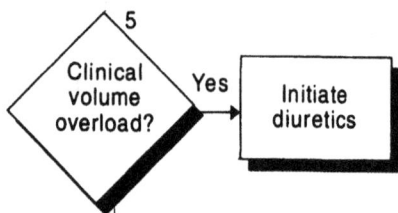

During initial evaluation, the clinician should determine if the patient manifests symptoms or signs of volume overload. Symptoms and signs of volume overload include orthopnea, paroxysmal nocturnal dyspnea, dyspnea on exertion, pulmonary rales, a third heart sound, jugular venous distention, hepatic engorgement, ascites, peripheral edema, and pulmonary vascular congestion or pulmonary edema on chest X-ray.

Patients suspected of heart failure with signs of significant volume overload should be started immediately on a diuretic. Patients with mild volume overload can be managed adequately on thiazide diuretics, while those with more severe volume overload should be started on a loop diuretic. Patients with severe volume overload may require intravenous loop diuretics and/or hospitalization.

## Left-Ventricular Function

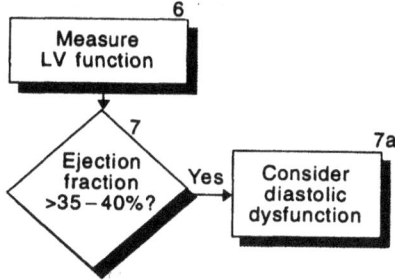

```
                  ┌──────────────┐  6
                  │   Measure    │
                  │  LV function │
                  └──────────────┘
                         │
                         ▼
              ╱─────────────╲        ┌──────────────┐ 7a
             ╱  Ejection     ╲  Yes  │   Consider   │
             ╲  fraction      ╱─────▶│  diastolic   │
              ╲ >35–40%?     ╱       │  dysfunction │
               ╲───────────╱         └──────────────┘
```

Measurement of left-ventricular performance is a critical step in the evaluation and management of almost all patients with suspected or clinically apparent heart failure. The combined use of history, physical examination, chest radiography, and electrocardiography does not appear to be reliable in determining whether a patient's symptoms and physical findings are due to dilated cardiomyopathy, left-ventricular diastolic dysfunction, valvular heart disease, or a noncardiac etiology. Therefore, echocardiography or radionuclide ventriculography can substantially improve diagnostic accuracy.

Patients with suspected heart failure should undergo echocardiography or radionuclide ventriculography to measure left-ventricular ejection fraction (if information about ventricular function is not available from previous tests). The exhibit, "Echocardiography and Radionuclide Ventriculography Compared," summarizes the advantages and disadvantages of echocardiography and radionuclide ventriculography in the evaluation of left-ventricular performance.

Most patients with signs and symptoms of heart failure are found to have EFs less than 40%. Patients with an EF of 40% or greater may still have heart failure on the basis of valvular disease or stiffness of the ventricular wall (diastolic dysfunction). The recommendations here are designed for patients with heart failure due to left-ventricular systolic dysfunction, ie, EFs less than 35% to 40%.

Screening for arrhythmias, such an ambulatory electrocardiographic (Holter) recording, is not warranted as part of the evaluation of patients with heart failure. Patients with a history of syncope or near-syncope should be referred immediately to a cardiologist with expertise in arrhythmias.

## General Counseling

```
                  ┌─────────────────┐ 8
                  │   Patient and   │
                  │family counseling│
                  └─────────────────┘
```

Patients with heart failure should be informed about their diagnoses including the prognosis, symptoms of worsening heart failure, and what to do if these symptoms occur. Information should also be provided concerning the benefits of regular activity, dietary restrictions, necessary medications, and the importance of compliance with recommendations. It is vital that patients understand their disease and be involved in developing the plan for their care. In addition, family members and other responsible caregivers should be included in counseling and decision making sessions.

**Activity.** Regular exercise such as walking or cycling should be encouraged for all patients with stable heart failure. Even short periods of bed rest result in reduced exercise tolerance and aerobic capacity, muscular atrophy, and weakness. Recent studies show that patients with heart failure can exercise safely, and regular exercise may improve functional status and decrease symptoms.

An explanation of the importance of exercise can help prevent patients from becoming afraid to perform daily activities that might provoke some shortness of breath. Patients should be advised to stay as active as possible.

There is insufficient evidence at this time to recommend the routine use of formal rehabilitation programs for patients with heart failure, although patients who are anxious about exercising on their own or are dyspneic at a low work level may benefit from such programs.

**Diet.** Dietary sodium should be restricted to as close to 2 grams per day as possible. In no case should sodium intake exceed 3 grams daily. Alcohol use should be discouraged. Patients who drink alcohol should be advised to consume no more than one drink per day. One drink equals a glass of beer or wine, or a mixed drink or cocktail containing no more than 1 ounce of alcohol. Patients with heart failure should be advised to avoid excessive fluid intake. However, fluid restriction is not advisable unless patients develop hyponatremia. Patients should be advised to keep a diary of their daily weights and to advise the clinicians if a weight gain of 3–5 pounds or more occurs within one week or since the previous visit with the clinician.

**ECHOCARDIOGRAPHY AND RADIONUCLIDE VENTRICULOGRAPHY COMPARED IN EVALUATION OF LEFT-VENTRICULAR PERFORMANCE**

| Test | Advantages | Disadvantages |
|---|---|---|
| Echocardiogram | Permits concomitant assessment of valvular disease, left-ventricular hypertrophy, and left-atrial size | Difficult to perform in patients with lung disease |
| | Less expensive than radionuclide ventriculography in most areas | Usually only semi-quantitative estimate of ejection fraction provided |
| | Able to detect pericardial effusion and ventricular thrombus | Technically inadequate in up to 18% of patients under optimal circumstances |
| | More generally available | |
| Radionuclide ventriculogram | More precise and reliable measurement of EF | Requires venipuncture and radiation exposure |
| | Better assessment of right-ventricular function | Limited assessment of valvular heart disease and left-ventricular hypertrophy |

Source: Konstam M, Dracup K, Baker D, et al. *Heart Failure: Management of Patients with Left-Ventricular Systolic Dysfunction. Quick Reference Guide for Clinicians No. 11.* AHCPR Publication No. 94-0613. Rockville, MD: Agency for Health Care Policy and Research, Public Health Service, U.S. Department of Health and Human Services. June 1994.

**Medications.** Medications are prescribed for patients with heart failure for two basic reasons: (1) to reduce mortality (angiotensin-converting enzyme [ACE] inhibitors, isosorbide dinitrate/hydralazine) and (2) to reduce symptoms and improve functional status (ACE inhibitors, diuretics, digoxin). Patients should be provided with complete and accurate information concerning the medications they are being asked to take, including the reasons the medications are being prescribed, dosing requirements, and possible side effects.

**Compliance.** Because noncompliance is a major cause of morbidity and unnecessary hospital admissions for heart failure, educational programs or support groups can be very helpful in the care of patients with heart failure. Noncompliance may reduce life expectancy (eg, if patients are not taking beneficial medications) and is also a major cause of hospitalizations. Practitioners should be aware of the problem of noncompliance and its causes and should discuss the importance of compliance at follow-up visits and assist patients in removing barriers to compliance (eg, cost, side effects, or complexity of the medical regimen).

**Prognosis.** Patients with heart failure must understand the serious implications of this diagnosis, including a five-year mortality rate approaching 50% in some studies. Patients should be encouraged to complete advance directives regarding their health care preferences. Patients, families, and caregivers must be provided with the accurate information necessary to make decisions and plans for the future, while maintaining hope and emphasizing that good quality of life is still possible.

The exhibit, "Suggested Topics for Patient, Family, and Caregiver Education and Counseling," summarizes many of the topics that should be discussed during counseling.

## Initial Pharmacological Management

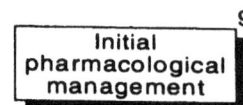

Initial pharmacological management 9

The exhibit, "Medications Commonly Used for Heart Failure," summarizes the usual dosing and potential adverse effects of the pharmacological agents commonly used to treat patients with heart failure.

**Diuretics.** Diuretics are extremely useful for reducing symptoms of volume overload, including orthopnea and paroxysmal nocturnal dyspnea. As noted above under Clinical Volume Overload (Algorithm Node 5), diuretics should be started immediately when patients present with symptoms or signs of volume overload.

## SUGGESTED TOPICS FOR PATIENT, FAMILY, AND CAREGIVER EDUCATION AND COUNSELING

**General Counseling**
Explanation of heart failure and the reason for symptoms
Cause or probable cause of heart failure
Expected symptoms
Symptoms of worsening heart failure
What to do if symptoms worsen
Self-monitoring with daily weights
Explanation of treatment/care plan
Clarification of patient's responsibilities
Importance of cessation of tobacco use
Role of family members or other caregivers in the
treatment/care plan
Availability and value of qualified local support group
Importance of obtaining vaccinations against influenza and
pneumococcal disease

**Prognosis**
Life expectancy
Advance directives
Advice for family members in the event of sudden death

**Activity Recommendations**
Recreation, leisure, and work activity
Exercise
Sex, sexual difficulties, and coping strategies

**Dietary Recommendations**
Sodium restriction
Avoidance of excessive fluid intake
Fluid restriction (if required)
Alcohol restriction

**Medications**
Effects of medications on quality of life and survival
Dosing
Likely side effects and what to do if they occur
Coping mechanisms for complicated medical regimens
Availability of lower cost medications or financial
assistance

**Importance of Compliance with the Treatment/Care Plan**

Source: Konstam M, Dracup K, Baker D, et al., *Heart Failure: Management of Patients with Left-Ventricular Systolic Dysfunction. Quick Reference Guide for Clinicians No. 11.* AHCPR Publication No. 94-0613. Rockville, MD: Agency for Health Care Policy and Research, Public Health Service, U.S. Department of Health and Human Services. June 1994.

Although initiation of diuretics is important in these patients, it is also important to avoid overdiuresis before starting ACE inhibitors. Volume depletion may lead to hypotension or renal insufficiency when ACE inhibitors are started or when the doses of these agents are increased to full therapeutic levels. After the ACE inhibitor is increased to full therapeutic levels, additional diuretic therapy may be necessary to optimize the patient's status.

**ACE Inhibitors.** Because of their beneficial effects on mortality risk and functional status, ACE inhibitors should be prescribed for all patients with left-ventricular systolic dysfunction unless specific contraindications exist (ie, history of intolerance or adverse reactions to these agents, serum potassium >5.5, or symptomatic hypotension). Patients with contraindications to ACE inhibitors or who cannot tolerate them should be placed on isosorbide dinitrate/hydralazine.

ACE inhibitors may be considered as sole therapy in patients who present with fatigue or mild dyspnea on exertion and who do not have any signs or symptoms of volume overload. Diuretics should be added if symptoms persist in these patients despite ACE inhibitors or if volume overload develops at a later time.

**Digoxin.** Digoxin increases the force of ventricular contraction in patients with left-ventricular systolic dysfunction. Although physical functioning and symptoms may be improved with digoxin, its effect on mortality is not known. Digoxin should be initiated along with ACE inhibitors and diuretics in patients with severe heart failure. Patients with mild to moderate heart failure will often become asymptomatic on optimal doses of ACE inhibitors and diuretics; these patients do not require digoxin. Digoxin should be added to the therapeutic regimen of those patients whose symptoms persist despite optimal doses of ACE inhibitors and diuretics.

**Anticoagulation.** Routine anticoagulation is not recommended. Patients with a history of systemic or pulmonary embolism or recent atrial fibrillation should be anticoagulated to a prothrombin time ratio of 1.2–1.8 times each individual control time (International Normalization Ratio of 2.0–3.0). Although there has never been a controlled trial of anticoagulation for patients with heart failure, the risks of routine treatment, including intracranial or gastrointestinal hemorrhage, do not appear warranted given the relatively low incidence of significant thromboembolic events in this population.

## MEDICATIONS COMMONLY USED FOR HEART FAILURE

| Drug | Initial Dose (mg) | Target Dose (mg) | Recommended Maximal Dose (mg) | Major Adverse Reactions |
|---|---|---|---|---|
| **Thiazide Diuretics** | | | | |
| Hydrochlorothiazide | 25 QD | As needed | 50 QD | Postural hypotension, hypokalemia, hyperglyce- |
| Chlorthalidone | 25 QD | As needed | 50 QD | mia, hyperuricemia, rash. Rare severe reaction includes pancreatitis, bone marrow suppression, and anaphylaxis. |
| **Loop Diuretics** | | | | |
| Furosemide | 10–40 QD | As needed | 240 BID | Same as thiazide diuretics. |
| Bumetanide | 0.5–1.0 QD | As needed | 10 QD | |
| Ethacrynic acid | 50 QD | As needed | 200 BID | |
| **Thiazide-Related Diuretic** | | | | |
| Metolazone | 2.5[a] | As needed | 10 QD | Same as thiazide diuretics. |
| **Potassium-Sparing Diuretics** | | | | |
| Spironolactone | 25 QD | As needed | 100 BID | Hyperkalemia, especially if administered with |
| Triamterene | 50 QD | As needed | 100 BID | ACE inhibitor; rash; gynecomastia (spironolac- |
| Amiloride | 5 QD | As needed | 40 QD | tone only). |
| **ACE Inhibitors** | | | | |
| Enalapril | 2.5 BID | 10 BID | 20 BID | Hypotension, hyperkalemia, renal insufficiency, |
| Captopril | 6.25–12.5 TID | 50 TID | 100 TID | cough, skin rash, angioedema, neutropenia. |
| Lisinopril | 5 QD | 20 QD | 40 QD | |
| Quinapril | 5 BID | 20 BID | 20 BID | |
| **Digoxin** | 0.125 QD | As needed | As needed | Cardiotoxicity, confusion, nausea, anorexia, visual disturbances. |
| **Hydralazine** | 10–25 TID | 75 TID | 100 TID | Headache, nausea, dizziness, tachycadia, lupus-like syndrome. |
| **Isosorbide Dinitrate** | 10 TID | 40 TID | 80 TID | Headache, hypotension, flushing. |

[a]Given as a single test dose initially.

*Note:* ACE = angiotensin-converting enzyme, BID = twice a day, QD = once a day, TID = three times a day.

Source: Konstam M, Dracup K, Baker D, et al. *Heart Failure: Management of Patients with Left-Ventricular Systolic Dysfunction. Quick Reference Guide for Clinicians No. 11.* AHCPR Publication No. 94-0613. Rockville, MD: Agency for Health Care Policy and Research, Public Health Service, U.S. Department of Health and Human Services. June 1994.

## Revascularization

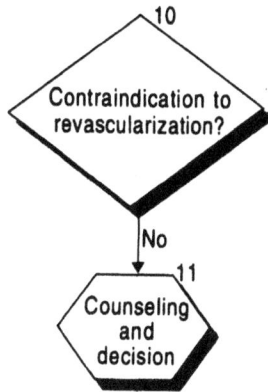

Coronary artery disease is currently the most common cause of heart failure in the United States, and some patients may benefit from revascularization. In particular, patients with viable myocardium subserved by substantially stenotic vessels may reasonably be expected to obtain longevity benefits and, perhaps, improved quality of life if the stenosis is successfully relieved. On the other hand, revascularization entails significant morbidity and mortality. Before studies are initiated to determine if patients are candidates for revascularization (ie, have viable myocardium subserved by stenotic arteries), it is important to determine first if any conditions exist that may preclude intervention or that could raise the risk of revascularization above any potential benefit. These may include:

- patient would not consider surgery or is unable to give informed consent
- severe comorbid diseases, especially renal failure, pulmonary disease, or cerebrovascular disease (eg, severe stroke)
- very low ejection fraction (ie, <20%)
- illnesses with a projected life expectancy less than or equal to one year. These include advanced cancer, severe lung or liver disease, chronic renal disease, advanced diabetes mellitus, and advanced collagen vascular disease.
- technical factors, including previous myocardial revascularization or other cardiac procedure, history of chest irradiation, and diffuse distal coronary artery atherosclerosis

Patients without contraindication to revascularization should be advised of the possibility of revascularization, including its potential benefits and harms.

Three parameters are important: (1) likelihood of surgically correctable lesions, (2) expected benefits of revascularization, and (3) expected risks and potential harms of revascularization. These parameters vary depending on several factors, including whether clinical evidence of myocardial ischemia is present and the patient's general state of health.

Counseling should be based on patients' particular characteristics, particularly on an assessment of patients' risk factors for coronary artery disease. Patients can be classified into three major subgroups: (1) patients who have neither angina nor a history of myocardial infarction, (2) patients without significant angina (angina that limits exercise or occurs frequently at rest), but who have a history of MI, and (3) patients with significant angina pectoris.

**No Angina and No MI.**

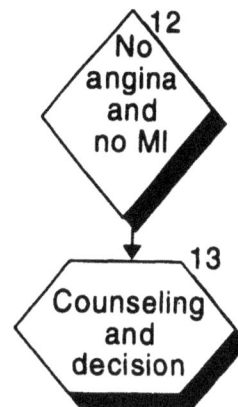

The likelihood of coronary disease in heart failure patients without angina or history of myocardial infarction varies depending on patient risk factors (eg, age, sex, smoking history, hyperlipidemia, hypertension, family history of premature coronary artery disease, and diabetes).

Patients should be counseled concerning the expected benefits and risks of evaluation for ischemia, including the fact that there is no evidence from controlled trials to show that revascularization benefits heart failure patients in the absence of angina.

It is unclear whether patients without a history of MI or significant angina should be routinely evaluated for ischemia. The decision about whether to perform physiological tests for ischemia or coronary angiography should be based on a consideration of patients' risk factors for coronary artery disease and the likelihood of alternative etiologies (eg, alcoholic cardiomyopathy).

**No Angina and History of MI.**

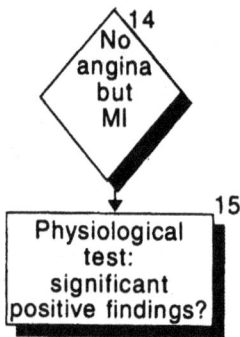

```
         /\  14
        /No\
       /angina\
       \ but  /
        \ MI /
         \/
          |
          v
   +------------------+ 15
   | Physiological    |
   | test:            |
   | significant      |
   | positive findings?|
   +------------------+
```

Available evidence suggests that as many as half of patients who suffer a myocardial infarction have clinically important myocardial ischemia in areas supplied by other coronary arteries. There are no data, however, to show that revascularization of these areas is beneficial, in terms of increased life expectancy or enhanced quality of life, in the absence of angina. Nevertheless, patients with large areas of ischemia may possibly benefit from revascularization.

Patients without angina but with a history of MI should undergo a physiological test for ischemia and should undergo cardiac catheterization if ischemic regions are detected. This strategy will miss a small number of patients with false negative physiological tests. However, in view of the lack of evidence that these patients benefit from surgery, together with a consideration of the morbidity, mortality, and the cost of catheterizing all patients in this group, this drawback is considered relatively minor. Although there are a number of acceptable physiological tests for ischemia, the most widely available and accepted procedure for determining the presence of ischemic myocardium is myocardial perfusion scintigraphy, such as thallium scanning, with poststress, redistribution, and rest reinjection imaging.

**Angina.**

```
         /\  16
        /  \
       /Angina\
       \      /
        \    /
         \/
          |
          v
   +------------------+ 17
   | Coronary         |
   | angiogram:       |
   | significant      |
   | positive findings?|
   +------------------+
```

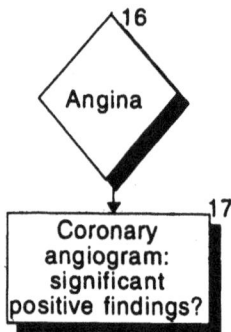

The potential benefit of revascularization is clearest and probably greatest in individuals with severe or limiting angina or angina-equivalent (eg, recurrent acute episodes of pulmonary edema despite appropriate medical management). Available evidence suggests that about 75% of heart failure patients with significant concomitant angina have operable disease. Although the three randomized trials of coronary artery bypass graft (CABG) surgery excluded patients with heart failure or severe left-ventricular dysfunction, several cohort studies and registries suggest that patients with angina and impaired left-ventricular function have improved functional status and survival if they undergo bypass surgery.

Heart failure patients without contraindications to revascularization and who have exercise-limiting angina, angina that occurs frequently at rest, or recurrent episodes of acute pulmonary edema should be advised to undergo coronary artery angiography as the initial test for significant coronary lesions. Some patients may need physiological testing for ischemia to interpret the significance of the findings from coronary artery angiography.

**Counseling and Decision.**

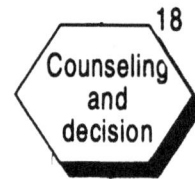

```
       _____  18
      /          \
     /  Counseling \
     |    and       |
     \  decision   /
      _____/
```

Based on the results of physiological testing and/or cardiac catheterization, the physician should give the patient a refined estimate of the risks and benefits of revascularization. The patient can then decide if he or she desires revascularization. No data are available that address the question of how much ischemia should be present to justify the risk of revascularization for the chance of an improvement in survival. In general, patients with severely depressed ejection fractions (EF <20%) should undergo revascularization only if large areas of ischemia are detected. Patients with less severely depressed ejection fractions may be willing to risk surgery for more modest-sized ischemic areas. The lack of data in this area makes it difficult to justify revascularization for small ischemic areas, except when severe angina is present.

**Continue Medical Management.**

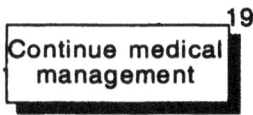

```
┌─────────────────────┐19
│ Continue medical    │
│    management       │
└─────────────────────┘
```

If (1) a patient is not a candidate for revascularization, (2) studies show insufficient evidence of reversible ischemia, or (3) surgery has been performed but the patient still has residual left-ventricular dysfunction, then the medical therapy stated under "Initial Pharmacological Management" (Algorithm Node 9) should be continued. As stated previously, an assessment of compliance is recommended at each visit. Use of a home health nurse or visiting nurse may be helpful for this purpose.

**Revascularize.**

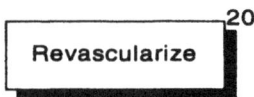

```
┌─────────────────────┐20
│   Revascularize     │
└─────────────────────┘
```

Coronary artery bypass grafting is the only revascularization procedure that has been shown to prolong life in patients with angina and left-ventricular dysfunction. The effect of coronary artery angioplasty on survival of heart failure patients has not been studied, nor are the risks of angioplasty in heart failure patients known at this time. The choice between CABG and angioplasty will depend on numerous considerations, including multiple technical factors (eg, coronary anatomy), relative risk of the two procedures in individual patients, and patient preferences.

*Follow-Up*

```
      21                              22
   ◇ Good  ◇ ──────▶  ┌──────────────┐
     outcome?         │   Followup    │
                      └──────────────┘
```

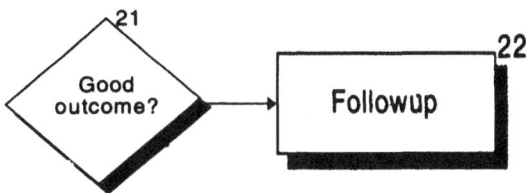

Careful history and physical examination should be the main guide to determining outcomes and directing therapy. A thorough history should include questions regarding physical functioning, mental health, sleep disturbance, sexual function, cognitive function, and ability to perform usual work and social activities.

On follow-up visits, patients should be asked about the presence of orthopnea, paroxysmal nocturnal dyspnea, edema, and dyspnea on exertion. It is im-portant to remember that patients are likely to experience changes in symptoms before there is evidence of deterioration by physical examination.

Patients should be encouraged to keep a record of their daily weights and to bring that record with them when visiting their practitioner. Patients should be instructed to call if they experience an unexplained weight gain greater than three to five pounds since their last clinical evaluation.

Family members or other caregivers can often contribute important additional information about the patient's status and compliance when asked similar questions. In some cases, it may be desirable to interview family members or other caregivers apart from the patient in order to validate the patient's report. If discrepancies do occur, additional measures need to be instituted for clarification.

In addition to questions about symptoms and activities, providers should ask about other aspects of patients' health-related quality of life, including sleep, sexual function, mental health (or outlook on life), appetite, and social activities. A worsening in any of these parameters may indicate the need to adjust therapy. To ensure optimal care for heart failure, the provider must view the disease in the broad context of the patient's life and see how the patient is coping with the disease.

Consultation with psychologists, dietitians, health educators, and clinical nurse specialists may be necessary to deal with specific problems such as depression, difficulties adhering to complicated dietary or medical regimens, or poor functional status.

The Heart Failure Guideline Panel recommends against the use of other tests (eg, echocardiography, exercise testing) for monitoring the response of heart failure patients to treatment. No data exist to suggest that the monitoring of these end points contributes information beyond that obtained by a careful history and physical examination. However, repeat testing may be useful in patients with a new heart murmur, a new myocardial infarction, or sudden deterioration despite compliance with medications. Repeat testing as part of the evaluation for transplantation may also be necessary.

*Additional Pharmacological Management*

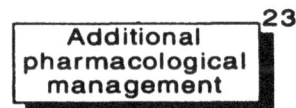

```
┌─────────────────────┐23
│    Additional       │
│  pharmacological    │
│    management       │
└─────────────────────┘
```

If patients remain symptomatic on a combination of a diuretic, an ACE inhibitor, and digoxin, they should be seen at least once by a cardiologist.

Patients with persistent volume overload despite initial medical management may require more aggressive administration of the current diuretic (eg, intravenous administration), more potent diuretics, or a combination of diuretics (see the exhibit, "Medications Commonly Used for Heart Failure").

Patients with persistent dyspnea after optimal doses of diuretics, ACE inhibitors, and digoxin should be given a trial of hydralazine and/or nitrates. The addition of a vasodilator to an ACE inhibitor may also relieve symptoms. Direct vasodilators may be particularly helpful in patients with hypertension or evidence of severe mitral regurgitation. Even patients with blood pressure in the usual normal range may benefit by reducing their blood pressure with direct vasodilators. Alternatively, if a patient primarily has symptoms of pulmonary congestion or has a low systolic blood pressure, nitrates are preferred over arterial vasodilators.

There is some evidence that gradually incremental therapy with low-dose beta-blockers may produce long-term improvements in symptoms and in natural history in patients with heart failure. However, because beta-blockers may also cause acute deterioration in patients with heart failure, this form of treatment should be considered experimental at this time.

## Heart Transplantation

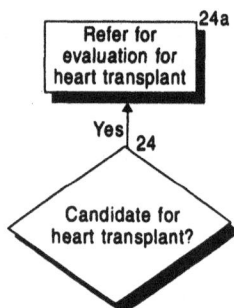

Consideration should be given to cardiac transplantation in patients with severe limitation and/or repeated hospitalization because of heart failure, despite aggressive medical therapy, and in whom revascularization is not likely to convey benefit. Patients with severe symptoms should be referred to a cardiologist to ensure that medical therapy is optimized prior to referral for possible transplantation. Practitioners should refer to existing documents concerning heart transplantation for further information on patient selection criteria.

Patients with poor systolic function whose symptoms are controlled on optimal medical management need not be referred for transplantation. Where appropriate, patients with severe symptoms uncontrolled by optimal medical management who are unable to obtain a heart transplant should be informed of the availability of experimental treatment protocols for which they may be eligible (eg, new drugs, mechanical assist devices).

## Prevention in Patients with Left-Ventricular Systolic Dysfunction

Asymptomatic patients who are found to have moderately or severely reduced left-ventricular systolic function (ejection fraction <35%–40%) should be treated with an ACE inhibitor to reduce the chance of developing clinical heart failure.

Probably the largest number of such patients will be those who have recently sustained a myocardial infarction. For this reason, the EF should be determined in most patients following a myocardial infarction unless they are at low risk for significant systolic dysfunction, ie, unless they meet all of the following criteria:

1. no previous myocardial infarction
2. inferior infarction
3. relatively small increase in cardiac enzymes (ie, <2–4 times normal)
4. no Q waves developing on electrocardiogram
5. uncomplicated clinical course (eg, no arrhythmia or hypotension)

Other asymptomatic patients without infarctions may be found to have reduced EF on evaluation of heart murmurs or cardiomegaly. These patients should also be treated with ACE inhibitors.

# GUIDELINES FOR MANAGING CONGESTIVE HEART FAILURE

## Congestive Heart Failure: A Clinical Quality Improvement Study*

Congestive heart failure (CHF) contributes more than $8 billion annually to the nation's health bill. More than 3 million Americans suffer from heart failure, with approximately 400,000 new cases being diagnosed each year. The condition has a high mortality rate: about 50 percent of CHF patients will not live beyond 5 years of their diagnosis.

At Advocate Health Care (a newly merged entity as of January 1995, formerly known as EHS Health Care and Lutheran General Health System), more than 1,800 patients with CHF are treated each year. Given the volume of patients, the cost of providing their care, and an interest on the part of several key internal stakeholders, the former EHS Health Care undertook CHF as its first systemwide (five hospitals) clinical quality improvement project.

The project began within a framework of clinical subgroups, each changed with development of a specific product. A 20-member implementation team and physician advisor group (comprising cardiologists, clinical nurse specialists, pharmacists, and quality management personnel) created a continuum of care for the treatment of CHF that consisted of the following:

- inpatient care, including a clinical path and discharge disposition guidelines
- drug therapy guidelines
- enhanced patient and family education
- a transitional care program for outpatient support
- home health follow-up for appropriate patients.

## Inpatient Management*

### Admission Guidelines

Patients with CHF present to the hospital with variable intensity of service needs. To assist those charged with

*Source: Cindy Welsh, BSN, MBA, RN, and Maureen McCafferty, MS, RN, CCRN, "Congestive Heart Failure: A Continuum of Care," *Journal of Nursing Care Quality,* Vol. 10:4, Aspen Publishers, Inc., © 1996.

determining the appropriate level of care, admission guidelines were developed. An objective assessment of service needs could be made to determine the appropriate level of treatment (see "Guidelines for Disposition of CHF Patients after Clinical Assessment: Three Options").

### Clinical Pathway

Clinical pathways or their equivalents have become commonplace in most hospitals. Our five hospitals were no exception. Many of them had existing pathways that needed to be revised to reflect changing length of stay expectations. When the subgroup charged with developing a standard pathway met, a few potential roadblocks surfaced:

- The hospitals that had pathways were quite attached to them.
- It was difficult to devise a prototype that would meet each hospital's needs.
- Some pathways were a part of the medical record, and some were not.
- All existing pathways had desirable aspects, but we could not find one model that fit across the board.
- Even what the tool was called varied by hospital.
- A wide variety of case management styles were in place.
- It was not the intention of this project to overhaul and standardize the case management process.

Consensus was reached on the development of a template. (See "Clinical Pathway for CHP"). The content was considered nonnegotiable, but how the pathway looked at each hospital was. This was an important step for us. Each operating unit had put time and effort into development of tools that fit its culture. We did not want to negate that by mandating a "cookie cutter" approach to care. Once we gave ourselves permission to vary a bit, it was not hard to agree on content.

Our clinical pathway is based on a 4-day length of stay with discharge on day 5. Because the majority of our patients are admitted through the emergency department, it is designed to be implemented there or on the floor. It is multidisciplinary in nature, and expectations of all staff are accounted for. Other aspects of the project were woven into the pathway. One example of this is the drug guidelines. High-risk screens for social service intervention with these patients would prepare them for a smooth exit from the hospital in a timely fashion.

**Guidelines for Disposition of CHF Patients after Clinical Assessment: Three Options**

| Option 1: Patient discharged/remains home | Option 2: Patient transferred/ admitted to observation bed | Option 3: Patient admitted to hospital |
|---|---|---|
| Indications | Indications | Indications |
| Extremely mild exacerbation of chronic CHF | Acute failure with benign or treatable precipitant | Presentation of new-onset CHF requiring comprehensive cardiac work-up to determine etiology |
| Emergency department visit for specific, uncomplicated intervention (intravenous [IV] diuretic/oxygen/ medication adjustment) | Absence of unstable comorbidity, other contraindications as listed below (see option 3) | High severity of illness or high intensity of service requirement |
| | Assessed high probability that short-term treatment will prove successful, allowing patient to be discharged safely home (i.e., patient "clearing up" well in period since IV diuretic administered, yet emergency physician uncomfortable releasing patient from the emergency department) | Severe hypoxia |
| | | Evidence of acute myocardial infarction |
| | | Life-threatening dysrhythmias |
| | | Hypotensive emergency |
| | | Cardiac tamponade |
| | | Respiratory failure requiring intubation |
| | | Serious precipitating event (e.g., pneumonia, sepsis, thyrotoxicosis) |
| | | Unstable major comorbidity (e.g., chronic renal failure, diabetes) |
| | Disposition: Discharge to home, extended care facility, other | Disposition: Admit to hospital |
| | Clinical conditions cleared | Clinical conditions fail to improve |
| | No serious disease found after full evaluation | Serious disease found after full evaluation of symptoms |

Source: Cindy Welsh, B.S.N., M.B.A., R.N., and Maureen McCafferty, M.S., R.N., C.C.R.N., "Congestive Heart Failure: A Continuum of Care," *Journal of Nursing Care Quality*, Vol. 10:4, Aspen Publishers, Inc., © 1996.

Clinical outcomes are at the bottom of the "Clinical Pathway for CHF." They are not meant to be all inclusive. A few vital outcomes were agreed upon. The staff were expected to address these objective/subjective issues on a daily basis. If "unmet" was the outcome, it would trigger the staff to modify the treatment plan.

## Drug Therapy

The increasing severity and incidence of CHF have created a market for research. Many studies have been conducted over the past decade. Primary end points of clinical trials have included reduction in mortality, improvement of symptoms, and decreased hospitalizations. The questions we faced were: How do we summarize all the current recommendations, and how do we get this information out to our medical staff?

A subgroup comprising primarily clinical pharmacists and physicians took charge of the issues. They conducted a comprehensive review of the clinical literature with the assistance of the Advocate Health Care Library Network. Because clinical research in CHF has been geared toward patients with systolic dysfunction, it soon became clear that our focus needed to be narrowed. We determined that, if we focused inpatient care on systolic dysfunction, we could affect the greatest number of patients and those with the worst prognoses.

The team developed two final documents. The first was a schematic matching the four main classes of drugs used in the treatment of CHF with the patients' symptoms (see "Drug Treatment Strategy for CHF Due to Systolic Dysfunction"). This schematic was designed to be placed on the front of the medical record of those patients admitted with CHF due to systolic dysfunction. A second, more detailed document summarized specific information from the literature. The guidelines were divided into the major classes of drugs vasodilators (including angiotensin-converting enzyme [ACE] inhibitors), diuretics, digoxin, and positive inotropic agents. Drug names, doses, indications, and goals for therapy were identified. This guideline was enlarged and posted on the patient care units. The two documents were color coded to make them stand out in the typical nurses' station clutter.

Before their release, the two guidelines and our baseline data were extensively reviewed at the local hospital level.

# CLINICAL PATHWAY FOR CHF

Etiology
NYHA Functional Class

| | Em. Dept/Day 0 | Patient Admitted | Day 2 | Day 3 | Day 4 | Day 4 |
|---|---|---|---|---|---|---|
| **Test** | CXR, EKG, BUN Crest, Lytes, Pulse Ox.ABG Magnesium Blood Sugar, if diabetic If on Digoxin—get Dig level see CHF Drug Guidelines | If tests not done in ED, should be done on admission to unit → ECHO if not done in last 6 months | K+ Follow-up on abnormal labs | BUN/Creat K+/Magnesium Follow-up on abnormal labs | Follow-up on abnormal labs | Follow-up on abnormal labs Final Baseline Dig level 1 day prior to discharge |
| **Assess Need For** | -Outpatient Care -Subacute Care -23 hr OBS -Inpatient Admission to Med Floor, Telemetry, ICU-CCU per condition | Protime if on Coumadin Advanced Directive Status Old chart(s) to floor | | | | |
| **Activity** | | Bed Rest with Bedside Commode | Up as tolerated | | | assess functional status |
| **Diet** | | Dietitian notified Sodium Restriction | | Diet instruction documented | | |
| **Medications** | | See CHF Drug Guidelines for Digoxin, ACE Inhibitors, Diuretics, Inotropes | | | Change to PO meds Discharge medication plan documented | |
| **Treatments/Intervention** | Heplock/IV → O2 → | If not done in ED Consider Fluid Restriction I/O Wt(Actual) _____ lbs | Consider Fluid Restriction I/O Wt _____ lbs | Consider switch to PO meds D/C O2 Consider Fluid Restriction I/O Wt _____ | Consider Fluid Restriction I/O Wt _____ lbs | Consider Fluid Restriction I/O Wt _____ lbs |
| **Discharge Plan** | Repeat ED Visit    Y/N Previous Home Care Agency    Y/N When? _____ | Social Service notified Repeat admission    Y/N Age > 65    Y/N Patient Compliance    Y/N Family Support    Y/N Follow-up Referral    Y/N | Social Work Assessment documented | Discharge Plan documented | Discharge Arrangements documented | If D/C to Home Care, D/C Record: Med Sheet initial documentation |
| **Teaching/Plan** | | | Teaching aids given to patient & family Encourage viewing of CHF Video | Physiology discussed | CHF Discharge Teaching documented | |
| **Desired Outcomes** | K+ WNL Met ( ) Not Met ( ) O>1 Met ( ) Not Met ( ) Improved Signs & Symptoms Met ( ) Not Met ( ) | K+ WNL Met ( ) Not Met ( ) O>1 Met ( ) Not Met ( ) Improved Signs & Symptoms Met ( ) Not Met ( ) | K+ WNL Met ( ) Not Met ( ) O>1 Met ( ) Not Met ( ) Improved Signs & Symptoms Met ( ) Not Met ( ) | K+ WNL Met ( ) Not Met ( ) O>1 Met ( ) Not Met ( ) Improved Signs & Symptoms Met ( ) Not Met ( ) | K+ WNL if ordered Met ( ) Not Met ( ) NA ( ) O>1 Met ( ) Not Met ( ) Improved Signs & Symptoms Met ( ) Not Met ( ) | K+ WNL if ordered Met ( ) Not Met ( ) NA ( ) O>1 Met ( ) Not Met ( ) Improved Signs & Symptoms Met ( ) Not Met ( ) |

Source: Cindy Welsh, BSN, MBA, RN, and Maureen McCafferty, MS, RN, CCRN, "Congestive Heart Failure: A Continuum of Care," *Journal of Nursing Care Quality,* Vol. 10:4, Aspen Publishers, Inc., © 1996.

Existing practice demonstrated a significant lag in the use of ACE inhibitor drugs (now considered first-line therapy for systolic dysfunction in those patients who can tolerate these drugs). This information was extremely helpful in demonstrating the need to summarize the latest research and have the information available to the physicians ordering the medications. Guideline approval was obtained from a variety of medical staff committees as well as from the pharmacy and therapeutics committees.

By the time we were ready to implement the entire project, a national summary of clinical guidelines for the treatment of systolic dysfunction was published by the Agency for Health Care Policy and Research. We were pleased to discover that the work of our group was in line with current recommended practice.

As CHF research continues, we are obligated to review and revise the drug therapy guidelines periodically to reflect the latest developments and recommendations.

## Discharge Guidelines

Many staff nurses believed that matching the patient with appropriate services after discharge was a weak area for them. Discharge guidelines for proper posthospitalization care were agreed upon and placed on the flip side of the clinical pathway for easy reference. The five levels of care were home unassisted (with a referral to our transitional care program), home with home care, subacute care, traditional extended care facility, and hospice (our use of hospice services for end-stage patients has grown with our understanding of the natural course of the disease (see "CHF Guidelines for Hospital Discharge").

## Patient Education

The patient education subgroup reviewed all existing internal teaching tools for the CHF patients. This subgroup also looked outside the system to search for the best and most current tools. This search included identifying tools that met the needs of populations in our hospitals whose primary language is not English. The subgroup also agreed upon a commercially prepared, patient-focused video. Patients and families can view this video on the unit and also on the patient education closed-circuit television channel.

Because patients often ignored their early warning signs or said that they did not want to 'bother the doctor," a reminder sheet was developed. Early warning signs of recurring CHF as well as instructions on when to call the physician were included. The sheet is meant to be posted in a prominent place in the home (e.g., the refrigerator). These early warning signs may be treated outside the hospital if reported in a timely manner. If inpatient admission is warranted, a lesser intensity of service or shorter stay may result if these signs are reported early.

A tool was develop to standardize the essential components of patient education. A copy of the tool is sent to the home care agency if applicable. This way, the home care nurse can continue to build on the teaching that was started in the hospital.

## Staff Education

A vital step in the implementation process was ensuring preparation of the staff caring for CHF patients. To ease the roll-out of such an extensive program, a comprehensive staff education plan was developed. Included in the curriculum was a review of CHF management, drug therapy, and teaching needs. Woven into these 3-hour sessions were the various aspects of the project (i.e., the drug guidelines, teaching tools, the clinical pathway, and discharge criteria). The classes were approved for continuing education hours as well.

This education was mandatory for all staff who cared for these patients. The classes were multidisciplinary, involving anyone who owned a part of the clinical pathway. Staff nurses were joined by dietitians, chaplains, echocardiology technicians, respiratory therapists, and home care coordinators. Each discipline's contribution to the best patient outcome was stressed. All the participants saw this as a positive step. They felt better prepared to incorporate the "finished products" into their daily practice.

# Continuity of Care*

## Transitional Care Program

To improve the health of our CHF population and to lower costs for treating these patients, EHS Health Care developed a transitional care program for CHF patients. The program's goal is to provide outpatient follow-up and educational support that enhances compliance with the regimen designed by each patient's physician.

Transitional care program patients are identified by a CHF care card. The card was developed to alert the health care provider to a preexisting diagnosis of CHF, thereby preventing duplication of previous work-ups during acute exacerbations. The three components of the transitional care program are telemanagement follow-up 48 hours after hospital discharge, individual follow-up visits for each patient 5 to 7 days after discharge, and subsequent structured follow-up support, including individual visits, group meetings, or continued telemanagement.

Under telemanagement, within 48 hours of discharge from the hospital, the patient is telephoned by a registered nurse

---

*Source: Cindy Welsh, BSN, MBA, RN, and Maureen McCafferty, MS, RN, CCRN, "Congestive Heart Failure: A Continuum of Care," *Journal of Nursing Care Quality,* Vol. 10:4, Aspen Publishers, Inc., © 1996.

**Drug Treatment Strategy for CHF Due to Systolic Dysfunction**

| NYHA Class 1 | NYHA Class II | NYHA Class III | NYHA Class IV |
|---|---|---|---|
| | | | (See Guidelines for Inotropes Selective Therapy) |
| | | Hydralazine & Isordil | |
| | ACE Inhibitors | | |
| | Digoxin | | |
| PO Diuretics | IV Diuretics (See Guidelines for Progressive Therapy) | | |

| NYHA Class I | NYHA Class II | NYHA Class III | NYHA Class IV |
|---|---|---|---|
| Patients with cardiac disease but without resulting limitation of physical activity. Ordinary physical activity does not cause undue fatigue, palpitation, dyspnea, or anginal pain. | Patients with cardiac disease resulting in slight limitation of physical activity. Patients are comfortable at rest. Ordinary physical activity results in fatigue, palpitation, dyspnea, or anginal pain. | Patients with cardiac disease resulting in marked limitation of physical activity. Patients are comfortable at rest. Less than ordinary physical activity causes fatigue, palpitation, dyspnea, or anginal pain. | Patients with cardiac disease resulting in inability to carry out any physical activity without discomfort. Symptoms of cardiac insufficiency or of the anginal syndrome may be present even at rest. If any physical activity is undertaken, discomfort is increased. |

Source: Cindy Welsh, BSN, MBA, RN, and Maureen McCafferty, MS, RN, CCRN, "Congestive Heart Failure: A Continuum of Care," *Journal of Nursing Care Quality*, Vol. 10:4, Aspen Publishers, Inc., © 1996.

from Health Advisor (a centrally located physician referral and triage service). Using a prompting script (developed by the implementation team and physician advisors), the nurse assesses the patient's understanding of CHF, medication compliance, diet, exercise, and daily weight measurements. He or she is also prepared to make referrals to social services, assist in arranging transportation, and schedule both medical and individual follow-up appointments. After the phone call, the patient is mailed a CHF care card. The phone call is summarized by the nurse, printed, and then mailed to the attending physician and CHF coordinator at the patient's local hospital.

Within 5 to 7 days after discharge, the patient is scheduled for an individual follow-up visit at the hospital site with the CHF coordinator. Each CHF coordinator is a nurse with advanced knowledge of the disease process. The patient's vital signs and weight are measured against the hospital baseline. Compliance and educational needs are also assessed by the nurse. The coordinator determines whether the patient should be referred for group follow-up or requires additional individual follow-up for continued reinforcement of the medical regimen. The results of the visit are communicated in writing to the attending physician.

Group follow-up provides the emotional and social support that many CHF patients need. Patients and their families say that they feel comforted in knowing that everyone at the session is there for the same reason. The hospital coordinator facilitates the meeting but seeks input from the participants

**CHF Guidelines for Hospital Discharge**

| Subacute/skilled care | Home care | Hospice | Extended care facility | Home without home care (unassisted) |
|---|---|---|---|---|
| Acute care clinical outcomes<br>• Electrolytes WNL for patient<br>• Edema (peripheral/ pulmonary) resolving<br>• Nonlethal dysrhythmias<br>• Hemodynamically stable<br>Requires rehabilitation under supervision for cardiac complications<br>Not candidate for acute rehabilitation<br>Potential for readmission because of overall deconditioning<br>Medication regulation<br>Intermittent inotropic agents, intravenous diuretics<br>Requires reinforcement of teaching regarding disease, medications, treatment plan | Acute care clinical outcomes<br>• Electrolytes WNL for patient<br>• Edema (peripheral/ pulmonary) resolving<br>• Baseline rhythm for patient<br>• Improved signs/ symptoms<br>Homebound<br>Poor support system<br>Readmission within 30 days<br>New chronic illness diagnosis (insulin-dependent diabetes mellitus, CHF, uncontrolled hypertension)<br>Potentially unstable medical conditions<br>Durable medical equipment | Acute care clinical outcomes<br>• Electrolytes WNL for patient<br>• Relief of presenting signs/ symptoms<br>End-stage heart failure (death expected within 6 months)<br>Functional class IV<br>Other terminal medical conditions<br>Patient/family desires comfort measures only | Acute care clinical outcomes<br>• Electrolytes WNL for patient<br>• Baseline rhythm for patient<br>• Hemodynamically stable<br>Not able to perform activities of daily living<br>Disoriented<br>Insufficient family/social support<br>Inability to care for self at home<br>Other medical conditions requiring skilled facility<br>No knowledge of disease<br>Frequent readmission because of noncompliance | Acute care clinical outcomes<br>• Electrolytes WNL for patient<br>• Edema resolved<br>• Effectively diuresed<br>• Baseline rhythm for patient<br>• Relief of shortness of breath<br>Demonstrates understanding of medications, diet, treatment plan<br>Demonstrates knowledge of disease process and understands long-term nature of disease<br>Can identify signs and symptoms of recurrent heart failure<br>Verbalizes when to seek medical attention<br>Independent in activities of daily living<br>Family/social support in place<br>No durable medical equipment |

Source: Cindy Welsh, BSN, MBA, RN, and Maureen McCafferty, MS, RN, CCRN, "Congestive Heart Failure: A Continuum of Care," *Journal of Nursing Care Quality*, Vol. 10:4, Aspen Publishers, Inc., © 1996.

on desired topics for discussion. Guest speakers are utilized to provide continuing education. Speakers to date have included nurses, cardiologists, dietitians, pharmacists, staff from patient support services, and staff from cardiac conditioning. If for some reason a patient cannot attend group meetings (i.e., there are distance or transportation problems). Health Advisor will conduct periodic telephone assessments and keep the patient's physician and CHF coordinator informed of the patient's status.

*Home Care*

For patients qualifying for home health care, a comprehensive educational program has been developed to enhance compliance with the medical regimen while increasing the patient's understanding of CHF. The home health nurse not only provides a thorough physical assessment but also continues the educational process started in the hospital, reports abnormal findings to the physician, and can administer intravenous diuretics, if ordered.

**Lessons Learned***

Lessons learned through implementation of the project include the following:

• Communicate, communicate, communicate! The work you are doing can never be presented to too many people too many times.

*Source: Cindy Welsh, BSN, MBA, RN, and Maureen McCafferty, MS, RN, CCRN, "Congestive Heart Failure: A Continuum of Care," *Journal of Nursing Care Quality*, Vol. 10:4, Aspen Publishers, Inc., © 1996.

**Disease Management in CHF**

*The information below depicts advantages for elderly patients, with substantial risk factors beyond age alone, whose CHF is managed using principles of disease management. The main outcomes are a reduction in the rate of readmission due to recurrent heart failure by 56.2 percent, and improved life quality scores.* \*

*Study design*
Randomized controlled trial

*Population*
Seniors older than 70 years ($N = 282$)
Risk factors in addition to age

*Duration*
90 days

*Care patterns*
Disease management (treatment group, $n = 142$)
Conventional management (control group, $n = 140$)

*Functional status measure*
Chronic Heart Failure Questionnaire
- Has shown responsiveness to improvement in health status
- Has demonstrated validity (e.g., in measuring shortness of breath)

$p = 0.03.$

*Treatment group interventions*
Cardiovascular nurse education
Booklet specific for geriatric patients with CHF
Diet instruction
Social services consultation
Medication analysis by geriatric cardiologist
Intensive postdischarge home care
- Visits
- Phone contacts

*Survival (for 90 days without readmission from subset of survivors of the initial hospitalization)*
Treatment group: 66.9%
Control group: 54.3%
$p = .04.$

*90-Day episode cost*
| | | |
|---|---|---|
| Treatment group: | $4,815 | $2,178 |
| Control group: | $5,275 | $3,236 |
| Difference: | $460 | $1,058* |

**Table 1** Disease Management in CHF

| Group | Readmissions | More Than One Readmission | Hospital Days | Drug Compliance | Daily Drug Doses | Quality of Life Scores | Understanding CHF |
|---|---|---|---|---|---|---|---|
| Treatment | 53 | 9 | 556 | 82.5% | 2.7 | Greater improvement | Greater |
| Control | 94 | 23 | 865 | 64.9% | 3.0 | — | — |
| p | .02 | .01 | .04 | .02 | .01 | .001 | .001 |

The two study groups were compared by students' t-test for normally distributed continuous variables, by the chi-square test for discrete variables, and by the Wilcox rank-sum test for categorical and abnormally distributed continuous variables.

*Source: Peter R. Kongstvedt, MD, FACP, *The Managed Health Care Handbook*, 3rd ed., Aspen Publishers, Inc., © 1996.

- Find a physician champion. Having a spokesperson who supports your improvement efforts can greatly accelerate acceptance by the peer group.
- Multiple mechanisms to disseminate information and educate are needed. The more methods used, the better.

- Implementation planning will make or break the project. Do not assume that, because your implementation group and physician advisor are fully vested in the project, others are as well. A thorough implementation plan, includ-ing checklists, time lines, responsibilities, and a designated "process owner" will be the key to successful implementation.

# HIGHLIGHTS OF AHCPR CLINICAL PRACTICE GUIDELINE— CARDIAC REHABILITATION AS SECONDARY PREVENTION*

## Abstract

The following conclusions and recommendations were derived from an extensive and critical review of the scientific literature pertaining to cardiac rehabilitation, as well as from the expert opinion of the panel. This summary addresses the role of cardiac rehabilitation and the potential benefits to be derived in the comprehensive care of the 13.5 million patients with coronary heart disease in the United States, as well as the 4.7 million patients with heart failure and the several thousand patients undergoing heart transplantation.

This summary also highlights the major effects of multifactorial cardiac rehabilitation services; medical evaluation; prescribed exercise; cardiac risk factor modification; and education, counseling, and behavioral interventions. The outcomes of and recommendations for cardiac rehabilitation services are categorized as to their effects on exercise tolerance, strength training, exercise habits, symptoms, smoking, lipids, body weight, blood pressure, psychological well-being, social adjustment and functioning, return to work, morbidity and safety issues, mortality and safety issues, and pathophysiologic measures. Patients with heart failure and after cardiac transplantation, as well as elderly patients, are specifically addressed. Alternative approaches to the delivery of cardiac rehabilitation services are presented.

## Purpose and Scope

Cardiovascular disease is the leading cause of morbidity and mortality in the United States, accounting for almost 50% of all deaths. Coronary heart disease (CHD) with its clinical manifestations of stable angina pectoris, unstable angina, acute myocardial infarction, and sudden death affects 13.5 million Americans. Nearly 1.5 million Americans sustain myocardial infarction each year, of which almost 500,000 episodes are fatal. Myocardial infarctions can occur at a young age: 5% occur in people younger than age 40, and 45% occur in people under age 65.

The almost 1 million survivors of myocardial infarction each year and the more than 7 million patients with stable angina pectoris are candidates for cardiac rehabilitation, as are patients following revascularization with coronary artery bypass graft (CABG) surgery (309,000 patients in 1993, 45% under age 65) or percutaneous transluminal coronary angioplasty (PTCA) and other transcatheter interventional procedures (362,000 in 1993, 54% under age 65). Although several million patients with CHD are candidates for cardiac rehabilitation services, only 11% to 20% have participated in cardiac rehabilitation programs. More recently, among patients with acute myocardial infarction enrolled in the Global Utilization of Streptokinase and t-PA for Occluded Coronary Arteries (GUSTO) Trial, 38% of U.S. patients and 32% of Canadian patients were subsequent participants in cardiac rehabilitation programs.

Heart failure is the most common discharge diagnosis for hospitalized Medicare patients and the fourth most common discharge diagnosis for all hospitalized patients in the United States. Application of cardiac rehabilitation services to patients with heart failure and after cardiac transplantation has gained increasing recognition and acceptance as their benefits and safety are documented. An estimated 4.7 million patients with heart failure may be candidates for cardiac rehabilitation.

Cardiac rehabilitation is characterized by comprehensive long-term services involving medical evaluation; prescribed exercise; cardiac risk factor modification; and education, counseling, and behavioral interventions. This multifactorial process is designed to limit the adverse physiologic and psychological effects of cardiac illness, reduce the risk of sudden death or reinfarction, control cardiac symptoms, stabilize or reverse the atherosclerotic process, and enhance the patient's psychosocial and vocational status. Provision of these services is physician-directed and implemented by a variety of health care professionals.

This summary is designed for use by health care professionals who provide care to patients with cardiovascular disease. These clinicians include physicians (primary care, cardiologists, and cardiovascular surgeons), nurses, exercise physiologists, dietitians, behavioral medicine specialists, psychologists, and physical and occupational therapists. The information can guide clinical decision making regarding referral and follow-up of patients for cardiac rehabilitation services, as well as administrative decisions regarding the availability of and access to cardiac rehabilitation.

The exhibit, "Decision Tree for Cardiac Rehabilitation Services," describes patient categories addressed herein as well as the patient assessment and treatment strategies involved in the delivery of cardiac rehabilitation services. The exhibits, "Summary of Evidence of Cardiac Rehabilitation Outcomes: Effects of Exercise Training" and "Effects of Education, Counseling, and Behavioral Interventions," display the outcomes pertaining to the two major components of

*Source: Wenger NK, Froelicher ES, Smith LK, et al. *Cardiac Rehabilitation as Secondary Prevention*. Clinical Practice Guideline. Quick Reference Guide for Clinicians, No. 17. Rockville, MD: U.S. Department of Health and Human Services, Public Health Service, Agency for Health Care Policy and Research and National Heart, Lung, and Blood Institute. AHCPR Pub. No. 96-0673. October 1995.

**DECISION TREE FOR CARDIAC REHABILITATION SERVICES**

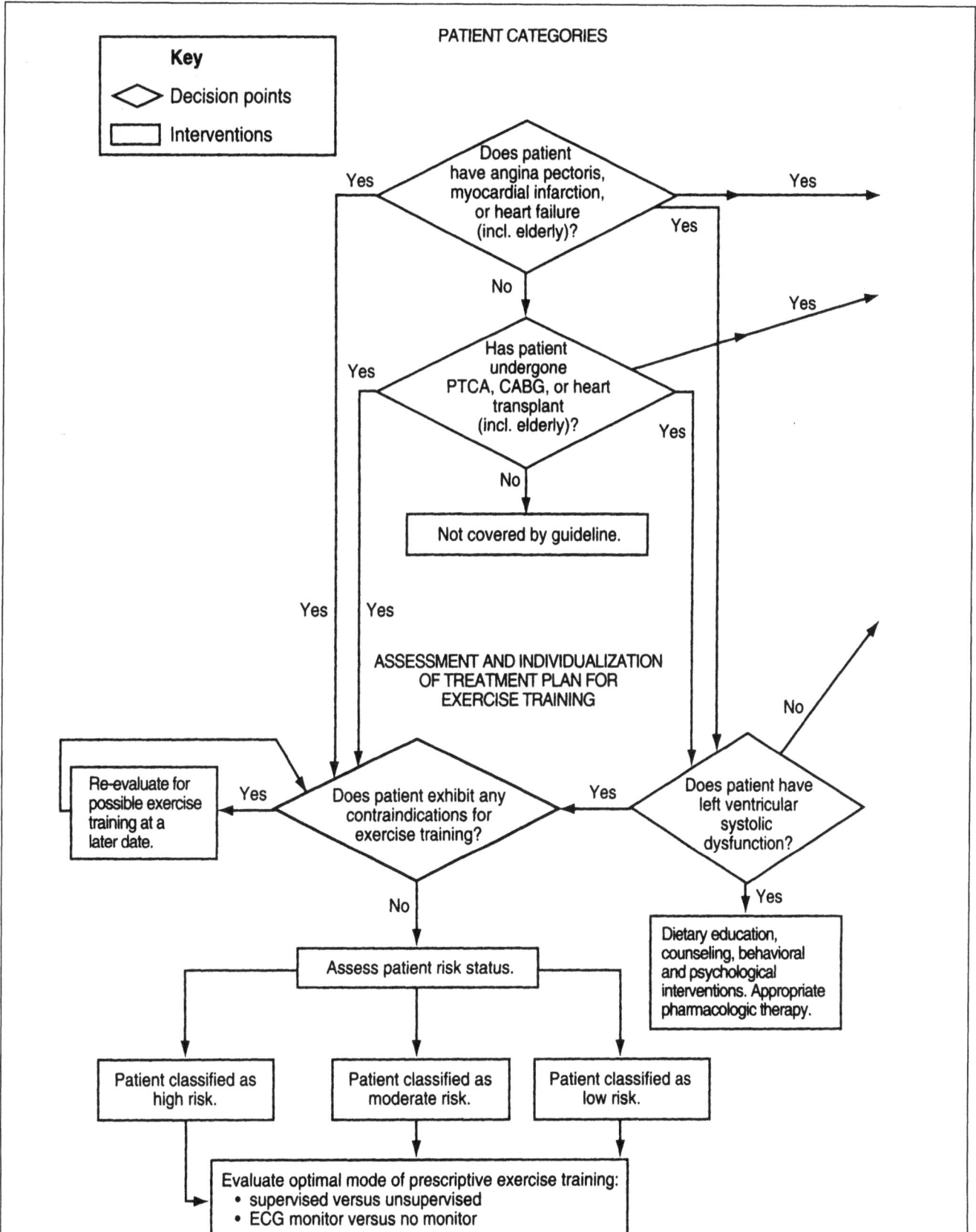

*continues*

**Decision Tree for Cardiac Rehabilitation Services** continued

ASSESSMENT AND INDIVIDUALIZATION
OF TREATMENT PLAN FOR RISK FACTOR
MODIFICATION, PSYCHOSOCIAL STATUS

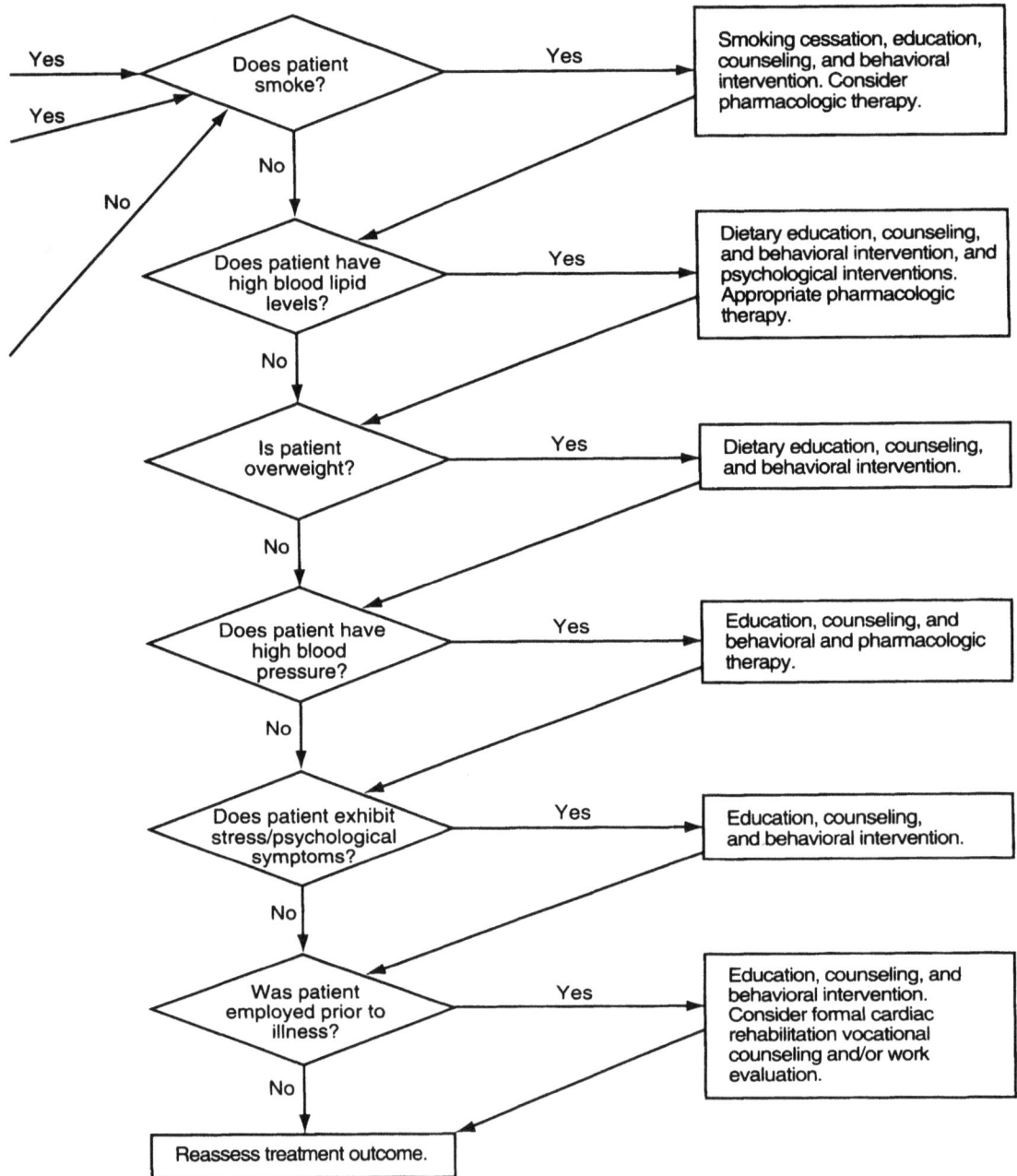

Yes →

Yes →

**Does patient smoke?** → Yes → Smoking cessation, education, counseling, and behavioral intervention. Consider pharmacologic therapy.

No ↓

No

**Does patient have high blood lipid levels?** → Yes → Dietary education, counseling, and behavioral intervention, and psychological interventions. Appropriate pharmacologic therapy.

No ↓

**Is patient overweight?** → Yes → Dietary education, counseling, and behavioral intervention.

No ↓

**Does patient have high blood pressure?** → Yes → Education, counseling, and behavioral and pharmacologic therapy.

No ↓

**Does patient exhibit stress/psychological symptoms?** → Yes → Education, counseling, and behavioral intervention.

No ↓

**Was patient employed prior to illness?** → Yes → Education, counseling, and behavioral intervention. Consider formal cardiac rehabilitation vocational counseling and/or work evaluation.

No ↓

Reassess treatment outcome.

Source: Adapted from material provided by Health Economics Research, Inc., Waltham, MA.

**SUMMARY OF EVIDENCE OF CARDIAC REHABILITATION OUTCOMES:
EFFECTS OF EXERCISE TRAINING**

| Outcome | Evidence Base[a] | | | | Strength of Evidence[b] |
|---|---|---|---|---|---|
| | Total Number of Studies | Randomized Studies | Nonrandomized Studies | Observational Studies | |
| Exercise tolerance | 114 | 46 | 25 | 43 | A |
| Exercise tolerance (strength training) | 7 | 4 | 3 | 0 | B |
| Exercise habits | 15 | 10 | 2 | 3 | B |
| Symptoms | 26 | 12 | 7 | 7 | B |
| Smoking | 24 | 12 | 8 | 4 | B |
| Lipids | 37 | 18 | 6 | 13 | B |
| Body weight | 34 | 11 | 7 | 16 | C |
| Blood pressure | 18 | 9 | 6 | 3 | B |
| Psychological well-being | 20 | 9 | 8 | 3 | B |
| Social adjustment and functioning | 6 | 2 | 2 | 2 | B |
| Return to work | 28 | 10 | 9 | 9 | A |
| Morbidity | 42 (+2 survey reports) | 15 | 14 | 13 | A |
| Mortality | 31 (+2 survey reports) | 17 | 8 | 6 | B |
| Pathophysiologic measures: | | | | | |
| Changes in atherosclerosis | 9 | 5 | 1 | 3 | A/B |
| Changes in hemodynamic measurements | 5 | 0 | 0 | 5 | B |
| Changes in myocardial perfusion/myocardial ischemia | 11 | 6 | 2 | 3 | B |
| Changes in myocardial contractility, ventricular wall motion abnormalities, and/or ventricular ejection fraction | 22 | 9 | 5 | 8 | B |
| Changes in cardiac arrhythmias | 5 | 4 | 0 | 1 | B |
| Heart failure patients | 12 | 5 | 3 | 4 | A |
| Cardiac transplantation patients | 5 | 0 | 1 | 4 | B |
| Elderly patients | 7 | 0 | 1 | 6 | B |

[a]Number of studies from scientific literature by type of study design.
[b]Rating for strength of evidence:
   **A** Scientific evidence from well-designed and well-conducted controlled trials (randomized and nonrandomized) provides statistically significant results that consistently support the guideline statement.
   **B** Scientific evidence is provided by observational studies or by controlled trials with less consistent results.
   **C** Guideline statement supported by expert opinion; the available scientific evidence did not present consistent results or controlled trials were lacking.

Source: Wenger NK, Froehlicher ES, Smith LK, et al. *Cardiac Rehabilitation as Secondary Prevention*. Clinical Practice Guideline. Quick Reference Guide for Clinicians, No. 17. Rockville, MD: U.S. Department of Health and Human Services, Public Health Service, Agency for Health Care Policy and Research and National Heart, Lung, and Blood Institute. AHCPR Pub. No. 96–0673. October 1995.

## SUMMARY OF EVIDENCE FOR CARDIAC REHABILITATION OUTCOMES: EFFECTS OF EDUCATION, COUNSELING, AND BEHAVIORAL INTERVENTIONS

| Outcome | Evidence Base[a] | | | | Strength of Evidence[b] |
|---|---|---|---|---|---|
| | Total Number of Studies | Randomized Studies | Nonrandomized Studies | Observational Studies | |
| Smoking | 7 | 5 | 1 | 1 | B |
| Lipids | 18 | 12 | 3 | 3 | B |
| Weight | 5 | 3 | 1 | 1 | B |
| Blood pressure | 2 | 0 | 2 | 0 | B |
| Exercise tolerance | 3 | 1 | 1 | 1 | C |
| Symptoms | 4 | 2 | 1 | 1 | B |
| Return to work | 3 | 2 | 0 | 1 | C |
| Stress/psychological well-being | 14 | 7 | 5 | 2 | A |
| Morbidity | 3 | 3 | 0 | 0 | B |
| Mortality | 8 | 8 | 0 | 0 | B |

[a]Number of studies from scientific literature by type of study design.
[b]Rating for strength of evidence:

  **A** Scientific evidence from well-designed and well-conducted controlled trials (randomized and nonrandomized) provides statistically significant results that consistently support the guideline statement.
  **B** Scientific evidence is provided by observational studies or by controlled trials with less consistent results.
  **C** Guideline statement supported by expert opinion; the available scientific evidence did not present consistent results or controlled trials were lacking.

Source: Wenger NK, Froehlicher ES, Smith LK, et al. *Cardiac Rehabilitation as Secondary Prevention*. Clinical Practice Guideline. Quick Reference Guide for Clinicians, No. 17. Rockville, MD: U.S. Department of Health and Human Services, Public Health Service, Agency for Health Care Policy and Research and National Heart, Lung, and Blood Institute. AHCPR Pub. No. 96–0673. October 1995.

cadiac rehabilitation services: (1) exercise training and (2) education, counseling, and behavioral interventions.

The components of cardiac rehabilitation services include exercise training; education, counseling, and behavioral interventions; and organizational issues, including consideration of alternative approaches to the delivery of cardiac rehabilitative care. The physiologic parameters targeted include improvement in exercise tolerance and exercise habits; optimization of risk factor status including improvement in blood lipid and lipoprotein profiles, body weight, blood glucose and blood pressure levels, and cessation of smoking. Emotional responses to living with heart disease must be addressed, including reduction of stress and anxiety and lessening of depression. Functional independence of patients, particularly at elderly age, is an essential goal. Return to appropriate and satisfactory occupation could benefit both patients and society.

The results of cardiac rehabilitation services, based on over 400 reports in the scientific literature, are summarized here. The most substantial benefits include:

- improvement in exercise tolerance
- improvement in symptoms
- improvement in blood lipid levels
- reduction in cigarette smoking
- improvement in psychosocial well-being and reduction of stress
- reduction in mortality

The outcomes of application of cardiac rehabilitation services are addressed on the following pages.

## Exercise Tolerance

Cardiac rehabilitation exercise training consistently improves objective measures of exercise tolerance, without significant cardiovascular complications or other adverse outcomes. Appropriately prescribed and conducted exercise training is recommended as an integral component of cardiac rehabilitation services, particularly for patients with decreased exercise tolerance. Continued exercise training is required to sustain improved exercise tolerance.

The beneficial effect of cardiac rehabilitation exercise training on exercise tolerance is one of the most clearly established favorable outcomes for coronary patients with angina pectoris, myocardial infarction, CABG, and PTCA and for patients with compensated heart failure or a decreased ventricular ejection fraction or following cardiac transplantation. This approach is particularly beneficial for patients with decreased functional capacity. The large number of studies that reported a favorable outcome revealed characteristics of exercise training that resulted in improved exercise tolerance. The most consistent benefit appeared to occur with exercise training at least three times weekly for 12 or more weeks' duration. The duration of aerobic exercise training sessions varied from 20 to 40 minutes, at an intensity approximating 70% to 85% of the baseline exercise test heart rate.

No increase in cardiovascular complications or other serious adverse outcomes were reported in any randomized controlled trial that evaluated exercise training in patients with CHD. These trials involved patients with various manifestations of CHD including 3,932 patients following myocardial infarction, 745 patients with catheterization-documented CHD, 215 patients following CABG, and 139 patients following PTCA. No deterioration in measures of exercise tolerance was reported in any patient undergoing exercise training, nor did any controlled study document significantly greater improvement in exercise tolerance in control patient groups compared with exercise patient groups.

Limited data fail to demonstrate the efficacy of education, counseling, and behavioral interventions as sole interventions, independent of cardiac rehabilitation exercise training, in improving exercise tolerance. Education and behavioral interventions may improve morale, self-esteem, and adherence to exercise.

## Strength Training

Strength training improves skeletal muscle strength and endurance in clinically stable coronary patients. Training measures designed to increase skeletal muscle strength can safely be included in the exercise-based rehabilitation of clinically stable coronary patients, when appropriate instruction and surveillance are provided.

Scientific data demonstrate the effectiveness of resistance exercise training in selected patients with CHD. The absence of signs or symptoms of myocardial ischemia, abnormal hemodynamic changes, and cardiovascular complications in these studies suggests that resistance exercise training is safe for selected coronary patients who have previously participated in rehabilitative aerobic exercise training. Improvement in muscle strength can benefit patients' performance of activities of daily living. The absence of cardiovascular and orthopedic complications in the three-year follow-up of strength training was largely attributed to strict preliminary screening and careful supervision. Most studies involved small numbers of low-risk male patients, 70 years or younger, with minimal functional aerobic impairment and with normal or near-normal left-ventricular function. The extent to which the safety and effectiveness demonstrated by these studies can be extrapolated to other populations of coronary or cardiac patients (eg, women, older patients of both genders with low aerobic fitness, patients at moderate to high cardiovascular risk) requires study.

## Exercise Habits

Cardiac rehabilitation exercise training promotes increased participation in exercise by patients after myocardial infarction and CABG. This effect does not persist long term after completion of exercise rehabilitation. Long term cardiac rehabilitation exercise training is recommended to provide the benefit of enhanced exercise tolerance and exercise habits.

There is suggestive evidence that exercise training enhances subsequent exercise habits. A limitation of the scientific data relating to continued exercise habits as a result of rehabilitative exercise training is the self-report nature of the information, which was typically based on questionnaire or physical activity diary data. Despite limited information in the cardiac rehabilitation literature, extensive studies and position statements in populations without apparent heart disease document that regular exercise, including a wide scope of physical activities with a broad range of intensity and duration, has beneficial effects on overall health, morbidity, and mortality. Patients should be encouraged to undertake exercise activities following cardiac exercise rehabilitation that are personally enjoyable and that can be sustained long term. The panel highlighted the need to encourage women, particularly older women, to participate in cardiac rehabilitation designed to enhance exercise capacity and physical activity.

The panel endorses the position statement of the American Heart Association regarding physical activity, that "regular aerobic physical activity increases exercise capacity and plays a role in both primary and secondary prevention of cardiovascular disease."

## Symptoms

Exercise rehabilitation decreases angina pectoris in patients with CHD and decreases symptoms of heart failure in patients with left-ventricular systolic dysfunction. Exercise training is recommended as an integral component of the symptomatic management of these patients. Symptoms of angina pectoris are also reduced by cardiac rehabilitation education, counseling, and behavioral interventions alone or as a component of multifactorial cardiac rehabilitation.

Improvement in cardiovascular symptomatic status, both angina pectoris and heart failure symptoms, occurs as a result of cardiac rehabilitation exercise training. Symptomatic outcomes in the scientific studies were confounded by inadequate information regarding changes in medication status, and by differing levels of exercise or physical activity, as well as by nonrehabilitation exercise activities of control patients. Change in symptomatic status of cardiac patients often results in changes in medication regimens.

Education and behavioral interventions, either alone or as components of multifactorial cardiac rehabilitation, are associated with a reduction in angina pectoris. Behavioral interventions are generally effective in reducing anginal pain.

## Smoking

A combined approach of cardiac rehabilitation education, counseling, and behavioral interventions results in smoking cessation and relapse prevention. Smoking cessation and relapse prevention programs should be offered to patients who are smokers to reduce their risk of subsequent coronary events. Smoking cessation is achieved by specific smoking cessation strategies.

Well-designed education, counseling, and behavioral interventions (relapse prevention) reduce cigarette smoking. Between 17% and 26% of patients can be expected to stop smoking, in addition to the spontaneously high smoking cessation rates in most populations soon after myocardial infarction. One effective model includes nurse-managed smoking cessation behavioral intervention with biochemical verification of smoking status. Whether biochemical verification should be recommended for clinical practice is unclear. Scientific evidence, consensus papers, and other scientific reviews in nonrehabilitation settings, including the Surgeon General's messages since 1965, lend strong support that education, counseling, and behavioral interventions are beneficial for smoking cessation. Given the documented benefit of smoking cessation in decreasing coronary risk, specific techniques of proven value in effecting smoking cessation should be incorporated into multifactorial cardiac rehabilitation.

There is little or no evidence of beneficial outcome in smoking cessation resulting from exercise training as a sole intervention.

## Lipids

Intensive nutrition education, counseling, and behavioral interventions improve dietary fat and cholesterol intake. Education, counseling, and behavioral interventions about nutrition, with and without pharmacologic lipid-lowering therapy, result in significant improvement in blood lipid levels and are recommended as a component of cardiac rehabilitation. Optimal lipid management requires specifically directed dietary and, as medically indicated, pharmacologic management, in addition to cardiac rehabilitation exercise training.

Efficacy is documented in noncardiac-rehabilitation settings of intensive nutrition education, counseling, and behavioral interventions on dietary fat intake and blood lipid levels. Results from a meta-analysis of 70 studies indicate that weight reduction through dietary modification can help normalize plasma lipid and lipoprotein levels in overweight individuals. *The Second Report of the Expert Panel on Detection, Evaluation, and Treatment of High Blood Cholesterol in Adults (Adult Treatment Panel II)* (NCEP II) recommended a low-density lipoprotein (LDL) cholesterol goal of less than 100 mg/dL for coronary patients. This requires high-intensity intervention that includes education, counseling, behavioral intervention, and adherence and motivational strategies as well as pharmacologic therapy for appropriate patients. Thus, independent effects of education and counseling may be impossible to ascertain.

Improvement in lipid profiles resulting from multifactorial cardiac rehabilitation is well established by review of the scientific literature. Most randomized controlled trials reported beneficial effects on total cholesterol, LDL cholesterol, high-density lipoprotein (HDL) cholesterol, and triglyceride levels in rehabilitation compared with control patients. Well-designed nonrandomized controlled trials reported similar beneficial outcomes. The rehabilitation studies that reported the most favorable impact on lipid levels were multifactorial, that is, providing exercise training, dietary education and counseling, and, in some studies, pharmacologic treatment, psychological support, and behavioral training. These favorable effects on lipid profiles involved patients who were both younger and older than 65 years of age. Cardiac rehabilitation exercise training as a sole intervention has inconsistent effects on lipid and lipoprotein levels.

The panel concurs with the recommendation of the NCEP II regarding the role of physical activity for lipid control, namely "the appropriate use of physical activity is considered an essential element in the nonpharmacologic therapy of elevated serum cholesterol." The panel also noted the results of a major randomized placebo-controlled trial of cholesterol lowering in coronary patients, most with prior myocardial infarction. Patients treated with a cholesterol-altering medication and a Step I diet showed a significant reduction in total mortality, coronary death, and major coronary events compared with diet-plus-placebo–treated patients. Favorable results occurred in both men and women patients younger and older than 60 years of age. The panel agreed with the trial conclusions that patients with CHD and diet-resistant cholesterol levels above 210 mg/dL should be considered for treatment with lipid-altering medication.

## Body Weight

Multifactorial cardiac rehabilitation that combines dietary education, counseling, and behavioral interventions designed to reduce body weight can help patients lose weight. Education as a sole intervention is unlikely to achieve and maintain weight loss. Cardiac rehabilitation exercise training as a sole intervention also has an inconsistent effect on controlling overweight and is not recommended as an isolated approach for weight loss. The optimal management recommended for overweight patients to promote maintenance of weight loss requires multifactorial rehabilitation including nutrition education, counseling, and behavioral modification, in addition to exercise training.

Education is a necessary component of a successful weight-reduction intervention but is not sufficient as a sole intervention to effect sustained weight loss. Nutrition education combined with behavioral interventions and prescribed exercise training can achieve modest and sustained weight loss. Results of meta-analysis of 70 studies indicate that weight reduction through dieting can also help normalize plasma lipid and lipoprotein levels in overweight individuals. The panel noted a review of the behavioral therapy literature involving obese patients; state-of-the-art weight loss programs that have been shown to be successful in nonrehabilitation settings are also likely to be successful in a cardiac rehabilitation setting. Expert opinion agrees that multifactorial interventions, with intensive education, counseling, and behavioral intervention, are effective to reduce weight.

Rehabilitative exercise training, as a component of multifactorial intervention, appears beneficial in improving body weight, excess body mass, or percentage of body fat. Exercise training as a sole intervention has no consistent effect, but no exercise-training study specifically targeted overweight coronary patients, and the definition of "overweight" varied among studies.

## Blood Pressure

Expert opinion supports a multifactorial education, counseling, behavioral, and pharmacologic approach as the recommended strategy for the management of hypertension. This approach is documented to be effective in nonrehabilitation populations. Neither education, counseling, and behavioral interventions nor rehabilitative exercise training as sole interventions have been shown to control elevated blood pressure levels.

Scientific evidence suggests that cardiac rehabilitation education alone fails to significantly decrease blood pressure. One of the most serious flaws in study designs includes the mixed sample of normotensive patients and a small proportion of hypertensive patients. The panel recommends the application of *The Fifth Report of the Joint National Committee on Detection, Evaluation and Treatment of High Blood Pressure* (JNC V) educational and behavioral recommendations as an important component of a multifactorial approach to reduce hypertension for the cardiac rehabilitation population. The JNC V recommendations, which were based on the opinion of recognized experts on hypertension, stated that "lifestyle modifications such as weight reduction, physical activity and moderation of dietary sodium are recommended as definitive or adjunctive therapy for hypertension." The JNC V also concluded that the scientific literature does not support use of stress management as a sole intervention for hypertension control and reiterated that relaxation and biofeedback techniques have little effect on hypertension control.

Review of the scientific evidence suggests that exercise-based cardiac rehabilitation has only modest effects in reducing blood pressure levels, but confounding variables include the effects of antihypertensive medications and medication changes. No study was specifically designed to address hypertension control in patients with elevated blood pressures participating in exercise-based cardiac rehabilitation. It is unlikely that hypertensive patients with CHD would be provided only exercise training without other appropriate therapies such as weight reduction, sodium restriction, moderation or abstinence from alcohol, or pharmacologic therapy, although these components may have been directed by the patient's treating physician.

Comprehensive educational programs should include information about weight management, exercise, and nutrition; they should also provide information about the purpose of medications, their potential side effects, and strategies to improve medication adherence.

## Psychological Well-Being

Education, counseling, and/or psychosocial interventions, either alone or as a component of multifactorial cardiac rehabilitation, result in improved psychological well-being and are recommended to complement the psychosocial benefits of exercise training.

Cardiac rehabilitation exercise training, with and without other cardiac rehabilitation services, results in improvement in measures of psychological status and functioning and is recommended to enhance psychological functioning, particularly as a component of multifactorial cardiac rehabilitation. Exercise training as a sole intervention does not consistently improve measures of anxiety and depression.

The scientific literature provides evidence of psychological improvement following education, counseling, and/or psychosocial interventions.

Training in behavioral modification, stress management, and relaxation techniques is effective in lowering levels of self-reported emotional stress and in modifying Type-A behavior.

Cardiac rehabilitation exercise training, either alone or as a component of multifactorial rehabilitation, often results in improvement in various measures of psychological status and functioning. This evidence from the scientific literature is consistent with the widespread belief among cardiac rehabilitation professionals that cardiac rehabilitation exercise training improves the sense of well-being among participants, particularly among individuals with high levels of distress at entry into the study. Patients tend to perceive themselves as improving in a number of psychosocial domains, although these perceptions may not be objectively documented. More sensitive tests may have to be developed to better ascertain changes in cardiac patients without specific psychiatric illness.

Studies of exercise rehabilitation as a sole intervention are confounded by the consequences of group interaction, formation of social support networks, peer and professional support, counseling, and guidance, all of which may affect depression, anxiety, and self-confidence.

## Social Adjustment and Functioning

Cardiac rehabilitation exercise training improves social adjustment and functioning and is recommended to improve social outcomes.

The scientific literature addressed various measures of social adjustment and functioning in patients following cardiac rehabilitation exercise training including the Sickness Impact Profile scores, leisure and social questionnaire scores, social activity scores, and scores of satisfaction with work and social satisfaction. Randomized controlled trials established that social benefits result from participation in exercise and in multifactorial cardiac rehabilitation. Only two reports involved patients over age 65; social outcomes for this age group may differ from those in the majority of patients studied, younger than 60–65 years.

## Return to Work

Cardiac rehabilitation exercise training exerts less of an influence on the rates of return to work than many nonexercise variables including employer attitudes, prior employment status, economic incentives, and the like. Exercise training as a sole intervention is not recommended to facilitate return to work, nor have education, counseling, and behavioral interventions resulted in improvement in rates of return to work. Many patients return to work without formal interventions. However, in selected patients, formal cardiac rehabilitation vocational counseling may improve rates of return to work.

Assessment of return to work as a result of exercise training must be considered within the context of social and political variables that are typically not addressed in the studies of cardiac rehabilitation; these include the political system and social policies of the country in which cardiac rehabilitation occurs. Additional factors include employment statistics for the years of the study, economic incentives or disincentives for patients to return to work, non-patient-related factors such as employer attitudes, and the pre-illness employment status of the patient, among others. Return to work as a measure of outcome of exercise-based cardiac rehabilitation may not be appropriate unless formal vocational rehabilitation services are provided to patients as part of the rehabilitative process.

Although multifactorial cardiac rehabilitation has not been shown to alter the rates of return to work, education and counseling may improve a patient's potential for return to work.

Better understanding (via education) of capabilities and limitations regarding work may influence a patient's self-efficacy for returning to previous employment or for seeking job retraining. A randomized controlled trial in a nonrehabilitation setting of the effects of occupational work evaluation on return to work, involving patients after myocardial infarction, documented a marked reduction in the duration of convalescence.

## Morbidity and Safety Issues

The safety of exercise rehabilitation is well established; the rates of myocardial infarction and cardiovascular complications during exercise training are very low.

Cardiac rehabilitation exercise training does not change the rates of nonfatal reinfarction.

Education, counseling, and behavioral interventions as components of multifactorial cardiac rehabilitation may decrease progression of coronary atherosclerosis and lower recurrent coronary event rates.

Appropriately designed and conducted exercise-based cardiac rehabilitation can safely be undertaken in appropriately selected patients undergoing individualized initial assessment and surveillance.

The randomized controlled trials reported in the scientific literature show no evidence for reduction in cardiac morbidity, specifically nonfatal reinfarction, as a result of exercise rehabilitation. No study documented an increase in morbidity comparing rehabilitation patients with control patients among 4,578 patients in the controlled trials reviewed.

A large survey of adverse experiences during rehabilitative exercise training in 142 US cardiac rehabilitation programs (1980–1984) reported a very low rate of nonfatal reinfarction of 1 per 294,000 patient-hours. These 1980–1984 survey data may not be applicable to the contemporary treatment of coronary patients, including the widespread use of risk stratification procedures following myocardial infarction, the more aggressive management techniques including thrombolytic therapy and myocardial revascularization, as well as current pharmacologic therapies for postinfarction patients (eg, beta-blockers, angiotensin-converting enzyme [ACE] inhibitors) that may further reduce reinfarction and morbidity in coronary patients. The current low nonfatal reinfarction rates may not be amenable to further reduction by exercise training as a sole intervention.

Based on the scientific literature, education, counseling, and behavioral interventions alone may have limited beneficial effect on cardiovascular event rates. Education, counseling, and behavioral interventions designed to encourage patients to adhere to therapies, as a component of multifactorial cardiac rehabilitation, have been associated with reduction in recurrent cardiovascular event rates, as well as with regression of atherosclerosis.

## Mortality and Safety Issues

Based on meta-analyses, total and cardiovascular mortality is reduced in patients following myocardial infarction who participate in cardiac rehabilitation exercise training, especially as a component of multifactorial rehabilitation. Education, counseling, and behavioral interventions reduce cardiac and overall mortality rates and are recommended in the multifactorial rehabilitation of patients with CHD.

A survival benefit among patients participating in exercise training as a component of multifactorial cardiac rehabilitation is suggested from review of the scientific data, but this benefit cannot be attributed solely to exercise training because many studies involved multifactorial rehabilitation. Because of the small number of patients in most randomized controlled trials, the panel used results of meta-analyses to gain additional information about mortality outcomes. Two meta-analyses of 21 randomized controlled trials of cardiac rehabilitation that included more than 4,000 patients with CHD established significant morality reduction, approximating 25% at three years, in rehabilitation patients compared with control patients. This mortality reduction is similar to that with other interventions for patients with CHD (eg, trials of beta-blocker drug therapy following myocardial infarction, ACE inhibitor therapy for left ventricular systolic dysfunction and heart failure). The beneficial mortality outcome was greater in the 15 trials that used multifactorial cardiac rehabilitation compared with the 7 trials that used exercise training as the sole intervention.

The randomized controlled trials in the panel's database that reported mortality rates included a total of 7,063 patients. In no trial was the rate of fatal events greater in the intervention group than in the control group.

Most studies involved principally male patients younger than age 65 years following myocardial infarction and excluded high-risk complex patients, limiting the generalizability of the data. The percentage of females, when enrolled, was 20% or less. Furthermore, subsequent to the research studies cited as scientific evidence, mortality has been further reduced by nonrehabilitation interventions such as myocardial revascularization procedures and newer pharmacologic agents that have far more powerful effects on survival.

Information obtained from two large surveys of cardiac rehabilitation program responses to questionnaires provided retrospective safety data regarding exercise training. Few fatal cardiac events occurred during or immediately following exercise training: 1 per 116,400 patient-hours of participation in supervised exercise training in the 1978 report and 1 per 784,000 patient-hours in the 1986 report. The data from both survey reports antedate the use of contemporary risk stratification procedures and contemporary medical and surgical therapies for CHD and heart failure. No mortality data were reported by gender or patient age, nor was definitive information available regarding the effect of levels of supervision and electrocardiographic (ECG) monitoring of exercise training.

A variety of education, counseling, and behavioral interventions are associated with reductions in total and cardiac mortality rates. The panel noted the consistency with which decreased mortality rates were reported in the randomized controlled trials of multifactorial cardiac rehabilitation involving education, counseling, and behavioral interventions The panel recognizes the potential for reducing mortality rates by education, counseling, and behavioral interventions that are designed to reduce cardiac risk, as components of multifactorial cardiac rehabilitation.

## Pathophysiologic Measures

### Coronary Atherosclerosis

Cardiac rehabilitation exercise training as a sole intervention does not result in regression or limitation of progression of angiographically documented coronary atherosclerosis. Exercise training, combined with intensive dietary intervention, with and without lipid-lowering drugs, results in regression or limitation of progression of angiographically documented coronary atherosclerosis and is recommended.

### Hemodynamic Measurements

Cardiac rehabilitation exercise training has no apparent effect on development of a coronary collateral circulation and produces no consistent changes in cardiac hemodynamic measurements at cardiac catheterization. Exercise training in patients with heart failure and a decreased ventricular ejection fraction produces favorable hemodynamic changes in the skeletal musculature and is recommended to improve skeletal muscle functioning.

### Myocardial Perfusion and/or Evidence of Myocardial Ischemia

Cardiac rehabilitation exercise training decreases myocardial ischemia as measured by exercise ECG, ambulatory ECG recording, and radionuclide perfusion imaging and is recommended to improve these measures of myocardial ischemia.

### Myocardial Contractility, Ventricular Wall Motion Abnormalities and/or Ventricular Ejection Fraction

Cardiac rehabilitation exercise training has little effect on ventricular ejection fraction and regional wall motion abnormalities and is not recommended to improve measures of ventricular systolic function. The effect of exercise training on left-ventricular function in patients after anterior Q-wave myocardial infarction with left-ventricular dysfunction is variable.

### Occurrence of Cardiac Arrhythmias

Cardiac rehabilitation exercise training has inconsistent effects on ventricular arrhythmias.

A number of scientific reports described the pathophysiologic outcomes of exercise training listed here. These stud-
ies explored and at times interrelated pathophysiologic mechanisms whereby exercise training may engender benefits or harms. All reports involved predominantly or exclusively male patients, typically of middle age, with few or no elderly patients studied; these demographic constraints limit the generalizability of the outcome data.

Multifactorial cardiac rehabilitation, including exercise training and dietary intervention, with and without the use of lipid-altering drugs, effected regression or limited progression of angiographically documented coronary atherosclerosis. The effect of exercise training as a sole intervention is not impressive. However, subsequent coronary events may be related to factors other than change in arterial luminal diameter, that is, factors promoting plaque stability versus rupture, which may be related to circulating lipid levels, among others.

Development of an angiographically documented coronary collateral circulation has not been demonstrated with exercise training; it occurred only with progression of the underlying coronary atherosclerosis. No prominent or consistent changes in cardiac hemodynamic measurements at cardiac catheterization occurred as a result of exercise training. In patients with heart failure and a decreased ventricular ejection fraction, improvement occurred in leg hemodynamic parameters with exercise, supporting the favorable effect of exercise training on the skeletal musculature.

The beneficial effects of exercise training on myocardial perfusion and/or measures of myocardial ischemia included less ischemic ECG abnormalities at exercise testing and during ambulatory ECG recording. Resolution of reversible thallium perfusion defects in the randomized controlled trials was also greater among exercising than nonexercising patients.

Most of the studies that examined the effect of usual rehabilitative exercise training on measures of myocardial function showed no significant difference in ejection fraction or regional wall motion abnormalities between exercising and control groups. Apparently spontaneous improvement in resting ejection fraction after myocardial infarction occurred in both exercise and control populations in several randomized clinical trials, rendering suspect described improvements in ejection fraction in observational studies. A nonrandomized controlled study of patients following anterior Q-wave myocardial infarction and decreased ejection fraction showed worsening of ejection fraction and wall motion asynergy in exercising compared with nonexercising patients. Two subsequent randomized controlled trials in patients following anterior Q-wave myocardial infarction with baseline decreased ejection fraction documented comparable spontaneous deterioration in global and regional left-ventricular function in exercising and control patients.

Studies that described changes in ventricular arrhythmias related to exercise rehabilitation provide inconsistent outcomes. No randomized controlled trial reported a significant arrhythmia-related adverse clinical outcome.

## Patients with Heart Failure and Cardiac Transplantation

Rehabilitative exercise training in patients with heart failure and moderate to severe left ventricular systolic dysfunction improves functional capacity and symptoms, without changes in left-ventricular function. Cardiac rehabilitation exercise training is recommended to attain functional and symptomatic improvement.

Rehabilitative exercise training in patients following cardiac transplantation improves measures of exercise tolerance and is recommended for this purpose.

In the early years of exercise rehabilitation, cardiac enlargement, decreased left-ventricular ejection fraction, and overt cardiac failure were considered relative or absolute contraindications to exercise training. Only in recent years has exercise training been undertaken in these patients; even these recent trials reflect only limited concomitant use of contemporary vasodilator drug therapies, particularly ACE inhibitors, which are now considered the standard of care for heart failure. The panel concurs with the recommendation of the AHCPR publication *Heart Failure: Evaluation and Care of Patients with Left-Ventricular Systolic Dysfunction, Clinical Practice Guideline No. 11*, that "patients with heart failure due to left-ventricular systolic dysfunction should be given a trial of ACE inhibitors unless specific contra-indications exist."

Most studies of exercise training of patients with heart failure and moderate to severe left-ventricular dysfunction do not demonstrate deterioration in left-ventricular function. Peripheral (skeletal muscle) adaptations appear to mediate the improvement in exercise tolerance. Exercise training augments the symptomatic and functional benefits of ACE inhibitor therapy. Low- to moderate-intensity exercise and home exercise regimens provide benefit, but adverse events may occur in this high-risk patient group.

In summary, although the studies of exercise training have been limited by small numbers and young populations consisting predominantly of men, and had CHD as the major etiology of heart failure, exercise training in patients with heart failure and decreased ventricular systolic function resulted in documented improvement in functional capacity. Data reinforce that the favorable training effects in these patients are due predominantly to adaptations in the peripheral circulation and skeletal musculature rather than adaptations in the cardiac musculature.

Cardiac transplantation, too, is a relatively recent surgical intervention; even more recent for cardiac transplantation patients is the frequent application of exercise training.

The few studies reported demonstrate improvement in exercise capacity in these medically complex patients, who are often markedly deconditioned prior to cardiac transplantation. Pretransplantation rehabilitative strength training may enhance preoperative status and operative recovery; effects of strength training after cardiac transplantation require study.

## Elderly Patients

Elderly coronary patients have exercise trainability comparable to younger patients participating in similar exercise rehabilitation. Elderly female and male patients show comparable improvement. Referral to and participation in exercise rehabilitation is less frequent at an elderly age, especially for elderly females. No complications or adverse outcomes of exercise training at an elderly age were described in any study. Elderly patients of both genders should be strongly encouraged to participate in exercise-based cardiac rehabilitation.

Elderly patients constitute a high percentage of those with myocardial infarction, CABG, and PTCA. Elderly patients are also at high risk of disability following a coronary event.

Although few studies and no randomized controlled trials addressed the efficacy and safety of exercise training and multifactorial rehabilitation of elderly patients, the available studies provide important new information of beneficial functional improvement from exercise training for current clinical practice.

Special effort is recommended to overcome the obstacles to entry and participation in cardiac rehabilitation services for elderly patients.

## Alternate Approaches to the Delivery of Cardiac Rehabilitation Services

Alternate approaches to the delivery of cardiac rehabilitation services, other than traditional supervised group interventions, can be implemented effectively and safely for carefully selected clinically stable patients. Transtelephonic and other means of monitoring and surveillance of patients can extend cardiac rehabilitation services beyond the setting of supervised, structured, group-based rehabilitation. These alternate approaches have the potential to provide cardiac rehabilitation services to low- and moderate-risk patients, who comprise the majority of patients with stable CHD, most of whom do not currently participate in structured supervised rehabilitation.

Recent studies have explored new approaches to deliver cardiac rehabilitation services, with the goals of increasing availability and decreasing costs, while preserving efficacy and safety. Case management approaches to exercise training, smoking cessation, diet-drug management of hyperlipidemia, and providing emotional support and guidance to patients as needed that rely on telephone contact can be provided to appropriately selected patients with CHD.

The generalizability of these case management systems to other treatment settings including university centers, public and community hospitals, and clinics will depend largely on formulas for reimbursement for services and the extent of physician support for this approach, as well as state regulations regarding medical and health care practices. Within each of these settings, managed care programs seeking optimal methods for coronary risk factor reduction and exercise rehabilitation may favor case management systems that provide convenient, individualized health care at low cost.

The feasibility, safety, efficacy, and economic impact of these alternate approaches have to be assessed in more diverse populations of patients with stable CHD, particularly elderly patients, those with ventricular dysfunction, and other patients of higher risk status.

## Adherence

Adherence to cardiac rehabilitation services may improve patient outcomes. Adherence to cardiac rehabilitation services may be enhanced by clear communication; emotional support; understanding the patient's (and family's) values, viewpoints, and preferences; and integration of the intervention into the patient's lifestyle.

## Cost

Limited data suggest that multifactorial cardiac rehabilitation is a cost-effective use of medical care resources.

A limited number of economic evaluations of cardiac rehabilitation in patients after coronary events demonstrated favorable economic outcomes. Although none of these studies provided comprehensive economic analyses, the costs of cardiac rehabilitation have to be considered in the perspective of benefits of such rehabilitation. At relatively low cost, clinical benefits are attained, as are favorable economic outcomes. Nonetheless, application of longer-term multifactorial cardiac rehabilitation services may entail increased costs.

## 4. Clinical Pathway and Care Planning Forms

# Inpatient Cardiopulmonary Progress Note

| Function | Status | Comments | Goal |
|---|---|---|---|
| Rolling | | | |
| Supine <-> Sit | | | |
| Sit <-> Stand | | | |
| Bed <-> Chair | | | |
| Ambulation: | | | |
| device | | | |
| distance | | | |
| 6-Minute Walk Test: # rests | | | |
| distance | | | |
| Stairs: | | | |
| device | | | |
| # steps | | | |
| Other: | | | |
| Other: | | | |

☑ = Goal revised

**CONTRIBUTING FACTORS**

Activity tolerance: _____ (See key)
Pacing: _____ (See key)
$O_2$ needs: _____
Clearing technique: _____
Breathing control:    Lateral costal _____
(See key)    Pursed lip _____
   Diaphragmatic _____
Hemodynamic responses: _____
Safety:    Asks for assistance if needed _____
(See key)    Negotiates environment safely _____
   Can negotiate $O_2$ line safely _____
Exercise knowledge:    _____/20
Patient/family teaching:    Initiated ___ Ongoing ___

*continues*

73

**Inpatient Cardiopulmonary Progress Note** continued

Self-monitoring (check one):    Perceived exertion ___    Independent ___    Dependent ___
                                 Dyspnea ___                Independent ___    Dependent ___
Home exercise program:          Independent ___            Dependent ___
Aide program:                   Date initiated ___         Ongoing ___        N.A. ___
Other:_____
_____
Assessment:_____
_____
_____
_____
Plan:_____
_____
Signature:_____ Date:_____

## KEY

Activity tolerance:

1 = Tolerates greater than or equal to 15 minutes high-level exercise (i.e., bike, treadmill) without rests.
2 = Tolerates 15 minutes high-level exercise (i.e., standing, bike, treadmill) with occasional rests.
3 = Tolerates 15 minutes moderate-level exercise (sitting and standing) with occasional rests.
4 = Tolerates 15 minutes low-level exercise (bed and sitting) with occasional rests.
5 = Tolerates 15 minutes low-level exercise (bed and sitting) with frequent rests.
6 = Cannot tolerate any active exercise.

Breathing control key:

1 = Performs independently, no cues needed.
2 = Dependent, needs occasional cues.
3 = Dependent, needs frequent cues.
4 = Unable to perform.

Pacing key (The ability to apply energy-conservation techniques during activity without causing undue fatigue or shortness of breath):

0 = No cues needed
1 = Cues needed 25% of the time
2 = Cues needed 50% of the time
3 = Cues needed 100% of the time
4 = N/A

Safety Scale Key:

0 = Never
1 = 25% of the time
2 = 50% of the time
3 = 75% of the time
4 = 100% of the time

Courtesy of Spaulding Rehabilitation Hospital, Boston, Massachusetts.

# Familial Hyperlipidemia
## Provider Pathway

| | Age 2 | Yearly | Yearly without Change in CHO | Yearly without Significant Change | Early Adulthood | Symptomatic Heart Disease |
|---|---|---|---|---|---|---|
| Date | | | | | | |
| Assessment | Height, weight, percentile for age, pulse, resp., BP ✓ murmur ✓ pulses | Height, weight, percentile for age, pulse, resp., BP ✓ murmur ✓ pulses ✓ carotid bruits | Height, weight, percentile for age, pulse, resp., BP ✓ murmur ✓ pulses ✓ bruits | Height, weight, pulse, resp., BP ✓ murmurs ✓ pulses ✓ bruits | Height, weight, pulse, BP ✓ murmurs, pulses, bruits Xanthelasmas, xanthomas, knuckles, elbow, Achilles tendon, corneal arcus | Height, weight, pulse, BP ✓ murmurs, pulses, bruits Xanthelasmas, xanthomas, knuckles, elbow, Achilles tendon, corneal arcus |
| Dietary | Low-fat milk Step I diet (15% calories from saturated fat) | Low-fat milk Step I diet | Step II diet (10% calories from saturated fat) | Step II ↑ fiber slowly to 30 g | Continue low-fat, ↑ fiber | Continue low-fat, ↑ fiber |
| Diagnostics and Treatment | Total cholesterol, HDL, LDL, TG, VLDL, APOA₁, APOB—fasting | Total cholesterol, HDL, LDL, TG, APOA, APOB, VLDL—fasting | TSH, total cholesterol, HDL, LDL, TG, VLDL, APOA₁, APOB—fasting (Try Step II diet before meds) | TSH, LFTs, total cholesterol, HDL, TG, VLDL, APOA₁, APOB—fasting | LFTs, total cholesterol, HDL, TG, VLDL, APOA₁, APOB—fasting ECG | Resting ECG, ECHO, stress test, stress-thallium Holter Cardioangiography |
| Activity | Encourage free play | Encourage activity ↑ play groups | Formalized exercise 3 days/week for 30 min—aerobic | Formalized exercise 3 days/week for 30 min Encourage two sports/semester and aerobics | Maintain exercise—aerobic | Exercise as exercise stress test permits |

*Note:* APOA₁, apollpoprotein A; APOB, apollpoprotein B.

*continues*

**Familial Hyperlipidemia Provider Pathway** continued

| | Age 2 | Yearly | Yearly without Change in CHO | Yearly without Significant Change | Early Adulthood | Symptomatic Heart Disease | |
|---|---|---|---|---|---|---|---|
| Date | | | | | | | |
| Teaching and Counseling | Discuss importance of diet and exercise Develop early patterns of exercise and good eating | Keep food diary Keep exercise diary | Slowly work up to four packs of Questran to limit gas Low-fat diet limits gas | Encourage to remain on good diet even though numbers will look better on Mevacor | No smoking Alcohol in moderation Avoid weight gain Behavior modification—stress ✔ oral contraceptives | No smoking Alcohol in moderation Avoid weight gain Behavior modification—stress ✔ oral contraceptives | |
| Medications | | | Cholestyramine Questran up to 2–4 packs/day | Lovastatin, Mevacor, or Lopid for ↑ TG | Lovastatin, Mevacor, or Lopid for ↑ TG | Lovastatin, Mevacor, or Lopid for ↑ TG | |
| Consults/Referrals | Dietary Physical exam | Dietitian/nutritionist Physical exam | Nutritionist Physical exam | Dietary Physical exam | Dietary Physical exam | Cardiology Dietary | |
| Comments | LDL = total cholesterol– (HDL + 1/5 TG) | Expect 10% drop with good diet; 12% Step II | Questran safe in child—not absorbed systemically SE: Constipation, flatus | LFTs with Mevacor | Monitor for hypertension <140/85 Discourage weight lifting for exercise | Maintain nutritional consult for encouragement | |
| Initials/Date | | | | | | | |

Source: Rufus S. Howe, *Clinical Pathways for Ambulatory Care Case Management*, Aspen Publishers, Inc., © 1996.

# Chest Pain Evaluation Center Patient Clinical Map

## CARDIAC SERVICES CLINICAL MAP

### CHEST PAIN EVALUATION CENTER PATIENTS

INTERNIST: _____

CARDIOLOGIST: _____

ED M.D.: _____

TIME OF ARRIVAL: ED _____ PCU _____

**PATIENT ADDRESSOGRAPH**

**DISCHARGE OUTCOMES\***    Yes   No

1. Oral temperature less than 100°F for 24 hr. prior to d/c.
2. Heart returns to baseline rhythm.
3. CE and ECG tracing non dx for acute MI.
4. Anxiety level is reduced.
5. Patient independent w/ADL or home help assured or a transfer to SNF arranged.
6. VS within acceptable d/c parameters.
7. Outcome criteria met, patient discharged home.
   If criteria not met - Alternative Clinical Map initiated:

  -Patient transferred to another facility.

\*Comment in Nursing Notes for outcomes not met.

R.N. Signature _____   Date _____   Date of DC _____

| DATE: | POINT OF ENTRY | 1ST 15' | 2ND 15' | 3RD 15' | 4TH 15' | 1ST 12° PCU | 2ND 12° PCU | D/C |
|---|---|---|---|---|---|---|---|---|
| | | | 1ST HR. | | | 1ST 12 HRS. | | 1ST 24 HRS. |
| **CONSULTS/ REFERRALS** | Notify Primary MD or Cardiologist of patient admission; Care Manager; Social Services; Financial Screen | Primary MD, Cardiologist, or ED MD to see patient. \*Initiate CPEC Protocol | If pt. doesn't have PMD, then ED MD to notify MD from call list | | Initiate CPEC Protocol/orders if appropriate | Cardiac assess & written plan of treatment; H&P dictated | Cardiac Rehab | |
| **ACTIVITY** | | BR - BSC if stable | | | | Advance as tolerated | Ambulate prior to DC | |
| **TREATMENTS** | O₂; Cardiac Monitor | ---> ; ---> | ---> ; ---> | ---> ; ---> | ---> ; ---> | ---> ; ---> | ---> ; ---> | |
| **MEDICATION** | As ordered: MS, NTG, Antiemetics, Rt & Cardiac meds; IV Protocol; Pain Mgmt Protocol | ---> ; ---> ; ---> ; ---> | ---> ; ---> ; ---> ; ---> | ---> ; ---> ; ---> ; ---> | ---> ; ---> ; ---> ; ---> | As ordered: Lax/stool softeners; HS & prn sed. | As ordered; PO analgesia | |
| **TESTS** | | \*ER Chem Panel; CBC, PCXR, EKG | EKG prn rhythm or status change | | | 12° post admit; CE & ISO's if CE ↑ (#2) | 24° post admit; CE & ISO's if CE ↑ (#3) | **TEST COMPLETE** ☐☐☐ ☐☐☐<br>Cardiac Cath<br>PTCA<br>ECHO<br>**STRESS TESTS:** ☐☐☐ ☐☐☐☐☐<br>- Cardiolyte<br>- Dobutamine<br>- Ergometer<br>- Low Level Stress<br>- Persantine Thallium<br>- Thallium<br>- Treadmill |
| **FLUIDS/NUTRITION** | IV or saline lock | ---> | ---> | ---> | ---> | Cardiac diet; IV TKO | IV ---> Saline lock | |
| **PATIENT/FAMILY TEACHING/DC PLAN** | D/C Planning | ---> | ---> | ---> | ---> | Stress Information; Angina Booklet | Videos: --- Risk Factors; --- Angina; --- Diet; --- Stress | --- Follow-up appt w/MD; --- Follow-up phone call |
| **SIGNATURE** | A.M. ☐ | | P.M. ☐ | | ☐ | ☐ | ☐ | |

*continues*

**Chest Pain Evaluation Center Patient Clinical Map** continued

| PATIENT PROBLEM | INTERMEDIATE OUTCOMES | DATE OUTCOMES ANTICIPATED | DATE OUTCOMES ACHIEVED | COMMENTS |
|---|---|---|---|---|
| **Anxiety: R/T Hospitalization, Insufficient Knowledge of Illness, Possible Threat of Life-Threatening Disease** | **Patient will:** <br>1. Verbalize fears, questions, anxieties <br>2. Be able to express anger, grief, depression to self and family <br>3. Begin to adapt to emotional stressors <br>4. Identify effective coping mechanisms | | | |
| **Alteration in Comfort: R/T Chest Discomfort** | **Patient will:** <br>1. Identify signs and symptoms of angina and importance of immediate reporting <br>2. Report duration and intensity of discomfort <br>3. Pain control as evidenced by verbal/non-verbal indicators <br>4. Pain is controlled by: <br>–IV analgesics <br>–SL, PO analgesics | | | |
| **Potential for Alteration in Cardiac Output: R/T Dysrhythmias, Impaired Contractility, EKG Changes, Abnormal Cardiac Enzymes** | **Patient will be:** <br>1. Electrophysiologically stable as evidenced by absence of dysrhythmias <br>2. Hemodynamically stable having SBP>100, HR >60 <120, usual mentation | | | |
| **Alteration in Mobility: R/T Insufficient Tissue Oxygenation** | **Patient will:** <br>1. Identify factors that ↑ workload on heart <br>2. Tolerate activity as evidenced by stable pulse, B/P, resp. rate <br>3. Ambulate in room without assistance <br>4. Ambulate in hall without assistance | | | |
| **Knowledge Deficit: R/T Home Care** | **Patient verbalizes understanding of:** <br>1. Risk factors <br>2. Dietary restrictions <br>3. Activity limitations <br>4. Pacing strategies <br>5. Reportable signs and symptoms <br>6. Medication administration <br>7. Follow-up care and availability of community resources | | | |
| | | | | |

*Nurse to initial date outcomes achieved and comments made.

Source: Clyde E. Wesp, Jr., and Donna E. Hartman, *Clinical Maps for Acute Care: Managing Care through Collaborative Practice*, Aspen Publishers, Inc., © 1996.

# Chest Pain
# Provider Pathway

| | Initial Assessment | 10–30 Minutes | 30 Minutes–4 Hours | 4–9 Hours |
|---|---|---|---|---|
| Date | | | | |
| Assessment | RN triage<br>VS<br>Admit to acute area | MD assessment or NP assessment | Remain in acute area<br>Triage to subacute or CCU or ICCU | MD will admit or DC patient |
| Medications | IVs × 2<br>O₂<br>NTG (sl, consider IV)<br>Monitor | Analgesia, ASA<br>Assess for thrombolysis | Analgesia PRN<br>Assess for thrombolysis | Analgesia PRN<br>Assess for thrombolysis |
| Tests | 12-lead ECG<br>CBC, SMAC, CK, CK-MB, PT, PTT | Chest X-ray<br>12-lead ECG PRN | | 12-lead ECG<br>CK, CK-MB |
| Results of Tests | 12-lead ECG (consider ischemic Δs) | | ECG<br>Chest X-ray | ECG, enzymes, and blood tests from initial assessment |
| Diet | NPO | NPO | Consider PO fluids | Consider PO fluids |
| Consultation | | Cardiology, if AMI | Cardiology, if unstable angina | Cardiology, if unstable angina |
| Disposition | Acute area of ED | Acute area of ED | Acute, subacute, or CCU or ICCU | Admit or DC |
| Teaching | Acute procedures | Medications<br>Procedures | Probable diagnosis<br>Meds | Follow-up instructions or information regarding unit |
| Physiological Outcomes | Hemodynamic and respiratory status assessed | Pain ↓ or relieved<br>VS stabilized<br>No dyspnea | Stabilized for transfer to unit, pain-free | Stabilized for DC home or admission |

*Note:* MS, morphine sulfate; NTG, nitroglycerin.

*continues*

**Chest Pain Provider Pathway** continued

| | Initial Assessment | 10–30 Minutes | 30 Minutes–4 Hours | 4–9 Hours |
|---|---|---|---|---|
| Date | | | | |
| Educational Outcomes | Importance of baseline 12-lead ECG stressed<br>Necessity to advise staff of change in chest pain communicated<br>Explain about NTG headache | Plan of care and methods of assessing potential cardiac damage explained | Results of lab, ECGs, chest X-ray shared with patient<br>Plan of care discussed with patient | If DC, patient instructed to return to ED if recurrence and to follow up with primary provider or clinic appointment |
| Psychosocial Outcomes | Reassure patient that he/she will be treated quickly, be calm | Establish rapport with patient and family | Include family in probable diagnosis and plan | Answer all questions from patient and family if patient is to be DC |
| Medication Outcomes | O₂ and NTG given | ASA and heparin given<br>MS PRN<br>Vasopressors PRN | Continue heparin<br>Assess thrombolysis eligibility<br>Maintain analgesia | If being DC, explain rationale for meds and possible side effects |
| Initials/Date | | | | |

Source: Rufus S. Howe, *Clinical Pathways for Ambulatory Care Case Management*, Aspen Publishers, Inc., © 1996.

# Unstable Angina—Rule Out Myocardial Infarction: Clinical Map

## DISCHARGE OUTCOMES*

| | Yes | No |
|---|---|---|
| 1. D/C temperature < 100°F for 24 hr. prior to discharge. | ☐ | ☐ |
| 2. Heart returns to baseline rhythm. | ☐ | ☐ |
| 3. Patient able to identify risk factors and symptoms of angina. | ☐ | ☐ |
| 4. Decrease in level of anxiety. | ☐ | ☐ |
| 5. Normal cardiac enzymes and baseline EKG. | ☐ | ☐ |
| 6. Pain control. | ☐ | ☐ |
| 7. Patient verbalizes understanding of diet. | ☐ | ☐ |
| 8. Patient independent w/ADL's, or assisted by home help or SNF. | ☐ | ☐ |
| 9. If criteria not met   - Alternative Clinical Map Initiated: | ☐ | ☐ |

    - Patient transferred to another facility.                    ☐          ☐

*Comment in Nursing Notes for outcomes not met.

R.N. Signature _____   Date _____   Date of DC _____

**CARDIAC SERVICES CLINICAL MAP**

**UNSTABLE ANGINA (R/O MI)**

PRIMARY M.D. _____
CARDIOLOGIST: _____
CONSULTANT: _____

PATIENT ADDRESSOGRAPH

| DATE:<br>HOSPITAL AREA: | DAY 1<br>ICU/PCU | DAY 2<br>PCU ---> DC | DAY 3 | DAY 4 |
|---|---|---|---|---|
| **CONSULTS/REFERRALS** | Cardiology as ordered<br>Care Manager<br>Social Services<br>Utilization Review | Outpatient Cardiac/Rehab prn<br>F&N prn | Nutrition Screen | |
| **ACTIVITY** | BR<br>BSC if stable | Advance as tolerated<br>Ambulate prior to D/C | | |
| **TREATMENTS** | O₂<br>Cardiac Monitor | ---><br>---> | | |
| **MEDICATION** | As ordered:<br>MS, NTG, Analgesics,<br>Antiemetics, Laxatives,<br>Routine & Cardiac meds<br>Gtts: Heparin/NTG<br>IV Protocol | ---><br>---><br>---><br>---> | | |
| **TESTS**<br>☐ Cath<br>☐ PTCA<br>☐ TST | ER Chem Panel<br>CBC, PCXR, EKG<br>Additional Enzymes and EKG as ordered | Diagnostic tests as ordered | | |
| **FLUIDS/NUTRITION** | IV or saline lock<br>Cardiac diet | ---><br>---> | | |
| **PATIENT/FAMILY<br>TEACHING/DC PLAN** | Orientation to Unit<br>Notify RN for chest pain<br>Explain tests<br>Family support<br>___ Education packet | Review pamphlets<br>Videos:<br>___ Diet<br>___ Risk Factors<br>___ Angina | Review DC Meds, Activity, Signs &<br>Symptoms Recognition, Risk<br>Factors<br>Nutrition education per physician<br>order | |
| **SIGNATURE**   A.M.<br>P.M. | ☐ ☐ ☐ ☐ | ☐ ☐ ☐ ☐ | ☐ ☐ ☐ ☐ | ☐ ☐ ☐ ☐ |

*continues*

**Unstable Angina—Rule Out Myocardial Infarction: Clinical Map** continued

| PATIENT PROBLEM | INTERMEDIATE OUTCOMES | DATE OUTCOMES ANTICIPATED (by Clin Path) | DATE OUTCOMES ACHIEVED/ INITIALED* | COMMENTS |
|---|---|---|---|---|
| **Anxiety: R/T Hospitalization, Insufficient Knowledge of Illness, Possible Threat of Life-Threatening Disease** | **Patient will:**<br>1. Verbalize fears, questions, anxieties<br>2. Be able to express anger, grief, depression to self and family<br>3. Begin to adapt to emotional stressors<br>4. Identify effective coping mechanisms | ———<br>———<br>———<br>——— | ———<br>———<br>———<br>——— | |
| **Alteration in Comfort: R/T Chest Discomfort** | **Patient will:**<br>1. Identify signs and symptoms of angina and importance of immediate reporting<br>2. Report duration and intensity of discomfort<br>3. Pain control as evidenced by verbal/non-verbal indicators<br>4. Pain is controlled by:<br>   –IV analgesics<br>   –SL, PO analgesics | | | |
| **Potential for Alteration in Cardiac Output: R/T Dysrhythmias, Impaired Contractility, EKG Changes, Abnormal Cardiac Enzymes** | **Patient will be:**<br>1. Electrophysiologically stable as evidenced by absence of dysrhythmias<br>2. Hemodynamically stable having SBP>100, HR >60 <120, usual mentation | | | |
| **Alteration in Mobility: R/T Insufficient Tissue Oxygenation** | **Patient will:**<br>1. Identify factors that ↑ workload on heart<br>2. Tolerate activity as evidenced by stable pulse, B/P, resp. rate<br>3. Tolerate getting up to BSC<br>4. Ambulate in room with assistance<br>5. Ambulate in room without assistance<br>6. Ambulate in hall with assistance<br>7. Ambulate in hall without assistance | ———<br>———<br>———<br>———<br>———<br>———<br>——— | ———<br>———<br>———<br>———<br>———<br>———<br>——— | |
| **Alteration in Nutrition: R/T to Hospitalization** | **Patient able to:**<br>1. Tolerate cardiac diet without nausea<br>2. Meet >50% of nutritional needs through oral intake by Day 5 (if not, consider nutrition support) | <br>DAY 5 | | |
| **Knowledge Deficit: R/T Home Care** | **Patient verbalizes understanding of:**<br>1. Risk factors<br>2. Dietary restrictions<br>3. Activity limitations<br>4. Pacing strategies<br>5. Reportable signs and symptoms<br>6. Medication administration<br>7. Follow-up care and availability of community resources | ———<br>———<br>———<br>———<br>———<br>———<br>——— | ———<br>———<br>———<br>———<br>———<br>———<br>——— | |

*Nurse to initial date outcomes achieved and comments made.

Source: Clyde E. Wesp, Jr., and Donna E. Hartman, *Clinical Maps for Acute Care: Managing Care through Collaborative Practice*, Aspen Publishers, Inc., © 1996.

# Myocardial Infarction—With/Without Thrombolytic Therapy: Acute Care Clinical Map

**DISCHARGE OUTCOMES***   Yes   No

1. D/C temperature < 100° for 24° prior to discharge.   ☐ ☐
2. Heart returns to baseline rhythm.   ☐ ☐
3. Patient able to identify risk factors and symptoms of angina.   ☐ ☐
4. Decrease in level of anxiety.   ☐ ☐
5. Normal cardiac enzymes and baseline EKG.   ☐ ☐
6. Pain control.   ☐ ☐
7. Patient verbalizes understanding of diet.   ☐ ☐
8. Patient tolerating diet.   ☐ ☐
9. Patient independent w/ADL's, or assisted by home help or SNF.   ☐ ☐

*Comment in Nursing Notes for outcomes not met.

R.N. Signature _____   Date _____   Date of DC _____

**CARDIAC SERVICES CLINICAL MAP**
**MYOCARDIAL INFARCTION**
**W/WO THROMBOLYTIC THERAPY**

PRIMARY M.D.: _____
CARDIOLOGIST: _____
CONSULTANT: _____

PATIENT ADDRESSOGRAPH

| ADM TIME: ____ DATE: ____ HOSPITAL AREA: | DAY 1: | DAY 2: | DAY 3: | DAY 4: | DAY 5: | DAY 6: |
|---|---|---|---|---|---|---|
| **CONSULTS/REFERRALS** | Care Manager / Cardiology / Social Services / Utilization Review | Heart/Mates | Nutrition Screen | Outpatient Cardiac Rehab as ordered | | |
| **ACTIVITY** | Bedrest | Advance as tolerated / BSC as tolerated | BRP as tolerated | ---> | ---> / Ambulate prior to DC | ---> |
| **TREATMENTS** | O₂ as ordered NC / CCS protocol / Stat EKG For CP | | O₂ prn | | | |
| **MEDICATION** THROMBOLYTICS: TPA ☐☐ Strepto ☐☐ N/A ☐☐ | As ordered: IV/TPA protocol / MS/NTG/Heparin/ASA / Lido/antiarrhythmics prn / RT & Card meds / Antiemetics/lax/stool softeners / HS & prn sed. | ---> / ---> / ---> / ---> / ---> | ---> / ---> / ---> / ---> / ---> | ---> / ---> / ---> / ---> / ---> | | |
| **TESTS:** CATH ____ PTCA ____ | ER Chem Panel / CSR, CBC / EKG ) Repeat / Enzymes ) as ordered / PT, PTT | Enzymes, EKG / PTT as ord. while on Heparin / *Inc. freq. of EKG & enzymes as ordered for chest pain | Enzymes, EKG / Cardiac tests as ordered | EKG / ---> | ---> | ---> |
| **FLUIDS/NUTRITION** | Cardiac diet / NPO for proc. as ord. / IV TKO | ---> / ---> / IV → Saline lock | ---> / ---> | ---> | | |
| **PATIENT/FAMILY TEACHING/DC PLAN** | Orientation to unit / Rationale for tests explained to pt/fam. / Fam. support/updates | Assess Rx for discharge teaching needs/learning readiness / ___ MI packet | Videos: / ___ Heart Attack / ___ Risk Factors / ___ Angina / ___ Diet Modifications / ___ Nutrition education | Other videos as needed / Reinforce teach. w/patient & family prn / Review MI packet | Outpatient Cardiac Rehab info: / Pacing activity / Pulse taking / Medication review | D/C instructions / Follow-up care / Pt. feedback |
| **SIGNATURE  A.M.  P.M.** | ☐☐☐☐ | ☐☐☐☐ | ☐☐☐☐ | ☐☐☐☐ | ☐☐☐☐ | ☐☐☐☐ |

*continues*

**Myocardial Infarction—With/Without Thrombolytic Therapy: Acute Care Clinical Map** continued

| PATIENT PROBLEM | INTERMEDIATE OUTCOMES | DATE OUTCOMES ANTICIPATED (by Clin Path) | DATE OUTCOMES ACHIEVED/ INITIALED* | COMMENTS |
|---|---|---|---|---|
| **Alteration in Comfort: R/T Angina, Nausea** | **Patient able to:**<br>1. Report duration and intensity of discomfort<br>**Pain control as evidenced by verbal/non-verbal indicators:**<br>1. IV NTG, MS<br>2. SL NTG, nitropatch<br>3. PO analgesics, antacids, anti-emetics | | | |
| **Potential for Decreased Cardiac Output: R/T Dysrhythmias, SOB, EKG Changes, Unstable Vital Signs** | **Patient will be:**<br>1. Electrophysiologically stable as evidenced by absence of dysrhythmias<br>2. Hemodynamically stable having SBP>100, HR >60 <120, usual mentation | | | |
| **Anxiety: R/T Unfamiliar Situation, Unpredictable Nature of Illness** | 1. Patient able to verbalize fears, questions, concerns<br>2. Patient and family able to share concerns about the effect of illness on normal functioning role and lifestyle<br>3. Patient exhibits effective coping mechanisms | | | |
| **Alteration in Mobility: R/T Insufficient Oxygenation for ADL** | **Patient will:**<br>1. Identify factors that will indicate when they may ↑ activity (as evidenced by stable pulse, B/P, respiratory rate)<br>**Patient tolerates:**<br>1. Getting up to BSC<br>2. Ambulate in room with assistance<br>3. Ambulate in room without assistance<br>4. Ambulate in hall with assistance<br>5. Ambulate in hall without assistance | | | |
| **Alteration in Nutrition: R/T to Hospitalization** | **Patient able to:**<br>1. Tolerate cardiac diet without nausea<br>2. Meet >50% of nutritional needs through oral intake by Day 5 (if not, consider nutrition support) | DAY 4 | | |
| **Alteration in Elimination: R/T ↓ Activity, Medication** | 1. Patient has stool without straining | | | |
| **Knowledge Deficit: R/T Home Care** | **Patient will:**<br>1. Identify cause of pain and rationales for medication, activity and diet restrictions<br>2. Identify reportable signs and symptoms<br>3. Describe self-administration of daily and prn meds.<br>4. Recognize symptoms of ↑ cardiac workload and identify pacing strategies<br>5. Verbalize understanding of diet<br>6. Verbalize follow-up of care needed, availability of community resources | | | |

*Nurse to initial date outcome achieved and comments made.

Source: Clyde E. Wesp, Jr., and Donna E. Hartman, *Clinical Maps for Acute Care: Managing Care through Collaborative Practice*, Aspen Publishers, Inc., © 1996.

# Percutaneous Transluminal Coronary Angioplasty (PTCA) Clinical Map for Acute Care

| DISCHARGE OUTCOMES* | Yes | No |
|---|---|---|
| 1. Oral temperature < 100°F. | ☐ | ☐ |
| 2. Pain controlled. | ☐ | ☐ |
| 3. Patient able to identify risk factors and symptoms of re-stenosis. | ☐ | ☐ |
| 4. Patient verbalizes understanding of diet. | ☐ | ☐ |
| 5. Patient able to demonstrate at home activities/restrictions. | ☐ | ☐ |
| 6. Patient states signs and symptoms to be reported to M.D. | ☐ | ☐ |
| * Comment in Nursing Notes for outcomes not met. | ☐ | ☐ |

R.N. Signature ____________ Date ________ Date of DC ________

**CARDIAC SERVICES CLINICAL MAP**

**PTCA**

PRIMARY M.D.: ____________

CARDIOLOGIST ____________

SURGEON: ____________

**PATIENT ADDRESSOGRAPH**

| DATE: HOSPITAL AREA: | PRE-PROC: ______ | PROC. DAY #1 ______ ICU | POST-PROC. DAY #2 ______ ICU/PCU/Discharge | POST-PROC. DAY #3 ______ |
|---|---|---|---|---|
| **CONSULTS/REFERRALS** | Care Manager<br>Surgical<br>Anesthesia | F&N Consult prn<br>Social Services | HeartMates<br>Cardiac Rehab | Nutrition Screen |
| **ACTIVITY** | Up ad lib | Ad lib pre-procedure<br>Bedrest 6 hrs., post-procedure, then ↑ HOB 30° | Bedrest × 6 hrs., post sheath d/c'd<br>Dangle → Chair → Ambulate → Discharge | |
| **TREATMENTS** | # 14 or #16 IV | Sheath removal<br>Post sheath removal care<br>VS/sheath checks/pulse checks<br>$O_2$ prn | ---> | |
| **MEDICATIONS** | Pre-op meds as ordered<br>IV Protocol | Heparinized solution to art/venus sheath<br>Heparin bolus/cath lab<br>IC NTG prn<br>NTG gtt prn<br>Sedation prn | Heparin gtt d/c'd - prior to sheath removal<br>Cardiac medications as ordered | |
| **TESTS:**<br>**Cath Results:** ______<br>**PTCA Results:** ______ | EKG<br>$SMA_{20}$<br>PT, PTT<br>CXR<br>T&C 2 units PC | EKG, Enzymes } PACU<br>PT, PTT<br>PTT at ____ hrs. | PTT, ACT } as ordered | |
| **FLUIDS/ NUTRITION** | NPO ___ hrs., before procedure | NPO<br>Cardiac diet post-procedure | ---> | |
| **PATIENT/FAMILY TEACHING/DC PLAN** | DC Planning<br>Videos/Booklets:<br>___ PTCA video<br>___ PTCA booklet<br>___ Stress packet<br>Pre/Post PTCA teaching to patient and family | Videos:<br>___ Risk Factor<br>___ Angina<br>___ Diet Modification | D/C instructions: diet, meds<br>Follow-up care - Cardiac Rehab<br>Nutrition education | |
| **SIGNATURE** A.M. P.M. | ☐ ______<br>☐ ______<br>☐ ______<br>☐ ______ | ☐ ______<br>☐ ______<br>☐ ______<br>☐ ______ | ☐ ______<br>☐ ______<br>☐ ______<br>☐ ______ | ☐ ______<br>☐ ______<br>☐ ______<br>☐ ______ |

*continues*

**Percutaneous Transluminal Coronary Angioplasty (PTCA) Clinical Map for Acute Care** continued

| PATIENT PROBLEM | INTERMEDIATE OUTCOMES | DATE OUTCOMES ANTICIPATED (by Clin Path) | DATE OUTCOMES ACHIEVED/ INITIALED* | COMMENTS |
|---|---|---|---|---|
| Anxiety/Fear R/T Health Status, Angioplasty Procedure, Routine Outcome and Possible Need for Cardiac Surgery | **Patient/Significant Other will:**<br>1. Verbalize fears concerning PTCA<br>2. Describe pre-angio routine<br>3. Describe procedure and expected sensations during procedure<br>4. Explain post-op routine | | | |
| Potential for Acute Coronary Occlusion, Dysrhythmias | **Patient will:**<br>1. Recognize signs and symptoms of angina and report them immediately | | | |
| Potential for Hemorrhage, Hematoma at Angio Site | **Patient will:**<br>1. Identify signs of pain as evidenced by pathological path, groin site pain or bleeding<br>2. Be hemodynamically stable as evidenced by stable B/P and pulse, UP > 30cc/hr. | | | |
| Impaired Mobility R/T Bedrest and Restricted Movement of Involved Extremity | **Patient will:**<br>1. State activity restrictions<br>2. Use log rolling techniques needed for turning<br>3. Keep involved leg immobilized<br>4. Gradually ↑ activity when prescribed | | | |
| Potential Altered Health Maintenance R/T Insufficient Knowledge of Care of Insertion Site, D/C Activities, Diet, Meds, Signs and Symptoms of Complications, Follow-up Care | **Patient will:**<br>1. Demonstrate care of insertion site<br>2. State restrictions regarding activity at home<br>3. Verbalize knowledge of risk factors<br>4. Verbalize knowledge of ↓ fat, ↓ cholesterol diet<br>5. Gradually resume daily activities<br>6. Identify signs and symptoms of re-stenosis, especially ↑ fatigue, angina, ↑ in anxiety<br>7. Understand need for follow-up appointment w/M.D., Cardiac Rehab as needed | | | |

*Nurse to initial date outcome achieved and comments made.

Source: Clyde E. Wesp, Jr., and Donna E. Hartman, *Clinical Maps for Acute Care: Managing Care through Collaborative Practice*, Aspen Publishers, Inc., © 1996.

# Coronary Artery Bypass Graft (CABG)/Valve
## Clinical Map for Acute Care

**CARDIAC SERVICES CLINICAL MAP**

**CABG/VALVE**

| DISCHARGE OUTCOMES* | Yes | No |
|---|---|---|
| 1. Stable cardiac rhythm. | ☐ | ☐ |
| 2. Oral temperature < 10°F for 24 hour period prior to d/c. | ☐ | ☐ |
| 3. HCT ≥ 24% - Hgb ≥ 8 gm/d. | ☐ | ☐ |
| 4. Absence of significant wound problem. | ☐ | ☐ |
| 5. Post-op pain controlled. | ☐ | ☐ |
| 6. Patient tolerates diet and verbalizes understanding of diet. | ☐ | ☐ |
| 7. Patient independent w/ADL's or assisted by home help/SNF. | ☐ | ☐ |
| 8. Patient/Family understanding discharge instructions. | ☐ | ☐ |

* Comment in Nursing Notes for outcomes not met.

R.N. Signature _____ Date _____

PRIMARY M.D.: _____
CARDIOLOGIST _____
SURGEON: _____
PERTINENT HISTORY: _____

PATIENT ADDRESSOGRAPH

Date of DC _____

| DATE: HOSPITAL AREA: | PRE-OP | DOS: OR/PACU/ICU | POD #1 ICU | POD #2 ICU/PCU | POD #3 PCU | POD #4 PCU | POD #5 PCU | POD #6 PCU |
|---|---|---|---|---|---|---|---|---|
| CONSULTS/ REFERRALS | Care Manager Surgical/Anesthesia Pulmonary as needed Social Services | - AVR - MVR - CABG X ___ | HeartMates | Physical Therapy as ordered | | CHC as ordered Outpatient Cardiac Rehab | | |
| ACTIVITY | Up ad lib or as ordered | Bedrest HOB ↑ 30° post extubation | Arm/leg exercises Dangle × 1 Chair as tolerated | ROM exercises Chair Amb. to BR w/assist once lines dc'd | Shower Ambulate × 2-3 using AHA guidelines | Shower Stairs w/assist Ambulate × 3-4 | ---> ---> ---> Discharge | |
| TREATMENTS | Clin prep Hiblclens shwr/scrub O₂ 40% venti-mask to OR | Vent Protocol Pulse oximeter Incision/vent care Hem. monitor'g N/G prn Ace wraps for 24° | Extubate: Venti-mask → O₂ N/C Pulse oximeter Incentive spirometer C&DB Chest Tube Protocol Wound Protocol TEDs as ordered | O₂ N/C ---> ---> ---> | O₂ Pulse oximeter if needed ---> | | | |
| MEDICATION | Pre-op per MD Antibiotic on call to Holding | IV Protocol Meds per orders, Analgesics, drug titration, sed/ antibiotics | Per routine PO meds post-extubation | Per routine | DC antibiotics 24° after CT removed unless valve LOC if no BM | | | |
| TESTS | TCM, EKG, CXR, SMA₂₀, CBC, PT, PTT, CABG Resp. Protocol Platelets as ord. Bleeding time as ord. **Report abnorm labs** | Intra-op tests ABGs, CBC, SMA20, PT/PTT, ACT, H&H K+, Mg+ prn CXR PACU | CXR, ECG @ 0530, ABGs/weaning param. CBC, SMA7, enzymes K+, Mg+ prn | CXR CBC, SMA7 @ 0530 | CXR, H&H as ordered | | | |
| FLUIDS/ NUTRITION | DAT - NPO after midnight | NPO, I/O Blood products Weight qd | Clear liquid NAS/2000cc fluid restrictions Progress diet ---> | Cardiac diet as tolerated ---> ---> | | | | |
| PATIENT/FAMILY TEACHING/DC PLAN | Consent Pre/Post-op teaching ___ CABG Packet ___ OHS Video ___ Valve Explain clinical map | Family support, Condition updates DC Planning | Reinf. prior teaching Pillow splinting | | Videos: ___ Open ♥ Recovery ___ Diet Modification ___ Risk Factors Nutrition education ---> ---> | ---> ---> ___ Surgery pkt ___ Printed DC Instr Schedule DC appt w/family | Review packet D/C prescrip. Home activity Community Resources | |
| SIGNATURE A.M. P.M. | ☐☐☐☐ | ☐☐☐☐ | ☐☐☐☐ | ☐☐☐☐ | ☐☐☐☐ | ☐☐☐☐ | ☐☐☐☐ | ☐☐☐☐ |

*continues*

**Coronary Artery Bypass Graft (CABG)/Value Clinical Map for Acute Care continued**

| PATIENT PROBLEM | INTERMEDIATE OUTCOMES | DATE OUTCOMES ANTICIPATED (by Clin Path) | DATE OUTCOMES ACHIEVED/ INITIALED* | COMMENTS |
|---|---|---|---|---|
| Knowledge Deficit: R/T Surgical Procedure | **Patient verbalizes understanding of:**<br>1. Pre-op tests<br>2. Surgical procedure<br>3. Post-op routine | PRE-OP<br>PRE-OP<br>PRE-OP | | |
| Potential for Cardiovascular, Renal, Respiratory Insufficiency | **Patient is:**<br>1. Electrophysiologically stable as evidenced by absence of dysrhythmias<br>2. Hemodynamically stable as evidenced by SBP > 90 w/o pressure support, UO > 30cc/hr, HR > 60 < 100<br>**Patient displays:**<br>3. Usual mentation<br>4. Demonstrated ability to C&DB and effectively use I.S. to clear lung secretions post extubation | | | |
| Alteration in Comfort: R/T Surgical Incisions | **Patient will:**<br>1. Notify nurse of need for pain med<br>2. Differentiate between surgical pain and angina | | | |
| Alteration in Mobility: R/T Surgical Procedure | **Patient will:**<br>1. Sit in chair for meals<br>2. Ambulate in hall w/assist<br>3. Ambulate in hall w/o assist<br>4. Tolerate sit down shower<br>5. Climb stationary stairs | | | |
| Alteration in Nutrition: R/T Surgical Procedure | **Patient will:**<br>1. Tolerate cardiac diet without nausea<br>2. Meet > 50% of nutritional needs through oral intake by Day 4 (if not, consider nutrition support | DAY 4 | | |
| Alteration in Elimination: R/T ↓ Activity/Medication | 1. Patient has stool w/o straining | | | |
| Potential for Altered Health Maintenance: R/T Insufficient Knowledge of Incisional Care, Signs and Symptoms of Complications, Risk Factors, Restrictions and Follow-up Care | **Patient/Significant Other will:**<br>1. Demonstrate incisional care<br>2. Verbalize knowledge of home care needs<br>3. Verbalize signs and symptoms to be reported to M.D.<br>4. Relate plan to reduce risk factors as indicated<br>5. Verbalize understanding of diet | | | |

*Nurse to initial date outcome achieved and comments made.

Source: Clyde E. Wesp, Jr., and Donna E. Hartman, *Clinical Maps for Acute Care: Managing Care through Collaborative Practice*, Aspen Publishers, Inc., © 1996.

# Congestive Heart Failure
## Provider Pathway

| | First Visit after Workup | Second Visit Second Week | Third Visit 4 Weeks | Fourth Visit 8 Weeks | Monthly for 3 Months Then Every 3 Months or PRN |
|---|---|---|---|---|---|
| Date | | | | | |
| Assessment | Apical and radial pulse RR, BP, pulsus alternans Postural signs Weight Complete physical exam: Cardiac, abdomen, pulmonary, peripheral vascular system, thyroid, skin Review activity level and symptoms: PND, edema, SOB, chest pain, palpitations | Apical and radial pulse RR, BP, pulsus alternans Postural signs Weight Complete physical exam: Cardiac, pulmonary, abdomen, peripheral vascular system, skin Review weight record Review activity level, symptoms, and aggravating or precipitating factors | Physical exam and VS same as in second visit Review weight and activity records Review symptoms and precipitating factors | Physical exam and VS same as in third visit Review weight and activity records Review symptoms and precipitating factors | Physical exam and VS same as in fourth visit Review activity and weight records Review symptoms and precipitating factors |
| Diagnostics and Treatments | Baseline ECG, chest X-ray Blood work may be dependent on medications: SMA 7, creatinine, Digoxin level, TSH, VA, $Mg^+$, $Ca^{++}$, PT/INR Flu and pneumococcus vaccines | PT/INR (if applicable) Consider SMA 7 Consider $K^+$ | PT/INR (if applicable) Consider SMA 7 Consider $K^+$ Creatinine, digoxin level (medication and prior value dependent) | PT/INR (if applicable) Consider SMA 7 Consider $K^+$ UA, digoxin level, and creatinine (medication and prior value dependent) | ECG and chest X-ray every 6 months Digoxin level: 4 times/year or PRN SMA 7 and creatinine: Every 3 months or PRN PT/INR: Every 4–8 weeks UA: Every 6 months TSH: Once a year $Mg^+$ and $Ca^{++}$: Every 6 months |

*Note:* CTA, clear to auscultation; PND, paroxysmal nocturnal dyspnea; RTC, return to clinic.

*continues*

**Congestive Heart Failure Provider Pathway** continued

| | First Visit after Workup | Second Visit Second Week | Third Visit 4 Weeks | Fourth Visit 8 Weeks | Monthly for 3 Months Then Every 3 Months or PRN |
|---|---|---|---|---|---|
| Date | | | | | |
| Teaching | Weight monitoring and weight record<br>Importance of follow-up and when to RTC or go to ED<br>Weight ↑ 3 lbs in 2 years, ↑ SOB, edema, PND<br>Diet: No added salt (2–4 g Na) ↓ cholesterol and weight reduction (if applicable)<br>Aggravating and precipitating factors<br>Fluid restriction (if applicable)<br>Risk factors and lifestyle modification: Smoking, stress<br>Activity: Depending on symptoms and functional class<br>Coumadin fact sheet (if applicable): Diet, BID testing, ↑ bleeding tendencies<br>Correct use of medications: Dose, importance of not skipping doses | Reinforce all teaching from first visit with patient and family: Diet, weight record, precipitating factors<br>Medications: Dose, side effects<br>Activity: Introduce activity log<br>Continue to reinforce importance of risk reduction: Smoking, stress<br>Review importance of follow-up and when to RTC or go to ED | Modify and review treatment plan<br>Continue reinforcing all teaching done on first and second visits | Modify and review treatment plan<br>Reinforce all teaching with patient and family | Modify and review treatment plan<br>Review all teaching with patient and family<br>Review importance of blood testing, follow-up appointments, and need to RTC or go to ED<br>Advise (as applicable) patient if he/she is responsible for adjusting diuretic dose depending on symptoms<br>Review the need for and encourage patient to continue weight and activity records |
| Medications | Determined by cause of CHF, functional class, physical assessment, and lab data: Digoxin, diuretics, angiotensin-converting enzymes, nitrates, vasodilators, potassium, oral anticoagulation | Continue medications<br>Adjust as needed depending on exam, lab data, symptoms, and weight record | Continue medications<br>Adjust as needed depending on exam, lab data, weight and activity records | Continue medications<br>Adjust as needed depending on exam, lab data, weight and activity records | Continue medications<br>Adjust as needed depending on exam, lab data, weight and activity records |

continues

**Congestive Heart Failure Provider Pathway** continued

| | First Visit after Workup | Second Visit Second Week | Third Visit 4 Weeks | Fourth Visit 8 Weeks | Monthly for 3 Months Then Every 3 Months or PRN |
|---|---|---|---|---|---|
| Date | | | | | |
| Consults/Referrals | Review records with cardiologist: EF, wall motion studies, chest X-ray, ECHO, treadmill studies<br>Social services: Home care, VNS | Dietitian: If continued need for teaching with patient and family<br>Physical therapy: For cardiac rehab, and/or endurance training<br>Social services: PRN | Dietitian: PRN<br>Physical therapy: PRN | | Cardiology: Yearly or PRN |
| Physiological Outcomes | Vital signs within baseline norm<br>Normal sinus rhythm<br>Lungs: CTA<br>⊖ JVD, edema (+1), ⊖ hepatosplenomegaly<br>Mild SOB on mild exertion<br>Two pillow PND<br>Additional physical exam WNL | Normal exam<br>⊖ edema<br>Baseline VS<br>Mild SOB on mild exertion<br>Two pillow PND<br>Blood testing WNL for patient<br>Diagnostic testing WNL for patient<br>Good weight record | Normal exam<br>Mild SOB on moderate exertion<br>Two pillow PND<br>Blood testing WNL for patient<br>Good weight and activity records | Normal exam<br>Mild SOB on moderate exertion<br>Two pillow PND<br>Blood testing WNL<br>Weight and activity records WNL | No additional clinic or ED visits<br>Mild SOB on moderate exertion<br>Two pillow PND |
| Educational Outcomes | Patient and family able to state when to RTC or when to go to ED<br>Patient able to state reason for weight record (and knows time of day to record weight) and fluid restrictions<br>Basic understanding of diet, medication, aggravating and precipitating factors | Patient and family able to follow diet and medication regimen<br>Patient and family able to state side effects of medication, need for blood testing, need to reduce risk factors, and precipitating factors<br>Patient able to maintain daily records of weight and activity | Patient and family following treatment plan<br>Risk factors reduced<br>Able to adjust weight recording to 4 times a week<br>Continue to keep activity record<br>Express knowledge and positive coping | Patient and family can do more self-care interventions<br>Continue to support and encourage | Patient and family understand and can express disease process and treatment regimen<br>Able to make proper diuretic adjustments with feedback from nurse practitioner or physician with progression to self-adjustments |

*continues*

**Congestive Heart Failure Provider Pathway** continued

| | First Visit after Workup | Second Visit Second Week | Third Visit 4 Weeks | Fourth Visit 8 Weeks | Monthly for 3 Months Then Every 3 Months or PRN |
|---|---|---|---|---|---|
| Date | | | | | |
| Psychosocial Outcomes | Begin patient and family knowledge base of disease control and treatment. Support patient and family with illness and possible changes in lifestyle and work and social habits | Increase knowledge base of disease process. Support patient and family with living with chronic disease. Encourage positive outcomes | Continual encouragement of positive outcomes and reduction in risk factors. Support patient and family as needed | Increase knowledge base and self-care | Adjusting well to living with chronic illness. Able to follow treatment regimen |
| Medication Outcomes | Review medications from referring cardiologist. Maintain or modify medications as needed | Review medications from last visit. Maintain or modify medications as needed | Review medications. Maintain or modify medications as needed | Maintain or modify medications as needed | Maintain and modify medications as needed with best weight, symptom management, and least adverse effects |
| Comments | | | | | |
| Initials/Date | | | | | |

Source: Rufus S. Howe, *Clinical Pathways for Ambulatory Care Case Management*, Aspen Publishers, Inc., © 1996.

# Congestive Heart Failure with Hypertension Provider Pathway

| | First Week after Initial Episode | Second Week | Third Week | Every Month | Yearly |
|---|---|---|---|---|---|
| **Date** | | | | | |
| **Assessment** | Weight<br>BP (sitting and standing)<br>TPR<br>Integumentary: Cyanosis, cold, clammy, pallor, edema, turgor, sweat<br>Ophthalmic: Optic fundi, papilledema<br>Respiratory: Observe, palpate, percuss, auscultate<br>Cardiovascular: JVD heart rate<br>Abdomen: Hepatomegaly, bruit<br>Extremities: BUE–BLE edema<br>Neurological: Anxiety, restlessness, confusion, memory lapse | Weight<br>BP<br>TPR<br>Integumentary<br>Respiratory (auscul-tate)<br>Cardiovascular<br>Extremities: Edema | Weight<br>BP<br>TPR<br>Integumentary<br>Respiratory (auscultate)<br>Cardiovascular<br>Extremities | Weight<br>BP<br>TPR<br>Integumentary<br>Respiratory<br>Cardiovascular<br>Extremities | Complete physical exam<br>Mini mental status exam |
| **Subjective** | Appetite, cough, hemoptysis, dyspnea, orthop-nea, dyspnea on exertion, bloating, chest pain, sweats | Same | Same | Same | Same |
| **Medications** | Diuretic<br>Antihypertensive (ACE)<br>Potassium supplement<br>Vitamins<br>Digoxin | Continue medication<br>Evaluate effectiveness | Same as second week | Same as second week | Pneumovax every 5 years<br>Flu vaccine yearly<br>Continue medication<br>Evaluate effectiveness |
| **Labs/Tests** | Electrolytes<br>Baseline:<br>• CBC with DIFF<br>• Digoxin level<br>• UA<br>• ECG<br>• Chest X-ray | None | None unless repeating those with abnormal values | q 3 months:<br>• Digoxin level<br>• Electrolytes | ECG<br>Chest X-ray<br>PPD q year<br>CBC with DIFF<br>UA |

*Note:* BUE–BLE, both upper extremities–both lower extremities.

*continues*

**Congestive Heart Failure with Hypertension Provider Pathway** continued

| | First Week after Initial Episode | Second Week | Third Week | Every Month | Yearly |
|---|---|---|---|---|---|
| Date | | | | | |
| Teaching | Medications:<br>• Hours of administration<br>• Check pulse before digoxin<br>• Side effects: Nausea and vomiting, anorexia, yellow vision/blur, palpitation, headache, fatigue, malaise, muscle cramps<br>Diet restrictions<br>Weight check<br>Rest periods<br>Wear nonconstricting garments<br>Importance of follow-up<br>↓ alcohol consumption<br>↓ or DC cigarette smoking | Ask if any side effects and teach accordingly<br>Teach re:<br>• Weight chart<br>• Pulse chart<br>Review instructions | Ask if any side effects and teach accordingly<br>Check weight and pulse charts<br>Review instructions with patient as needed<br>Recheck diet restrictions<br>Teach if patient not keeping follow-up visits<br>Reinforce teaching regarding alcohol and cigarette use | Ask if any side effects and teach accordingly<br>Check weight and pulse charts<br>Teach if patient not keeping follow-up visits<br>Offer counseling for smoking cessation/ reduced alcohol consumption PRN | Teach as need arises<br>Review 2-g sodium diet<br>Teach if patient not keeping follow-up visits<br>Offer counseling for smoking cessation/ reduced alcohol consumption PRN |
| Consults/Referrals | Physician for change in digoxin<br>Cardiologist, if complications occur<br>Dietitian, regarding 2-g sodium diet | PRN | PRN | PRN | PRN |
| Physiological Outcomes | BP ↓ 150/90<br>Weight stable<br>RR WNL<br>Pulse WNL<br>Skin: No edema, no cyanosis<br>Lungs clear, no dyspnea, no pulmonary edema<br>Cardiac: JVD, adequate cardiac output<br>Abdomen: No hepatomegaly, no bruits<br>Extremities: Minimal or no edema, no infection | BP stable<br>Weight stable<br>RR WNL<br>Pulse WNL<br>Skin: No edema, no cyanosis<br>Lungs clear<br>Cardiac: Adequate cardiac output<br>Extremities: No edema | Skin: No edema, no cyanosis | Skin: No edema, no cyanosis | Complete physical exam WNL for patient this age<br>Mini mental status exam |
| Medication Outcomes | No side effects<br>Adequate diuresis<br>BP WNL | Patient compliant<br>No side effects<br>Adequate diuresis<br>BP WNL | No side effects<br>Adequate diuresis<br>BP WNL | No side effects<br>Adequate diuresis<br>BP WNL | No side effects<br>No digoxin toxicity<br>Lasix: No electrolyte imbalance<br>BP WNL |
| Diet Outcomes | Diet (2-g sodium diet) helping in control of high blood pressure and edema | Patient compliant<br>No edema<br>BP WNL | Patient compliant<br>No edema<br>BP WNL | Patient compliant<br>No edema<br>BP WNL | Patient compliant<br>Minimal edema<br>BP WNL |

continues

Congestive Heart Failure with Hypertension Provider Pathway continued

| | First Week after Initial Episode | Second Week | Third Week | Every Month | Yearly |
|---|---|---|---|---|---|
| Date | | | | | |
| Lab Outcomes | WNL | | | q 3 months Electrolytes WNL Digoxin level WNL with no toxicity | ECG: No acute changes Chest X-ray WNL PPD: Induration <10 cm CBC with DIFF: No evidence of infection SMA 7: No imbalances UA: No evidence of UTI |
| Educational Outcomes | Correct administration of medications and aware of side effects. Patient knows how to check pulse and check weight. Patient will ↓ alcohol consumption. Patient will ↓ or DC smoking | Patient checks pulse accurately. Patient checks weight accurately. Patient understands importance of reporting weight gain. Patient understands and agrees to ↓ alcohol and cigarettes | Patient keeping accurate chart of pulse and weight | Patient keeping accurate chart of pulse and weight | Continue with education as needed |
| Psychosocial Outcomes | Patient is able to continue self-care at home OR Patient is able to continue at home with home care helper | Patient is gaining strength and independence. Patient is starting to resume contacts with friends | Patient is gaining strength and independence. Patient is starting to resume contacts with friends | Patient resumes former activities—church, senior citizens club, and so forth—with adequate rest | Patient maintains independence in ADL with help of home care helper |
| Comments | | | | | |
| Initials/Date | | | | | |

Source: Rufus S. Howe, *Clinical Pathways for Ambulatory Care Case Management*, Aspen Publishers, Inc., © 1996.

# Clinical Pathway for CHF Clinic

Patient Name _____  Clinic Admit Date: _____  Level: _____

Diagnosis: <u>Congestive Heart Failure (Clinic)</u>  LOS <u>4 WEEKS</u>

INPATIENT:  OUTPATIENT:

| | INITIAL INTERVIEW | WEEK 1 VISIT 1 | WEEK 1 VISIT 2 | WEEK 2 VISIT 3 | WEEK 2 VISIT 4 |
|---|---|---|---|---|---|
| Nursing interventions | <u>Assessment:</u> Introduce concept of CHF clinic<br><br>Assess family support/transportation needs<br><br>Schedule first clinic visit<br><br>Provide basic handout regarding signs and symptoms of CHF<br><br>Take basic history | *Follow-up phone call to confirm first visit day prior<br><br><u>Assessment:</u> Signs and symptoms of CHF & appropriate follow-up<br><br><u>Teaching:</u> Signs and symptoms of CHF<br><br>Dietary opportunities<br><br>Medication information/schedules | <u>Assessment:</u> Signs and symptoms of CHF<br><br><u>Teaching:</u> To call appropriate contact person in physician's office with signs and symptoms of CHF<br><br>Introduce concept of patient exercise | <u>Assessment:</u> Signs and symptoms of CHF<br><br>Validate patient's assessment<br><br><u>Teaching:</u> Encourage patient to interact with other CHF patients<br><br>Potential of exercise discussed | <u>Assessment:</u> Signs and symptoms of CHF<br><br>Validate patient's assessment<br><br><u>Teaching:</u> Consultation with registered dietitian to address compliance and provide support with dietary guidelines for patient and family |
| Patient outcomes | Commits to clinic Visit 1<br><br>Identifies a support system/person | Makes contract to participate in self-care<br><br>Helps identify needs<br><br>Sets mutual goals for 1 month of clinic visits 2x week | Verbalizes signs and symptoms of CHF<br><br>Agrees to contact physician's office with signs and symptoms<br><br>Observes CHF clients exercising or begins program according to readiness | Participates in exercise if appropriate | Patient verbalizes changes made in sodium and fluid intake<br><br>Patient acknowledges improvement in functional capacity due to regular exercise |

*continues*

**Clinical Pathway for CHF Clinic** continued

INPATIENT:     OUTPATIENT:

| | WEEK 3 | | WEEK 4 | | POST CLINIC DISCHARGE 2 WEEKS |
|---|---|---|---|---|---|
| | VISIT 5 | VISIT 6 | VISIT 7 | VISIT 8 | |
| Nursing interventions | Assessment: Signs and symptoms of CHF Validate patient's assessment Counseling: Body image, grief/loss addressed— encourage patient to vent and make appropriate referrals Involve family with patient's permission | Assessment: Signs and symptoms of CHF Validate patient's assessment Teaching: Handouts given with overview of physiology of CHF and precipitating illness | Assessment: Validate patient's assessment regarding signs and symptoms of CHF Give survey Teaching: Consultation with exercise physiologist to outline alternating periods of rest and exercise | Assessment: Validate patient's assessment regarding signs and symptoms of CHF Collect survey Counseling: Encourage patient to verbalize further grief/loss; discuss terminal nature of illness; emphasize patient's locus of control | Assessment: Follow-up phone call to ascertain patient progress Patient verbalizes progress in concrete terms regarding weight and fluid retention, dietary sodium and fluid intake, and signs and symptoms of CHF |
| Patient outcomes | Acknowledges loss, verbalizes examples of available support | Patient asks appropriate questions to verify information received Patient may continue grief/loss discussion | Patient verbalizes appropriate levels and types of exercise, ways of recognizing problems | Patient verbalizes/ shows signs of acceptance | Patient outlines continued exercise plans |

*Source:* Gail Hafferkamp Venner and Jeanne Silitro Seelbinder, "Team Management of Congestive Heart Failure Across the Continuum," *The Journal of Cardiovascular Nursing*, Vol. 10:2, Aspen Publishers, Inc., © 1996.

# Congestive Heart Failure Home Care Clinical Pathway

| | Week 1 | Week 2 | Week 3 | Week 4 | Week 5 | Week 6 | Week 7 | Week 8 | Week 9 | Week 10 | Week 11 | Week 12 |
|---|---|---|---|---|---|---|---|---|---|---|---|---|
| **CLINICAL RESOURCE USE** | Skilled Nursing Visits (visit1, visit2) | Skilled Nursing Visits (visit1, visit2) | Skilled Nursing Visits (visit1, visit2) | Skilled Nursing Visits (visit1, visit2) | Skilled Nursing Visits (visit1, visit2) | Skilled Nursing Visits (visit1, visit2) | Skilled Nursing Visits (visit1) | Skilled Nursing Visits (visit1) | Skilled Nursing Visits (visit1) | Skilled Nursing Visits (visit1) | Skilled Nursing Visits (visit1) | Skilled Nursing Visits (visit1) |
| | Home Health Aide (assess need for HHA) | Home Health Aide (Supervise HHA) | Home Health Aide (Supervise HHA) | Home Health Aide (Supervise HHA) | Home Health Aide (Supervise HHA) | Home Health Aide (Supervise HHA) | Home Health Aide (Supervise HHA) | Home Health Aide (Supervise HHA) | Home Health Aide (Supervise HHA) | Home Health Aide (Supervise HHA) | Home Health Aide (Supervise HHA) | Home Health Aide (Supervise HHA) |
| | Physical Therapy (assess need for P.T.) | | | | | | | | | | | |
| | Social Services (assess need for S.W.) | | | | | | | | | | | |
| **PATIENT ASSESSMENT** | Lung Sounds (visit1, visit2) | Lung Sounds (visit1, visit2) | Lung Sounds (visit1, visit2) | Lung Sounds (visit1, visit2) | Lung Sounds (visit1, visit2) | Lung Sounds (visit1, visit2) | Lung Sounds (visit1, visit2) | Lung Sounds (visit1, visit2) | Lung Sounds (visit1, visit2) | Lung Sounds (visit1, visit2) | Lung Sounds (visit1, visit2) | Lung Sounds (visit1, visit2) |
| | Temperature (on admission) | Temperature (PRN) | Temperature (PRN) | Temperature (PRN) | Temperature (PRN) | Temperature (PRN) | Temperature (PRN) | Temperature (PRN) | Temperature (PRN) | Temperature (PRN) | Temperature (PRN) | Temperature (PRN) |
| | Respiration Rate (visit1, visit2) | Respiration Rate (visit1, visit2) | Respiration Rate (visit1, visit2) | Respiration Rate (visit1, visit2) | Respiration Rate (visit1, visit2) | Respiration Rate (visit1) | Respiration Rate (visit1) | Respiration Rate (visit1) | Respiration Rate (visit1) | Respiration Rate (visit1) | Respiration Rate (visit1) | Respiration Rate (visit1) |
| | Blood Pressure (visit1, visit2) | Blood Pressure (visit1, visit2) | Blood Pressure (visit1, visit2) | Blood Pressure (visit1, visit2) | Blood Pressure (visit1, visit2) | Blood Pressure (visit1) | Blood Pressure (visit1) | Blood Pressure (visit1) | Blood Pressure (visit1) | Blood Pressure (visit1) | Blood Pressure (visit1) | Blood Pressure (visit1) |
| | Pulse (visit1) | Pulse (visit1) | Pulse (visit1) | Pulse (visit1) | Pulse (visit1) | Pulse (visit1) | Pulse (visit1) | Pulse (visit1) | Pulse (visit1) | Pulse (visit1) | Pulse (visit1) | Pulse (visit1) |
| | Dyspnea (visit1, visit2) | Dyspnea (visit1, visit2) | Dyspnea (visit1, visit2) | Dyspnea (visit1, visit2) | Dyspnea (visit1, visit2) | Dyspnea (visit1, visit2) | Dyspnea (visit1) | Dyspnea (visit1) | Dyspnea (visit1) | Dyspnea (visit1) | Dyspnea (visit1) | Dyspnea (visit1) |
| | Cognitive Capacity (visit1) | Cognitive Capacity (visit1) | Cognitive Capacity (visit1) | Cognitive Capacity (visit1) | Cognitive Capacity (visit1) | Cognitive Capacity (visit1) | Cognitive Capacity (visit1) | Cognitive Capacity (visit1) | Cognitive Capacity (visit1) | Cognitive Capacity (visit1) | Cognitive Capacity (visit1) | Cognitive Capacity (visit1) |
| | Weight (visit1, visit2) | Weight (visit1, visit2) | Weight (visit1, visit2) | Weight (visit1, visit2) | Weight (visit1, visit2) | Weight (visit1, visit2) | Weight (visit1) | Weight (visit1) | Weight (visit1) | Weight (visit1) | Weight (visit1) | Weight (visit1) |
| | Peripheral Edema (visit1, visit2) | Peripheral Edema (visit1) | Peripheral Edema (visit1) | Peripheral Edema (visit1) | Peripheral Edema (visit1) | Peripheral Edema (visit1) | Peripheral Edema (visit1) | Peripheral Edema (visit1) | Peripheral Edema (visit1) | Peripheral Edema (visit1) | Peripheral Edema (visit1) | Peripheral Edema (visit1) |
| **DIAGNOSTIC TESTS** | Electrolytes (Assess need for order/results) | Electrolytes (results) | Electrolytes (results) | Electrolytes (results) | Electrolytes (results) | Electrolytes (results) | Electrolytes (results) | Electrolytes (results) | Electrolytes (results) | Electrolytes (results) | Electrolytes (results) | Electrolytes (results) |
| | Creatinine Level (Assess need for order/results) | Creatinine Level (results) | Creatinine Level (results) | Creatinine Level (results) | Creatinine Level (results) | Creatinine Level (results) | Creatinine Level (results) | Creatinine Level (results) | Creatinine Level (results) | Creatinine Level (results) | Creatinine Level (results) | Creatinine Level (results) |

continues

Congestive Heart Failure Home Care Clinical Pathway   continued

| | Week 1 | Week 2 | Week 3 | Week 4 | Week 5 | Week 6 | Week 7 | Week 8 | Week 9 | Week 10 | Week 11 | Week 12 |
|---|---|---|---|---|---|---|---|---|---|---|---|---|
| **DIAGNOSTIC TESTS** | BUN (assess need for order/results | BUN (results | BUN (results | BUN (results | BUN (results | BUN (results | BUN (results | BUN (results | BUN (results | BUN (results | BUN (results | BUN (results |
| | CBC (Assess need for order/results | CBC (results | CBC (results | CBC (results | CBC (results | CBC (results | CBC (results | CBC (results | CBC (results | CBC (results | CBC (results | CBC (results |
| | Digoxin/digitoxin Blood Level (Assess need for order/results | Digoxin/digitoxin Blood Level | Digoxin/digitoxin Blood Level | Digoxin/digitoxin Blood Level | Digoxin/digitoxin Blood Level | Digoxin/digitoxin Blood Level | Digoxin/digitoxin Blood Level | Digoxin/digitoxin Blood Level | Digoxin/digitoxin Blood Level | Digoxin/digitoxin Blood Level | Digoxin/digitoxin Blood Level | Digoxin/digitoxin Blood Level |
| | Prothrombin Time (Assess need for order/results | Prothrombin Time (results | Prothrombin Time (results | Prothrombin Time (results | Prothrombin Time (results | Prothrombin Time (results | Prothrombin Time (results | Prothrombin Time (results | Prothrombin Time (results | Prothrombin Time (results | Prothrombin Time (results | Prothrombin Time (results |
| **TREATMENTS** | Oxygen Therapy (Assess need for order/obtain Pulse Oximetry as needed | Oxygen Therapy (SaO2 PRN | Oxygen Therapy (SaO2 PRN | Oxygen Therapy (SaO2 PRN | Oxygen Therapy (SaO2 PRN | Oxygen Therapy (SaO2 PRN | Oxygen Therapy (SaO2 PRN | Oxygen Therapy (SaO2 PRN | Oxygen Therapy (SaO2 PRN | Oxygen Therapy (SaO2 PRN | Oxygen Therapy (SaO2 PRN | Oxygen Therapy (SaO2 PRN |
| **MEDICATION USAGE** | Diuretic Therapy (Assess visit1 | Diuretic Therapy (Assess visit1 | Diuretic Therapy (Assess visit1 | Diuretic Therapy (Assess visit1 | Diuretic Therapy (Assess visit1 | Diuretic Therapy (Assess visit1 | Diuretic Therapy (Assess visit1 | Diuretic Therapy (Assess visit1 | Diuretic Therapy (Assess visit1 | Diuretic Therapy (Assess visit1 | Diuretic Therapy (Assess visit1 | Diuretic Therapy (Assess visit1 |
| | Digoxin (Assess visit1 visit2 | Digoxin (Assess visit1 visit2 | Digoxin (Assess visit1 visit2 | Digoxin (Assess visit1 visit2 | Digoxin (Assess visit1 visit2 | Digoxin (Assess visit1 visit2 | Digoxin (Assess visit1 | Digoxin (Assess visit1 | Digoxin (Assess visit1 | Digoxin (Assess visit1 | Digoxin (Assess visit1 | Digoxin (Assess visit1 |
| | Potassium Supplement (Assess visit1 | Potassium Supplement (Assess visit1 | Potassium Supplement (Assess visit1 | Potassium Supplement (Assess visit1 | Potassium Supplement (Assess visit1 | Potassium Supplement (Assess visit1 | Potassium Supplement (Assess visit1 | Potassium Supplement (Assess visit1 | Potassium Supplement (Assess visit1 | Potassium Supplement (Assess visit1 | Potassium Supplement (Assess visit1 | Potassium Supplement (Assess visit1 |
| **NUTRITION AND FLUIDS** | Fluids (Assess low NA diet/fluids visit1 visit2 | Fluids (assess fluids/diet visit 1 | Fluids (assess fluids/diet visit 1 | Fluids (assess fluids/diet visit 1 | Fluids (assess fluids/diet visit 1 | Fluids (assess fluids/diet visit 1 | Fluids (assess fluids/diet visit 1 | Fluids (assess fluids/diet visit 1 | Fluids (assess fluids/diet visit 1 | Fluids (assess fluids/diet visit 1 | Fluids (assess fluids/diet visit 1 | Fluids (assess fluids/diet visit 1 |
| **ACTIVITY** | Ambulation (assess tolerance/safety visit1 visit2 | Ambulation (assess tolerance/safety visit1 visit2 | Ambulation (assess tolerance/safety visit1 visit2 | Ambulation (assess tolerance/safety visit1 visit2 | Ambulation (assess tolerance/safety visit1 visit2 | Ambulation (assess tolerance/safety visit1 visit2 | Ambulation (assess tolerance/safety visit 1 | Ambulation (assess tolerance/safety visit 1 | Ambulation (assess tolerance/safety visit 1 | Ambulation (assess tolerance/safety visit 1 | Ambulation (assess tolerance/safety visit 1 | Ambulation (assess tolerance/safety visit 1 |

*continues*

**Congestive Heart Failure Home Care Clinical Pathway** continued

| | Week 1 | Week 2 | Week 3 | Week 4 | Week 5 | Week 6 | Week 7 | Week 8 | Week 9 | Week 10 | Week 11 | Week 12 |
|---|---|---|---|---|---|---|---|---|---|---|---|---|
| **CONTINUITY OF CARE** | Discharge Planning (begin on admission) | | | | | | | | | Discharge Planning (Discuss discharge plan) | Discharge Planning (Discuss discharge plan) | Discharge Planning (Discuss discharge plan) |
| **PATIENT OUTCOMES** | Patient Will Demonstrate/maint Maximum Level Of Adls ( | Patient Will Demonstrate/maint Maximum Level Of Adls ( | Patient Will Demonstrate/maint Maximum Level Of Adls ( | Patient Will Demonstrate/maint Maximum Level Of Adls ( | Patient Will Demonstrate/maint Maximum Level Of Adls ( | Patient Will Demonstrate/maint Maximum Level Of Adls ( | Patient Will Demonstrate/maint Maximum Level Of Adls ( | Patient Will Demonstrate/maint Maximum Level Of Adls ( | Patient Will Demonstrate/maint Maximum Level Of Adls ( | Patient Will Demonstrate/maint Maximum Level Of Adls ( | Patient Will Demonstrate/maint Maximum Level Of Adls ( | Patient Will Demonstrate/maint Maximum Level Of Adls (dc continue) |
| **PATIENT EDUCATION** | Diet And Fluid Restrictions (Initiate teaching visit1); How To Weigh Self (Assess ability visit2); Medication Education (Instruct visit1 visit2); Signs And Symptoms Of Heart Failure (Instruct visit1); Home Safety (Assess visit1); What Is Expected Of Patient (Review patient rights/responsibilities visit1) | Diet And Fluid Restrictions (Assess/reinstruct as needed visit1 visit2); How To Weigh Self (Instruct importance of monitoring weight visit1 visit2); How To Take Pulse (Instruct visit1 visit2); Medication Education (Instruct visit1 visit2); Home Safety (Teach home safety visit2); About Disease Condition (Teach complications of CHF visit2) | Diet And Fluid Restrictions (Assess/reinstruct as needed visit1 visit2); How To Take Pulse (Assess ability visit1); Medication Education (Instruct visit1 visit2); About Disease Condition (Teach energy conservation techniques visit2) | Importance Of Medical Follow-up (Instruct when to contact practioner visit1); Medication Education (Instruct visit1 visit2); Signs And Symptoms Of Heart Failure (Instruct visit1 visit2); Signs And Symptoms Of Infection (Instruct visit1) | Medication Education (Instruct visit1 visit2); Signs And Symptoms Of Heart Failure (Instruct visit1 visit2); Signs And Symptoms Of Infection (Instruct visit1) | Medication Education (Instruct visit1 visit2) | How To Take Pulse (Assess ability visit2); Medication Education (Instruct visit1); What Is Expected Of Patient (Review visit1) | Diet And Fluid Restrictions (Assess/reinstruct as needed visit1); About Disease Condition (Instruct importance of rest/activity visit1) | Importance Of Medical Follow-up (Instruct when to contact practioner visit1); Medication Education (Reassess compliance visit1); Signs And Symptoms Of Heart Failure (Instruct visit1) | How To Take Pulse (Assess ability visit2); Home Safety (Assess/reinstruct visit1) | Medication Education (Instruct visit1); Signs And Symptoms Of Infection (Instruct visit1) | Diet And Fluid Restrictions (Assess/reinstruct as needed visit1); Importance Of Medical Follow-up (Instruct when to contact practioner visit1); Signs And Symptoms Of Heart Failure (Reassess knowledge base and reinstruct as needed visit 1) |

Source: Deborah J. Plotkin, Lisa A. Smart, and Gail E. Russell, "Congestive Heart Failure Home Care Critical Path," *Inside Case Management*, Vol. 2:10, Aspen Publishers, Inc., © 1996.

# CHF Interdisciplinary Plan of Care for Skilled Nursing Facility

| PROBLEM | GOALS | INTERVENTIONS | DISCIPLINES |
|---|---|---|---|

**PROBLEM**

**Congestive Heart Failure or Potential or Actual Cardiac Output Decreased and/or Comfort, Alteration in, and/or Electrolyte Imbalance and/or Fluid Volume Excess and/or Gas Exchange Impaired and/or Self-Care Deficit**

**R/T**

___ CHF

___ _____

_____

**AEB**

___ Anorexia
___ Anxiousness
___ Ascites
___ Blood pressure, low
___ Chest pains
___ Cough
   ___ Persistent
   ___ Productive (sputum)
      ___ Blood tinged
      ___ Frothy
___ Edema
   ___ Dependent
   ___ Generalized
___ Exercise intolerance
___ Fatigue
___ Mental status, altered
___ Pulse
   ___ Rate increased
   ___ Thready
   ___ Weak

**GOALS**

___ Will function at optimal level within limitations imposed by congestive heart failure and complications R/T treatment AEB:

_____
_____
_____
_____
_____
_____
_____

by/through: _____

**And/or**

___ _____
_____
_____
_____

by/through: _____

**INTERVENTIONS**

___ Assess/record/report to MD prn: CHF
___ Anorexia
___ Anxiousness
___ Ascites
___ Blood pressure, low
___ Chest pains
___ Cough
   ___ Persistent
   ___ Productive (sputum)
      ___ Blood tinged
      ___ Frothy
___ Edema
   ___ Dependent
   ___ Generalized
___ Exercise intolerance
___ Fatigue
___ Mental status, altered
___ Pulse
   ___ Rate increased
   ___ Thready
   ___ Weak
___ Respirations
   ___ Difficult (dyspnea)
   ___ Noisy
   ___ Orthopnea
   ___ Rate increased
   ___ SOB
   ___ Wheezes, audible
___ Restlessness
___ Skin
   ___ Clammy
   ___ Cold
   ___ Diaphoresis
   ___ Pale
___ Urine output, decreased
___ Vein distention
   ___ Neck
___ Weight gain

**DISCIPLINES**

N

Resident's name: _____ Date: _____

*continues*

**CHF Interdisciplinary Plan of Care for Skilled Nursing Facility** continued

| PROBLEM | GOALS | INTERVENTIONS | DISCIPLINES |
|---|---|---|---|
| ___ Respirations | | ___ See care plans for problems associated with CHF | ALL |
|    ___ Difficult (dyspnea) | |    ___ Cardiac output, decreased | |
|    ___ Noisy | |    ___ Comfort, alteration in | |
|    ___ Orthopnea | |    ___ Electrolyte imbalance | |
|    ___ Rate increased | |    ___ Fluid volume excess | |
|    ___ SOB | |    ___ Gas exchange impaired | |
|    ___ Wheezes, audible | |    ___ Self-care deficit | |
| ___ Restlessness | | | |
| ___ Skin | | ___ Hospice referral | S |
|    ___ Clammy | | | |
|    ___ Cold | | ___ Elevate HOB ___ degrees | N NA |
|    ___ Diaphoresis | | | |
|    ___ Pale | | ___ Provide ___ pillows | N NA |
| ___ Urine output, decreased | | | |
| ___ Vein distention | | ___ Oxygen: Administer/monitor effectiveness | N |
|    ___ Neck | |    ___ See physician order sheet, or | |
| ___ Weight gain | |    ___ List (amount/route/ frequency): | |
| ___ _____ | |    _____ | |
|    _____ | | | |
| | | ___ Weight q ___; monitor results | N NA D |
| | | ___ Provide/serve/monitor intake of diet: _____ | D N NA |
| | | _____ | |
| | | _____ | |
| | |    ___ Fat/cholesterol restriction | |
| | |    ___ Fluid restriction | |
| | |    ___ Sodium restriction | |
| | |    ___ Weight reduction, if obese | |
| | | ___ Meet with resident/family discuss any concerns R/T CHF Meet with resident ___ times per _____ Discuss: _____ | S N |
| | | _____ | |

*continues*

**CHF Interdisciplinary Plan of Care for Skilled Nursing Facility** continued

| PROBLEM | GOALS | INTERVENTIONS | DISCIPLINES |
|---|---|---|---|
| | | ___ Provide a program of activities that accommodates resident's problem: _____ _____ | A |
| | | Invite/escort to: _____ _____ | |
| | | ___ Lab/diagnostic work: Monitor/report results to MD ___ Digoxin level ___ Electrolytes ___ ECG ___ _____ | N D |
| | | ___ Date/frequency/result: _____ _____ ___ See lab section of chart | |
| | | Make recommendations for dietary change to nursing/MD prn: _____ | |
| | | ___ Meds: Administer/monitor effectiveness/side effects ___ See physician order sheet, or ___ List: _____ _____ _____ | N |
| | | ___ Resident education ___ Diet/fluids ___ Disease process ___ Energy conservation techniques ___ Foods to avoid ___ Stress reduction techniques ___ _____ | N D S |
| | | ___ _____ _____ _____ _____ | __ __ __ __ |

Source: Janie L. Krechting and Victoria E. Koper, *Interdisciplinary Care Plans for Long-Term Care*, Aspen Publishers, Inc., © 1996.

# CAD Interdisciplinary Plan of Care for Skilled Nursing Facility

| PROBLEM | GOALS | INTERVENTIONS | DISCIPLINES |
|---|---|---|---|

**Coronary Artery Disease or Actual or Potential Cardiac Output Decreased and/or Comfort Alteration in and/or Tissue Perfusion Alteration in**

___ Will be free of s/s of coronary artery disease
AEB no
___ Discomfort below the breastbone
  ___ Burning
  ___ Crushing tightness
  ___ Squeezing
___ Extremities
  ___ Cool
___ Fainting
___ Nausea
___ Pain
  ___ Arm
  ___ Chest
  ___ Jaw
  ___ Neck
  ___ Shoulder
___ Palpitations
___ Sweating
___ Syncope
___ Vomiting
___ Weakness
___ _____

by: _____

___ Assess/monitor/record/report to RN/MD prn: Coronary artery disease s/s      N
___ Discomfort below the breastbone
  ___ Burning
  ___ Crushing tightness
  ___ Squeezing
___ Extremities
  ___ Cool
___ Fainting
___ Nausea
___ Pain
  ___ Arm
  ___ Chest
  ___ Jaw
  ___ Neck
  ___ Shoulder
___ Sweating
___ Syncope
___ Vomiting
___ Weakness

**R/T**

___ Coronary artery disease
___ _____
    _____

**AEB**

___ Discomfort below breastbone
  ___ Burning
  ___ Crushing tightness
  ___ Squeezing
___ Extremities
  ___ Cool
___ Fainting
___ Nausea
___ Pain
  ___ Arm
  ___ Chest
  ___ Jaw
  ___ Neck
  ___ Shoulder
___ Palpitations
___ Sweating
___ Syncope
___ Vomiting
___ Weakness
___ _____
    _____
    _____
    _____

**And/or**

___ Vital signs WNL
Pulse 60–100 q ___

by: _____

**And/or**

___ _____
    _____
    _____
    _____

by/through: _____

___ Weigh q ____; monitor results and report to RN/MD prn      N NA D

___ Provide/serve/monitor intake      N NA D
Diet: _____
_____
  ___ Avoid heavy, large meals
  ___ Caffeine restriction
  ___ Calorie restriction
  ___ Fat/cholesterol restriction
  ___ Fluid restriction
  ___ Sodium restriction
  ___ Weight reduction, if obese

___ I&O q _____      N NA

___ Promote rest (if chest pain is severe)      N NA A
  ___ Comfortable chair for upright sleep
  ___ Extra pillows/HOB elevated

Resident's name: _____  Date: _____

*continues*

**CAD Interdisciplinary Plan of Care for Skilled Nursing Facility** continued

| PROBLEM | GOALS | INTERVENTIONS | DISCIPLINES |
|---------|-------|---------------|-------------|
| | | ___ Frequent rest periods | |
| | | ___ _____ | |
| | | ___ Describe activity limitations/ accommodations | A |
| | | ___ Avoid overexertion | |
| | | ___ Encourage regular exercise within tolerance Describe: _____ | |
| | | _____ | |
| | | ___ Exercise restrictions | |
| | | ___ Notify nursing if chest pain occurs | |
| | | Invite/escort to: _____ | |
| | | _____ | |
| | | _____ | |
| | | ___ Assist with ADLs Describe: _____ | N NA |
| | | _____ | |
| | | ___ Oxygen | N |
| | | ___ L/min: _____ | |
| | | ___ Route: _____ | |
| | | ___ Frequency: _____ | |
| | | ___ Rationale: _____ | |
| | | ___ Lab/diagnostic work: Monitor/report results to MD | N D |
| | | ___ Chest X-ray | |
| | | ___ ECG | |
| | | ___ Electrolytes | |
| | | ___ _____ | |
| | | Date/frequency: _____ | |
| | | Make appropriate dietary change recommendations to nursing/MD | |
| | | ___ Meet with resident/family to discuss any concerns R/T coronary artery disease | S |

*continues*

**CAD Interdisciplinary Plan of Care for Skilled Nursing Facility** continued

| PROBLEM | GOALS | INTERVENTIONS | DISCIPLINES |
|---|---|---|---|
| | | Meet with resident ____ times per ____ | |
| | | Discuss: _____ <br> _____ <br> _____ | |
| | | ___ Take/monitor vital signs <br>   ___ BP q _____ <br>   ___ Pulse q _____ <br>   ___ Respirations q _____ | N |
| | | ___ Meds: Administer/monitor effectiveness/side effects <br>   ___ See physician order sheet, or <br>   ___ List: _____ <br>   _____ <br>   _____ | N |
| | | ___ Resident education <br>   ___ Disease process <br>   ___ Factors that precipitate chest pain <br>     ___ Diet <br>     ___ Exercise (strenuous) <br>     ___ Smoking <br>     ___ Stress/strong emotion <br>     ___ Temperature <br>       ___ Extreme cold <br>   ___ Stress management techniques <br>   ___ _____ | N D S |
| | | ___ _____ <br> _____ <br> _____ <br> _____ | __ __ <br> __ __ |

Source: Janie L. Krechting and Victoria E. Koper, *Interdisciplinary Care Plans for Long-Term Care*, Aspen Publishers, Inc., © 1996.

# PART II

## Self-Management of Coronary Artery Disease and Related Conditions: Patient Education

## 5. Overview of Coronary Artery Disease

---

# Facts about Coronary Heart Disease

## INTRODUCTION

Seven million Americans suffer from coronary heart disease, the most common form of heart disease. This type of heart disease is caused by a narrowing of the coronary arteries that feed the heart.

Coronary heart disease (CHD) is the number one killer of both men and women in the U.S. Each year, more than 500,000 Americans die of heart attacks caused by CHD.

Many of these deaths could be prevented because CHD is related to certain aspects of lifestyle. Risk factors for CHD include high blood pressure, high blood cholesterol, smoking, obesity, and physical inactivity—all of which can be controlled. Although medical treatments for heart disease have come a long way, controlling risk factors remains the key to preventing illness and death from CHD.

---

### Who Is at Risk for CHD?

Risk factors are conditions that increase your risk of developing heart disease. Some can be changed (left column), and some cannot (right column). Although these factors each increases the risk of CHD, they do not describe all the causes of coronary heart disease; even with none of these risk factors, you might still develop CHD.

**Controllable**
- High blood pressure
- High blood cholesterol
- Smoking
- Obesity
- Physical inactivity
- Diabetes
- Stress*

**Uncontrollable**
- Gender
- Heredity (family history of CHD)
- Age

*Although stress **may** be a risk factor for CHD, scientists still do not know exactly how stress might be involved in heart disease.

---

*continues*

continued

**Front View of Heart Showing Cross Sections of Arteries**

Normal

Diseased—Narrowed

Diseased—Blocked

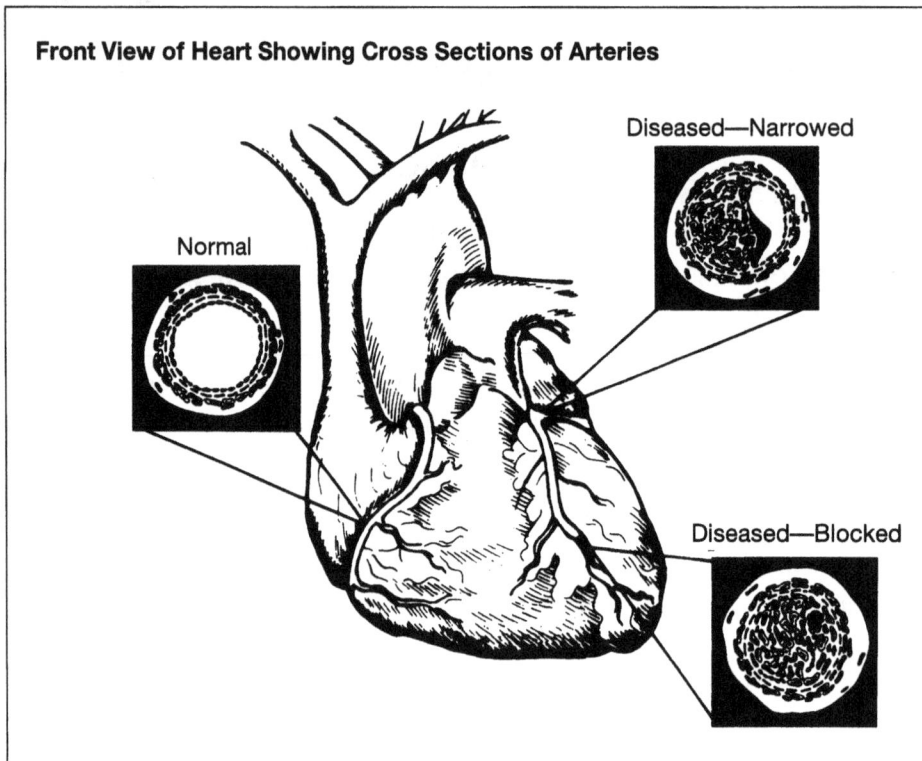

## WHAT IS CORONARY HEART DISEASE?

Like any muscle, the heart needs a constant supply of oxygen and nutrients that are carried to it by the blood in the coronary arteries. When the coronary arteries become narrowed or clogged and cannot supply enough blood to the heart, the result is CHD.

If not enough oxygen-carrying blood reaches the heart, the heart may respond with a pain called angina. The pain is usually felt in the chest or sometimes in the left arm and shoulder. (However, the same inadequate blood supply may cause no symptoms, a condition called silent angina.)

When the blood supply is cut off completely, the result is a heart attack. The part of the heart that does not receive oxygen begins to die, and some of the heart muscle may be permanently damaged.

*continues*

continued

## WHAT CAUSES CHD?

### High Blood Cholesterol

CHD is caused by a thickening of the inside walls of the coronary arteries. This thickening, called atherosclerosis, narrows the space through which blood can flow, decreasing and sometimes completely cutting off the supply of oxygen and nutrients to the heart.

Atherosclerosis usually occurs when a person has high levels of cholesterol, a fat-like substance, in the blood. Cholesterol and fat, circulating in the blood, build up on the walls of the arteries. This buildup narrows the arteries and can slow or block the flow of blood. When the level of cholesterol in the blood is high, there is a greater chance that it will be deposited onto the artery walls. This process begins in most people during childhood and the teenage years, and worsens as they get older.

### High Blood Pressure and Smoking

In addition to high blood cholesterol, high blood pressure and smoking also contribute to CHD. On the average, each of these doubles your chance of developing heart disease. Therefore, a person who has all three risk factors is eight times more likely to develop heart disease than someone who has none.

### Being Overweight or Inactive

Obesity and physical inactivity are other factors that can lead to CHD. Being overweight increases the likelihood of developing high blood cholesterol and high blood pressure, and physical inactivity increases the risk of heart attack. Regular exercise, good nutrition, and smoking cessation are key to controlling the risk factors for CHD.

## WHAT ARE THE SYMPTOMS OF CHD?

Chest pain (angina) or shortness of breath may be the earliest signs of CHD. A person may feel heaviness, tightness, pain, burning, pressure or squeezing, usually behind the breastbone but sometimes also in the arms, neck, or jaws. These signs usually bring the patient to a doctor for the first time. Nevertheless, some people have heart attacks without ever having any of these symptoms.

*continues*

continued

It is important to know that there is a wide range of severity for CHD. Some people have no symptoms at all, some have mild intermittent chest pain, and some have strong and steady pain. Still others have CHD that is severe enough to make normal everyday activities difficult.

Because CHD varies so much from one person to another, the way a doctor diagnoses and treats CHD will also vary a lot. The following descriptions are general guidelines to some tests and treatments that may or may not be used, depending on the individual case.

## ARE THERE TESTS FOR CHD?

There is no one simple test—some or all of the following procedures may be needed. These diagnostic procedures are used to establish CHD, to determine its extent and severity, and to rule out other possible causes of the symptoms.

After taking a careful medical history and doing a physical examination, the doctor may use some tests to see how advanced the CHD is. The only certain way to diagnose and assess the extent of CHD is coronary angiography (see below); other tests can indicate a problem but do not show exactly where it is.

An examination for CHD may include the following tests:

- An **electrocardiogram** (ECG or EKG) is a graphic record of the electrical activity of the heart as it contracts and rests. Abnormal heartbeats and some areas of damage, inadequate blood flow, and heart enlargement can be detected on the records.
- A **stress test** (also called a treadmill test or exercise ECG) is used to record the heartbeat during exercise. This is done because some heart problems only show up when the heart is working hard. In the test, an ECG is done before, during, and after exercising on a treadmill; breathing rate and blood pressure may be measured as well. Exercise tests are useful but are not completely reliable; false positives (showing a problem where none exists) and false negatives (showing no problem when something is wrong) are fairly common.
- **Nuclear scanning** is sometimes used to show damaged areas of the heart and expose problems with the heart's pumping action. A small amount of radioactive material is injected into a vein, usually in the arm. A scanning camera records the nuclear material that is taken up by heart muscle (healthy areas) or not taken up (damaged areas).
- **Coronary angiography** (or arteriography) is a test used to explore the coronary arteries. A fine tube (catheter) is put into an artery of an arm or leg and passed through this blood vessel to the heart. A fluid that shows up on x-rays is injected through the tube into the arteries of the heart. The heart and blood vessels are then filmed while the heart pumps. The picture that is seen, called an angiogram or arteriogram, will show problems such as a blockage caused by atherosclerosis.

*continues*

continued

## HOW IS CHD TREATED?

Coronary heart disease is treated in a number of ways, depending on the seriousness of the disease. For many people, CHD is managed with lifestyle changes and medications. Others with severe CHD may need surgery. In any case, once CHD develops, it requires lifelong management.

## WHAT KIND OF LIFESTYLE CHANGES CAN HELP A PERSON WITH CHD?

Although great advances have been made in treating coronary heart disease, changing one's habits remains the single most effective way to stop CHD from progressing.

### Changing Your Diet

If you know that you have CHD, changing your diet to one low in fat, especially saturated fat, and cholesterol will help reduce high blood cholesterol, a primary cause of atherosclerosis. In fact, it is even more important to keep your cholesterol low after a heart attack to help lower your risk of having another one. Eating less fat should also help you lose weight. If you are overweight, losing weight can help lower blood cholesterol and is the most effective lifestyle way to reduce high blood pressure, another risk factor for atherosclerosis and heart disease.

### Exercising

People with CHD can also benefit from exercise. Recent research has shown that even moderate amounts of physical activity are associated with lower death rates from CHD. However, people with severe CHD may have to restrict their exercise somewhat. If you have CHD, check with your doctor to find out what kinds of exercise are best for you.

### Quitting Smoking

Smoking is one of the three major risk factors for CHD. Quitting smoking dramatically lowers the risk of a heart attack and also reduces the risk of a second heart attack in people who have already had one.

*continues*

continued

## WHAT MEDICATIONS ARE USED TO TREAT CORONARY HEART DISEASE?

Medications are prescribed according to the nature of the patient's CHD and other problems.

The symptoms of angina can generally be controlled by "beta-blocker" drugs that decrease the workload on the heart, by nitroglycerin and other "nitrates" and by "calcium-channel blockers" that relax the arteries, and by other classes of drugs.

The tendency to form clots is reduced by aspirin or by other platelet inhibitory and anticoagulant drugs.

Beta-blockers are given to decrease the recurrence of heart attack.

For those with elevated blood cholesterol that is unresponsive to dietary and weight loss measures, cholesterol-lowering drugs may be prescribed, such as lovastatin, colestipol, cholestyramine, gemfibrozil, and niacin.

Impaired pumping function of the heart may be treated with digitalis drugs or ACE inhibitors.

If there is high blood pressure or fluid retention, these conditions are also treated.

Ask your doctor which medication you are taking, what it does, and whether there are any side effects. Knowing more about this will help you stick to the schedule that has been prescribed for you.

## WHAT TYPES OF SURGERY ARE USED TO TREAT CHD?

Many patients can control CHD with lifestyle changes and medication. Surgery may be recommended for patients who continue to have frequent or disabling angina despite the use of medications, or people who are found to have severe blockages in their coronary arteries.

**Coronary angioplasty** or **balloon angioplasty** begins with a procedure similar to that described under angiography. However, the catheter positioned in the narrowed coronary artery has a tiny balloon at its tip. The balloon is inflated and deflated to stretch or break open the narrowing and improve the passage for blood flow. The balloon-tipped catheter is then removed.

Strictly speaking, angioplasty is not surgery. It is done while the patient is awake and may last one to two hours. If angioplasty does not widen the artery or if complications occur, bypass surgery may be needed.

*continues*

continued

**Front View of Coronary Bypass Graft**

Aorta

Vein Bypass

Blockage

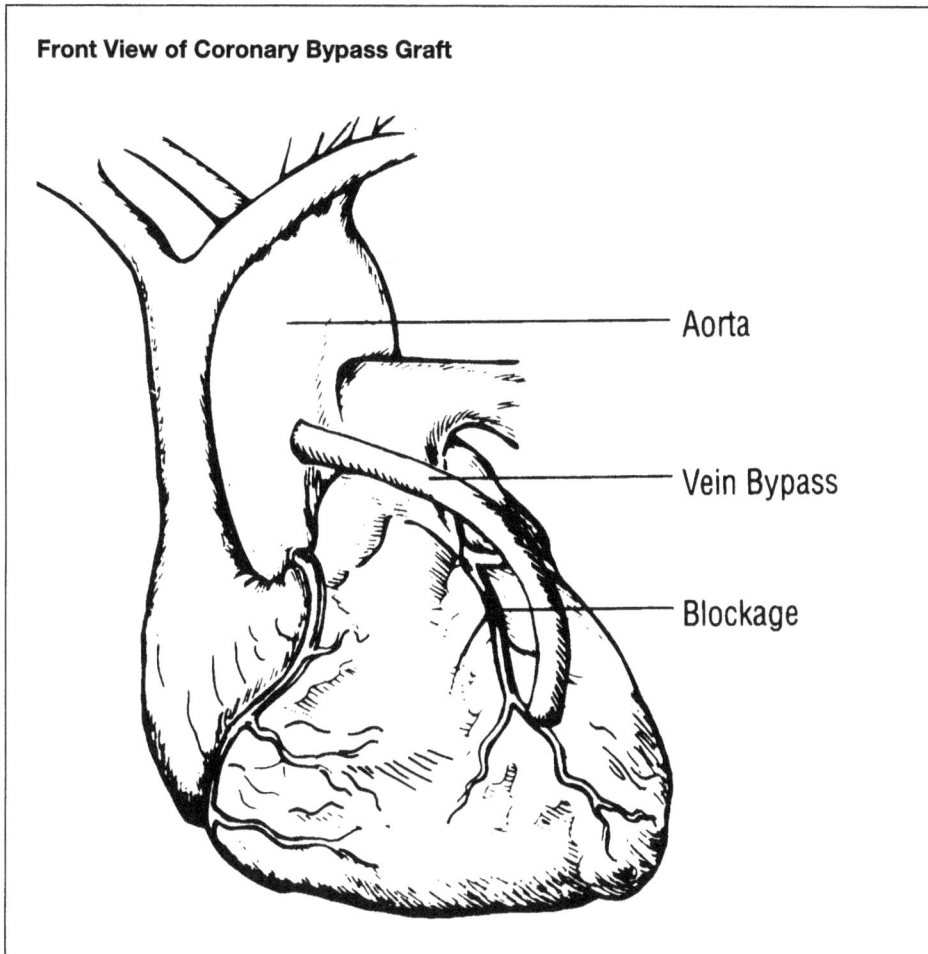

In a **coronary artery bypass operation**, a blood vessel, usually taken from the leg or chest, is grafted onto the blocked artery, bypassing the blocked area. If more than one artery is blocked, a bypass can be done on each. The blood can then go around the obstruction to supply the heart with enough blood to relieve chest pain.

Bypass surgery relieves symptoms of heart disease but does not cure it. Usually you will need to make a number of changes in your lifestyle after the operation. If your normal lifestyle includes smoking, a high-fat diet, or no exercise, changes are advised.

Several experimental catheter-surgical procedures for unblocking coronary arteries are under study; their safety and effectiveness have not yet been established. They include:

*continues*

continued

- **Atherectomy,** a procedure in which surgeons shave off thin strips of the plaque blocking the artery and remove these strips.
- **Laser angioplasty;** instead of using a balloon to open up the blocked artery, doctors insert a catheter with a laser tip that burns or breaks down the plaque.
- Insertion of a **stent,** a metal coil that can be permanently implanted in a narrowed part of an artery to keep it propped open.

## NOTES:

Source: Coronary Heart Disease, Public Health Service, National Institutes of Health, Publication No. 92–2265, U.S. Department of Health and Human Services, National Heart, Lung and Blood Institute, 1992.

# Women and Coronary Heart Disease

*If you're a woman who has or thinks she has coronary heart disease, this fact sheet is for you. It explains the causes, symptoms, detection, and treatments of coronary heart disease.*

*Coronary heart disease is a chronic condition—it will not disappear—and you may need to make some changes. But caring for your heart is worth the effort—your heart will thank you every day.*

## A LONG PROCESS

Coronary heart disease, the most common form of heart disease, develops over many years. It can begin as far back as childhood. In a process known as atherosclerosis, fatty substances build up inside the walls of blood vessels. Blood components also stick on the surface inside vessel walls. The vessels narrow and "harden," becoming less flexible.

The buildup and narrowing proceed gradually and result in decreasing blood flow and, eventually, the development of symptoms. But the buildup, or "plaque," may break open and suddenly produce a blood clot, limited blood flow, and symptoms.

When blood flow to the heart is reduced, chest pain, or "angina," can result. If blood flow is nearly or completely blocked, a heart attack can occur and cause muscle cells in the heart to die. Because the cells cannot be replaced, the result is permanent heart damage.

## WHO GETS CORONARY HEART DISEASE?

Coronary heart disease rarely affects young women. Instead, it usually develops after menopause. Before menopause, the ovaries make estrogen, which helps protect the heart.

Being over age 55 is a "risk factor" that affects the development of coronary heart disease. There are other risk factors (see "Factors That Put Your Heart At Risk"). They are: family history of early heart disease, cigarette smoking, high blood pressure, high blood cholesterol, being overweight, physical inactivity, and diabetes.

The risk factors do not add their effects in a simple way. Rather, they multiply each other's effects. For example, if you smoke and have high blood pressure and high blood cholesterol, you're eight times more likely to develop coronary heart disease than a woman with no risk factors.

You can have coronary heart disease without being aware of it. The best way to protect your heart is to know whether you have coronary heart disease and treat it as early as possible. You need to talk to your doctor about your coronary heart disease and any symptoms you may be experiencing (*see* "Talking with Your Doctor").

*continues*

continued

## DO YOU HAVE ANGINA?

The first symptom of coronary heart disease may be chest pain, or "angina." The chest pain, which is caused by reduced blood flow to the heart, typically occurs behind the breastbone and may travel down your left arm or up your neck, or be a squeezing, pressing sensation that does not change with breathing. It is usually caused and made worse by exercise and eased by rest. The pain usually lasts 2 to 5 minutes. If you have this kind of chest pain, you should contact your doctor.

A reduced blood flow to the heart can cause symptoms other than chest pain. For example, some women get a less typical angina. The chest pain may linger, occur in a different location than behind the breastbone, or not be worsened by exertion and eased by rest. Some women have shortness of breath or indigestion. If you have such symptoms, you should talk with your doctor. If treated, the outlook is good. Without treatment, however, the symptoms may recur and worsen and can become unstable and even lead to a heart attack.

Women who have coronary heart disease need to talk to their doctor about the symptoms of a heart attack and the appropriate steps to take to get emergency care. It is important to know the telephone number to call to get emergency transportation to the hospital. In most areas, this will be 9-1-1 or a 7-digit emergency number.

Getting to the hospital fast allows use of thrombolytic therapy—a clot-dissolving agent is injected to restore blood flow through an artery. This therapy saves lives and reduces damage to the heart muscle. But it must be done as soon as possible.

Doctors also have a new fast test for a heart attack. It detects changed levels of an enzyme (creatine kinase MB) produced by the heart. It once took up to a day to test the levels and tell if someone has had a heart attack—but now it can be done within 6 hours. So doctors can give fast care to those who need it and send the others home.

## WHAT ARE THE TESTS FOR CORONARY HEART DISEASE?

Diagnostic tests are usually needed to confirm the presence and assess the severity of coronary heart disease. Your doctor will know whether you need any of them. Often more than one test is needed because different tests supply different information. Also, patients vary in their symptoms and so may need more than one test to find out the heart's condition.

The main tests used to diagnose coronary heart disease are described below. Many are not "invasive" procedures—they are done outside the body—and are painless.

*continues*

continued

---

### Factors That Put Your Heart At Risk

One in ten American women ages 45 to 64 has some form of heart disease. That increases to one in five for women over age 65. Some of the factors that increase the risk to your heart cannot be controlled—but most can. You'll protect your heart by controlling those that can be changed. Here's a rundown of both types of risk factors:

Unchangeable Risk Factors

- Being age 55 or older
- Having a family history of early heart disease (this means having a mother or sister who has been diagnosed with heart disease before age 65, or a father or brother diagnosed before age 55)

Changeable Risk Factors

- Cigarette smoking
- High blood pressure
- High blood cholesterol
- Overweight
- Physical inactivity
- Diabetes

---

The tests are:

- Electrocardiogram (ECG or EKG) makes a graphic record of the heart's electrical activity as it beats. This can show abnormal heartbeats, muscle damage, blood flow problems, and heart enlargement.
- Stress test (or treadmill test or exercise ECG) records the ECG during exercise, usually on a treadmill or exercise bicycle. Some heart problems show up only when more effort is asked of the heart, as happens during increased activity. So the exercise ECG may be done even if the resting ECG is normal.

    Other exercise tests may be done with an ECG or a nuclear scan (see below) to assess heart muscle contraction or blood flow in the heart.

    Older women may not be able to exercise due to arthritis or another condition. For them, a stress test can be done without exercise by using a drug that increases blood flow.
- Echocardiography converts sound waves, bounced off the heart, into images that show heart size, shape, and movement. The sound waves also can be used to see how much blood is pumped out by the heart when it contracts.

*continues*

continued

## Talking with Your Doctor

Caring for a chronic condition like coronary heart disease is a partnership—you and your doctor should work as a team. That means good communication.

Here are some pointers to help you talk with your doctor:

### Before Your Office Visit

- Write down your concerns.
- Keep a diary of your symptoms, so you can describe them accurately.
- Note any past treatments.
- Gather any drugs you are taking and bring them or a list of them to the office visit.

### During Your Office Visit

- Be open.
  You will only hurt yourself if you're not. For instance, if you have trouble breathing or have pain, *tell* your doctor.
- Briefly describe all symptoms.
  Tell when each started, how often it happens, and if it has been getting worse.
- Note any causes of stress in your life.
  For instance, say if you are the caregiver for a sick parent or husband, or have other stressful responsibilities.
- Ask questions.
  Be sure you understand what the doctor says. Ask for an explanation of any term you do not understand. Be sure you know the instructions for any medication—when to take it; what to do if you forget and skip a dose; what other drug, food, or activity to avoid while taking it; and what side effects may occur with it.
- Write notes.
  This will help you remember what the doctor says.
- Bring a friend or relative with you if necessary.
  If you are worried about understanding what the doctor says or have trouble hearing, have someone with you during the discussion.
- Share your views.
  If something bothers you, say so. The doctor needs to know if something is working or not, or if you're having trouble following a treatment. For instance, if you're having trouble fixing low-saturated fat meals, say so. You may be referred to a dietitian for help. Dietitians are health care professionals who can help design an eating plan for you.

*continues*

continued

## If a Diagnostic Test is Ordered

- Ask the reason and find out what will be learned from the test.
- Ask when results will be ready.
- Know what the test involves and how to get ready for it.
- Ask who will do the test.
- Find out if you will need help getting home after the test.
- Find out if the test poses any dangers or side effects.

## If You Need a Special Procedure

- Find out the benefits and risks of the procedure.
- Ask what kind of doctor you need for it and get a referral.
- Ask if you will need to be hospitalized and for how long.
- Ask what kind of pain or discomfort you may feel.
- Ask about the recovery period, how long it will last, and what it will involve.

- Nuclear scan assesses heart muscle contraction as blood flows through the heart. A small amount of radioactive material is injected into a vein, usually in the arm, and a scanning camera then records how much is taken up by the heart muscle.
- Coronary angiography (or anrteriography) displays blood flow problems and blockages. A fine, flexible tube (or "catheter") is threaded through an artery of an arm or leg up into the heart. A fluid that shows up on x ray is then injected, and the heart and blood vessels are filmed as the heart pumps. The picture is called an angiogram or arteriogram.

## TREATING YOUR HEART RIGHT

You can reduce your risk of complications of coronary heart disease. But you must do your part.

There are three main types of treatment: lifestyle, medication, and special procedures for advanced atherosclerosis. A discussion of each of these follows.

## LIFESTYLE

Since you have coronary heart disease, you will need to take five key steps to keep your heart as healthy as possible: stop smoking, lower high blood pressure, lower high blood cholesterol, lose any extra weight, and become physically active.

*continues*

continued

---

### Diabetes—The Self-Help Disease

Diabetes mellitus increases the risk to your heart. It also is the single most common cause of kidney disease.

If you have diabetes, you will need to control it. Because those with it must manage their condition day-by-day, diabetes is sometimes called the "self-help disease."

In diabetes, the body cannot properly convert foods into energy. This causes a buildup in the blood of a form of sugar called glucose. The buildup produces symptoms and damages organs.

Women should have a routine test for diabetes. The doctor will test for too much sugar in the urine or blood.

Symptoms of diabetes include: a vague sick feeling, being "run down," increased thirst, frequent urination, unexplained weight loss, blurred vision, skin infections or itching, and slow healing of cuts, bruises, and gum and urinary tract infections.

Controlling diabetes can help keep your heart healthy. For more information on diabetes, contact:

- National Diabetes Information Clearinghouse
  Box NDIC
  9000 Rockville Pike
  Bethesda, MD 20892
  (301) 654-3327

---

In fact, these steps are so crucial for good health that they should be adopted by all people, even the young. So as a plus, do them with your family and friends. Studies show that such support makes lifestyle changes easier. You'll improve more if others join you in your new behavior. And teaching your children or grandchildren heart-healthy habits is a gift that will last them a lifetime.

Here's more on the five steps:

1. Stop smoking cigarettes
   There is no safe way to smoke. Smoking accelerates atherosclerosis. If you smoke, you are two to six times more likely to have a heart attack than a nonsmoker, and your risk increases with the number of cigarettes you smoke each day.

*continues*

continued

But if you quit, then the risk to your heart drops sharply, even in the first year, no matter what your age.

Even if you've had a heart attack, you'll benefit from quitting—some women's risk of having a second heart attack is cut by 50 percent or more after they stop smoking.

The National Heart, Lung, and Blood Institute (NHLBI) has information to help you kick the habit or ask your doctor for advice.

**2.** Lower high blood pressure

Also called hypertension, high blood pressure usually has no symptoms. It has no cure but can and must be controlled. High blood pressure makes the heart work harder and, uncontrolled, can lead to heart disease, stroke, heart failure, kidney problems, and other conditions.

Blood pressure is given as two numbers—the systolic pressure over the diastolic pressure, and both are important. A measurement of 140/90 mm Hg or above means you have high blood pressure. But even pressures slightly under that can put your heart at greater risk.

Most American women over age 60 have high blood pressure—nearly 80 percent of black women over age 60 have it.

However, blood pressure does not have to increase with age—hypertension can be prevented. And controlling your blood pressure will reduce your chance of suffering a first or repeat heart attack. Discuss your blood pressure with your doctor.

A normal blood pressure level is around 120/80. Often, this can be reached through lifestyle changes. If necessary, a medication will be used. If a drug is prescribed, you must take it as instructed, even if you feel fine because, if you stop, your blood pressure probably will rise again. (See the medication section for drugs that treat high blood pressure.) If you make lifestyle changes, however, your doctor may be able to decrease your medication.

The lifestyle steps that prevent and control high blood pressure are: losing excess weight, becoming physically active, choosing foods low in salt and sodium, and limiting alcohol intake. (The first two are described separately.)

Salt and sodium both affect blood pressure and must be watched. Salt (sodium chloride) is only one source of sodium, and there are others. You should consume no more than 6 grams (about 1 teaspoon) of salt a day, which equals 2.4 grams of sodium. This includes ALL salt—that in processed foods or added in cooking or at the table. A good way to keep track of sodium is by reading food labels.

If you drink alcohol, you should have no more than one drink a day. One drink equals 1.5 ounces of 80-proof whiskey, or 5 ounces of wine, or 12 ounces of beer (regular or light).

Recently, news stories have said that alcohol may lower the risk of having a heart attack. But this has yet to be proved. And too much alcohol has dangers. So if you don't drink, it's best not to start.

*continues*

continued

3. Lower high blood cholesterol

Why is cholesterol so important? The body makes all the cholesterol it needs. Extra cholesterol and fat in the diet cause the atherosclerotic buildup inside blood vessels. So, a high blood cholesterol leads to coronary heart disease.

And, once you have coronary heart disease, an elevated blood cholesterol increases your risk of a future heart attack. But you can take steps to keep your blood cholesterol from rising.

Cholesterol travels through the blood in protein-fat packages called lipoproteins. The two main types are: low-density lipoprotein, or LDL, which causes deposits and is termed the "bad" cholesterol; and high-density lipoprotein, or HDL, which helps remove cholesterol from the blood and is referred to as the "good" cholesterol.

Women who have coronary heart disease should have an LDL level of 100 mg/dL or less.

A low level of HDL (less than 35 mg/dL) is a major risk factor for coronary heart disease. Physical activity, weight loss if you're overweight, and stopping smoking help raise the level of HDL.

Women with coronary heart disease need to have a "lipoprotein analysis" done to check their levels of total cholesterol, HDL, and LDL, as well as triglycerides, which is another type of fat in the bloodstream. Lipoprotein tests should be taken on two occasions and the results averaged. The level of LDL is usually the main target of treatment.

Many women with coronary heart disease can lower their high blood cholesterol enough through lifestyle changes. However, cholesterol-lowering drugs may be needed as well. Hormone replacement therapy (see "Hormone Replacement Therapy—New Findings") also may improve blood cholesterol.

---

**Tips for Having Your Blood Pressure Taken**

A blood pressure test is painless. Here are some tips to assure that you get a good reading:

- Before the test, sit for 5 minutes with your feet flat on the ground, arm resting on a table at the level of your heart
- Wear short sleeves so your arm is exposed
- If you know your arm requires a large adult cuff, say so
- Get two readings, taken at least 2 minutes apart, and average the results

---

*continues*

continued

The lifestyle changes call for adopting a healthy eating plan, becoming physically active, and losing excess weight (the latter two described below). For healthy eating, have:

- Less than 7 percent of your day's total calories from saturated fat
- 30 percent or less of your day's total calories from fat
- Less than 200 milligrams of dietary cholesterol a day
- Just enough calories a day to achieve and maintain a healthy weight

Foods high in total fat and in saturated fat are also high in calories and often in cholesterol. Saturated fat, which raises blood cholesterol more than anything else in the diet, is found mainly in foods that come from animals—dairy products, meat, and poultry skin. Some vegetable fats—coconut oil, cocoa butter, palm kernel oil, and palm oil—also are high in saturated fat. Cholesterol is found only in foods that come from animals—egg yolks, liver, and kidney, for example.

A few pointers: To cut down on saturated fat, total fat, and cholesterol, choose fish, poultry, and lean cuts of meat; choose low-fat foods; choose low-fat or no-fat milk and other dairy products; and eat plenty of fruits and vegetables. Breads, rice, and pasta made from enriched or whole grains also are good choices. Broil, bake, roast, or poach, instead of frying, and be sure any sauce is also low in fat.

4. Lose excess weight
America is becoming heftier—and older women are among those gaining weight. More than half of American women ages 50 to 59 are overweight—30 years ago, only 35 percent of them were. This is a dangerous trend, because being overweight increases the risk of coronary heart disease, even if there are no other risk factors.

But being overweight also increases the chance of developing several other risk factors, which would compound the danger.

Losing excess weight is critical for good health. But weight loss must be viewed as a change of lifestyle, not as a temporary effort to drop pounds quickly. Such quick fixes are just that—temporary. The weight soon returns.

To lose weight, follow a heart-healthy eating plan and become physically active. Eat a variety of low-calorie, nutritious foods in moderate amounts. Keep to the eating pattern outlined for high blood cholesterol. Do not try to lose more than one-half to one pound a week.

Remember: When it comes to weight loss, take it slow and steady—learn a new way of eating to get to and stay at a healthy weight.

5. Become physically active
Physical activity is one of the best ways to control coronary heart disease. It is vital for good health and well-being. It helps lower LDL and raise HDL. Even if you're overweight, you'll have a lower blood pressure if you're active.

*continues*

continued

---

### Hormone Replacement Therapy—New Findings

At menopause, the ovaries essentially stop all production of the hormone estrogen. Menopause can occur naturally or surgically.

Hormone replacement therapy (HRT) supplies the estrogen the body no longer makes. It has been used to relieve the symptoms of menopause, such as hot flashes and flushes, sweats, disturbed sleep, and increased rate of bone loss.

New information from the Postmenopausal Estrogen/Progestin Intervention Trial (PEPI) suggests that HRT may also improve coronary heart disease risk factors after menopause. The research found that estrogen given alone or with a natural or synthetic progesterone increased HDL and decreased LDL. Progesterone is also a hormone made by the ovaries until menopause; it helps control the growth of cells that line the uterus. None of the HRT therapies tested significantly affected blood pressure or weight. But estrogen taken alone caused abnormal cell growth of the lining of the uterus.

PEPI's findings offer these guidelines:

- If you have a uterus, you may want to consider a combination therapy that uses both estrogen and a progesterone. If you have a uterus and take estrogen alone, you need to have a yearly endometrial biopsy.
- If you don't have a uterus, you may want to consider taking estrogen without a progesterone.

However, uncertainties remain, including the effects of HRT on breast cancer risk. So far, studies have had conflicting findings and more research is ongoing. Current evidence suggests that there is a small increased risk of breast cancer from HRT but that, for most women, the benefits of HRT probably outweigh the risk.

You should discuss these questions with your doctor.

---

You may worry that "becoming physically active" requires a lot of time and effort. Not so. Research shows that even a little exercise can improve your heart's health. And "exercise" can mean going up a flight of stairs (instead of taking the elevator) or gardening or walking at the mall. Walk with a friend or your husband, or get your whole family moving together.

Try to do some type of activity for at least 30 minutes on most days. But, if 30 minutes is too long a period, break up the time into shorter sessions done throughout the day. Incorporate exercise into your other daily activities too.

*continues*

*continued*

Since you have coronary heart disease, you should consult with your doctor before starting a physical activity program. This is especially important if you're over age 55, have been inactive, or have diabetes or another medical problem. Your doctor can help you prevent problems from overexertion.

It also is important to exercise in a way that will help you without hurting you. If you've been inactive, start slowly. Walking 10–15 minutes, three times a week, makes a good start.

If you've had a heart attack, you'll benefit greatly from exercise. Many hospitals have a "cardiac" (heart) rehabilitation program. Ask your doctor about your ability to exercise and about a suitable program for you.

If you have arthritis or another limiting condition, you may benefit from exercises that help keep you as flexible and healthy as possible. Again, ask your doctor about a suitable exercise.

## MEDICATIONS

A healthy lifestyle will improve your heart's condition. But you may need medication too, especially if you have chest pain, or if you have high blood pressure or high blood cholesterol that was not lowered enough with lifestyle changes.

Drugs can have side effects, so none should be taken without first seeing your doctor. If you take a drug, follow the dose instructions carefully and report any troublesome side effects to your doctor. Often a change in dose or type of drug can stop the side effect. Your doctor may even prescribe a combination of drugs to treat your coronary heart disease.

The following list will briefly introduce you to some medications used to treat coronary heart disease and its risk factors. If you need a medication, discuss it with your doctor and be sure you understand how and why it should be taken.

- *Aspirin*—helps prevent heart attacks when taken regularly in a low dose on a doctor's orders.
- *Digitalis*—makes the heart contract harder and is used when the heart's pumping function has been weakened; it also slows some fast heart rhythms.
- *ACE inhibitor*—stops production of a chemical that makes blood vessels narrow and is used for high blood pressure and heart muscle that has been damaged.
- *Beta-blocker*—reduces how hard the heart must work and is used for high blood pressure, chest pain, and to prevent a repeat heart attack.
- *Nitrate (including nitroglycerine)*—relaxes blood vessels and alleviates chest pain.
- *Calcium-channel blocker*—relaxes blood vessels; used for high blood pressure and chest pain.
- *Diuretic*—decreases fluid in the body and is used for high blood pressure.
- *Blood cholesterol-lowering agents*—HMG CoA reductase inhibitors (or "statins"), nicotine acid, bile acid sequestrants, fibric acid derivatives, and probucol.

*continues*

continued

## SPECIAL PROCEDURES

If you have advanced atherosclerosis, you may need a special procedure to open an artery and improve blood flow. This is usually done to ease severe chest pain or clear major or multiple blockages in blood vessels.

The two main procedures are:

1. Coronary angioplasty—also called "balloon" angioplasty. A fine tube is threaded through an artery to the narrowed heart vessel, where a tiny balloon at its tip is inflated. The balloon flattens the buildup and stretches the artery, improving blood flow. It is then deflated and removed, along with the tube.
2. Coronary artery bypass graft surgery—also known as "bypass surgery." A piece of blood vessel is taken from the leg or chest and is stitched onto the narrowed heart artery, making a bypass around the blockage. Sometimes, more than one bypass is needed.

Bypass surgery is used when blockages in an artery can't be reached by, or are too long or hard for, angioplasty. A bypass requires about 1 week in the hospital and several weeks of recuperation at home.

Remember: Take action and take charge!

**NOTES:**

Source: "Heart Disease and Women: So You Have Heart Disease," NIH Publication No. 95–2645, National Heart, Lung, and Blood Institute, National Institutes of Health, September 1995.

# 6. Unstable Angina and Myocardial Infarction

---

# Unstable Angina

## WHAT IS UNSTABLE ANGINA?

Unstable angina is a type of coronary artery disease. Because your heart is a muscle, it needs oxygen to work well. The coronary arteries bring oxygen-rich blood to your heart. In coronary artery disease, one or more of these arteries may be partially or even completely blocked.

The type of coronary artery disease you have usually depends on the amount of blockage in your arteries. A heart attack, called a myocardial infarction, means the heart muscle has been damaged by not getting enough blood. Stable angina usually does not damage the heart. Unstable angina is worse than stable angina and may progress to a heart attack if not treated.

Angina is caused by a lack of oxygen in the heart muscle. The symptoms of angina include pain or discomfort in the chest, arms, back, neck, or jaw. Sometimes, anginal pain may feel like a tightness or crushing sensation, or it may be a stabbing pain or seem like numbness. Some people mistake anginal pain as indigestion or gas pain.

Having either stable or unstable angina does not always mean you will have a heart attack. But, unstable angina can be serious and should be treated by a doctor.

## HOW ARE STABLE AND UNSTABLE ANGINA DIFFERENT?

Anginal discomfort may be different for different people. Some people have anginal discomfort when they overexert themselves (for example, when they shovel snow).

Other people feel anginal pain when they get very upset or exited. Over time, they can usually tell which activities will give them discomfort. Usually, the discomfort will go away in a few minutes. This type of chest discomfort is called stable angina.

Stable angina attacks usually have a regular pattern. But in some people the pattern of angina is different—it becomes unstable.

*continues*

---

continued

---

**People with Unstable Angina**

- Have anginal discomfort when they are resting or that awakens them from sleep.
- Suddenly develop moderate or severe discomfort on exertion when they have never had angina before.
- Have a marked increase in the frequency or severity of their discomfort.

---

Unstable angina is more serious than stable angina because the risk of having a heart attack is greater.

## WHAT CAUSES UNSTABLE ANGINA?

In coronary artery disease, blockages—made up of fats, such as cholesterol, and other debris—form on the inside walls of the coronary arteries. In patients who have stable angina, the blockages may not seriously block the flow of blood.

In stable angina, the blockages may be large. Sometimes, the blockage cracks open. When this happens, your body tries to heal the crack in the blockage by making a blood clot around the damage. If the clot is big enough to block the artery, the clot will keep blood from flowing through. This can cause a heart attack.

## CHEST PAIN CAN BE AN EMERGENCY

Here are some signs that your angina is very serious, and you should go to the hospital right away:

- pain or discomfort that is very bad, gets worse, and lasts longer than 20 minutes
- pain or discomfort along with weakness, feeling sick to your stomach, or fainting
- pain or discomfort that does not go away when you take three nitroglycerin tablets
- pain or discomfort that is worse than you have ever had before

If you live in an area where ambulance service is not quickly available, have someone drive you to the nearest hospital. You should not drive yourself to the hospital.

It is a good idea to talk with your family, friends, or neighbors about your heart condition and have them read this handout. They should be familiar with warning signs that signal when you should go to the hospital. You also may want to tell them which medicines you are taking and where you keep them.

Source: "Managing Unstable Angina," Consumer Version, Clinical Practice Guideline Number 10, U.S. Department of Health and Human Services, Public Health Service, Agency for Health Care Policy and Research, AHCPR Publications No. 94–0604, March 1994.

# La angina de pecho inestable

## EL PROPÓSITO DE ESTA GUÍA

Esta guía describe lo que es la angina de pecho y cómo se relaciona con otras enfermedades cardíacas. Responde a las preguntas más comunes sobre esta condición y describe los tratamientos principales.

La guía es para las personas que padecen de angina de pecho, que han recibido tratamiento para enfermedades cardíacas, o que creen padecer de una enfermedad del corazón. También está dirigida a las personas que tienen un familiar o amigo que padece de angina estable o inestable.

Finalmente, se sugieren algunas preguntas que podrían ayudarle en sus conversaciones con el médico, y el momento oportuno para presentarlas.

## ¿QUÉ ES LA ANGINA DE PECHO INESTABLE?

La angina de pecho inestable es una forma de enfermedad de las arterias coronarias. El corazón es un músculo que se encarga de irrigar la sangre a todo el cuerpo. Como cualquier otro músculo, el corazón necesita oxígeno para funcionar adecuadamente y las coronarias son las que le llevan sangre rica en oxígeno. Cuando una persona padece de enfermedad de las coronarias, una o varias de estas arterias se encuentran parcial o totalmente obstruídas.

Normalmente, el tipo de enfermedad de las coronarias que padece cada paciente depende del grado de obstrucción de las coronarias. Un ataque cardíaco, conocido también como infarto miocárdico, sucede cuando el músculo del corazón ha sufrido daño debido a la falta de sangre oxigenada. La angina estable normalmente no deteriora al corazón. En cambio, la angina de pecho inestable es más grave, así es que si no se da tratamiento adecuado, puede resultar en un ataque cardíaco.

La falta de oxígeno al músculo del corazón causa la angina de pecho. Sus síntomas incluyen dolor o molestias en el pecho, los brazos, la espalda, el cuello, o la mandíbula. Algunas veces el dolor de angina se manifiesta como una sensación de opresión o presión en el tórax, o puede ser un dolor punzante o un adormecimiento (falta de sensación). Algunas personas confunden el dolor de angina con molestias de indigestión o gases.

*continúa*

continuación

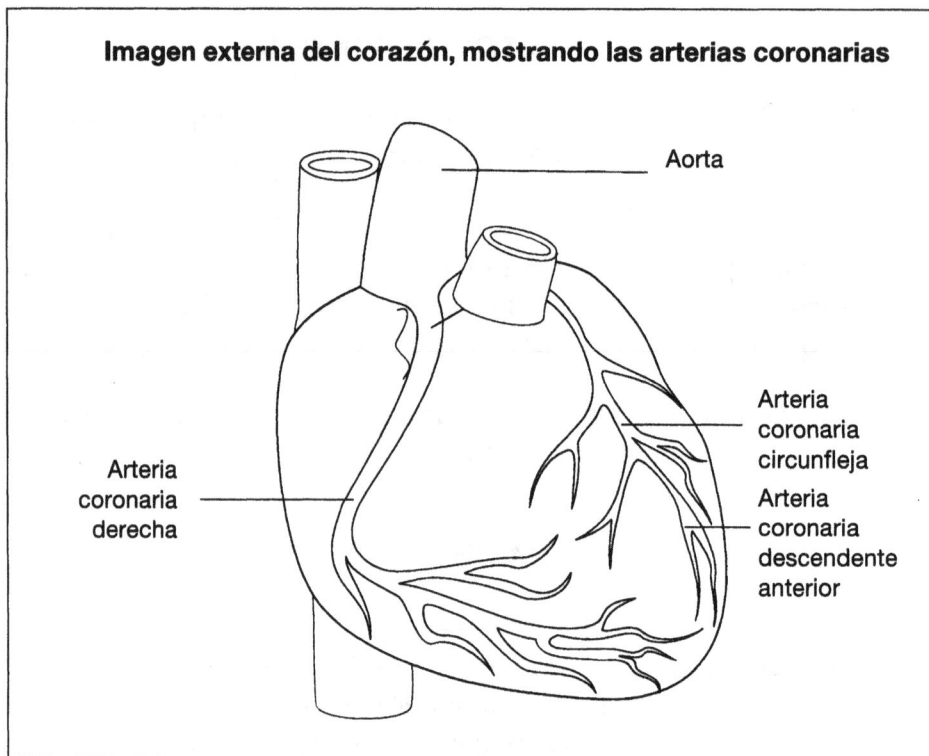

**Imagen externa del corazón, mostrando las arterias coronarias**

Aorta

Arteria coronaria circunfleja

Arteria coronaria descendente anterior

Arteria coronaria derecha

El padecer de angina de pecho estable o inestable no necesariamente quiere decir que tendrá un ataque cardíaco. Sin embargo, la angina de pecho inestable es una condición grave para la cual necesitará recibir atención médica.

## ¿CUÁL ES LA DIFERENCIA ENTRE LA ANGINA DE PECHO ESTABLE E INESTABLE?

Las molestias de la angina de pecho varían de un paciente a otro. Para algunos pacientes las molestias se presentan cuando realizan un esfuerzo físico (como cavar, o subir muchas escaleras). Otras personas sienten el dolor cuando se irritan o enfadan. Con el tiempo, los pacientes pueden predecir las situaciones o actividades que probablemente les van a provocar molestias. Normalmente estas molestias desaparecen en unos pocos minutos y se conocen como angina de pecho estable.

Los ataques de angina de pecho estable siguen un patrón (ritmo) regular. Sin embargo, para algunos pacientes estos patrones cambian y entonces la condición se conoce como angina de pecho inestable.

*continúa*

continuación

---

**Los pacientes con angina de pecho inestable son aquellos que:**

- sienten molestias de angina de pecho cuando se encuentran descansando, o las molestias los despiertan del sueño
- sin haber presentado síntoma alguno de angina de pecho, de momento tienen dolor entre moderado a severo y se sienten muy cansados (fatigados)
- tienen un marcado aumento en la frecuencia o la intensidad de las molestias

---

La angina de pecho inestable es una condición más grave que la angina de pecho estable, y el riesgo de que el paciente tenga un ataque al corazón es mayor.

## ¿QUÉ PROVOCA LA ANGINA DE PECHO INESTABLE?

El paciente padece de una enfermedad de las coronarias cuando las paredes de estas arterias se obstruyen (estrechan) con depósitos de grasas u otras sustancias tales como el colesterol. Estas obstrucciones no son tan severas entre las personas que padecen de angina de pecho estable, así es que no alteran el flujo sanguíneo.

En los pacientes con angina de pecho inestable, estas obstrucciones llegan a ser tan grandes que tapan la arteria casi totalmente. Algunas veces la obstrucción se rompe y el cuerpo intenta cicatrizar (reparar) esta fisura produciendo un coágulo alrededor de la zona dañada. Cuando el coágulo es lo suficientemente grande para tapar el orificio de la arteria totalmente, puede interrumpir el flujo de sangre y causar un ataque cardágulo que es lo suficientemente grande para tapar el orificio de la arteria totalmente, puede interrumpir el flujo de sangre y causar un ataque cardíaco.

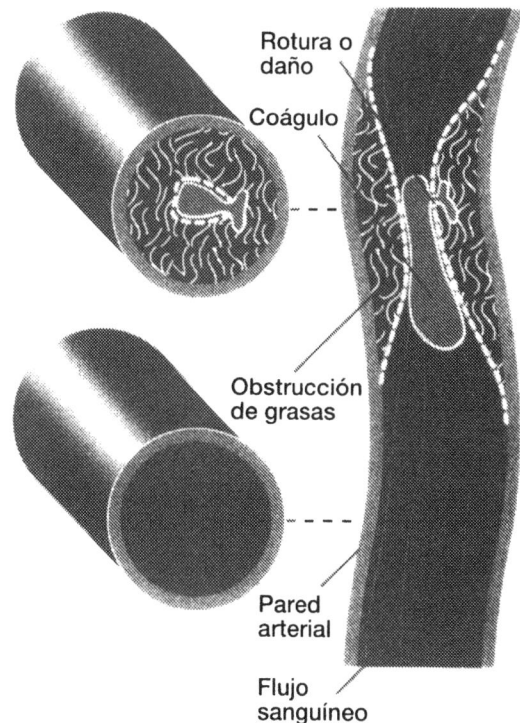

**Imagen de un corte de una arteria coronaria mostrando segmentos normales y obstruídos (bloqueados)**

Rotura o daño

Coágulo

Obstrucción de grasas

Pared arterial

Flujo sanguíneo

*continúa*

continuación

# ¿NECESITO VISITAR AL MÉDICO?

Esto depende si su médico le ha dicho alguna vez que padece de una enfermedad de las coronarias.

**Si siente dolor como el que se describe en la sección "La angina de pecho puede ser una emergencia médica," debe llamar una ambulancia de inmediato y después llamar a su médico.**

## Las personas que no tienen antecedentes de enfermedad de las coronarias

La angina de pecho inestable frecuentemente se presenta entre personas que no sabían que tenían enfermedad de las coronarias. Cualquier dolor de pecho severo o nuevo que no se pueda explicar como el resultado de un accidente o golpe (tal como un músculo lesionado) podría ser angina de pecho inestable o un ataque cardíaco.

La angina de pecho no es una condición grave para las personas que reciben atención médica inmediata; pero puede ser muy seria si no se presta cuidado médico. Incluso el dolor de angina que desaparece cuando el paciente descansa puede ser serio. Solamente el médico puede decidir si sus molestias son el resultado de una condición seria y lo que se debe hacer al respecto.

## Las personas que tienen antecedentes de enfermedad de las coronarias

Para los pacientes con antecedentes de enfermedad de las coronarias, los síntomas en el pasado son la mejor manera de juzgar si es necesario llamar al médico al presentar nuevos síntomas. Llámelo si las molestias son más severas o duran más tiempo que antes; si las molestias ocurren con mayor frecuencia o con menor esfuerzo físico; o si siente molestias cuando está descansando o durmiendo.

## La angina de pecho puede ser una emergencia médica

Presentar cualquiera de los siguientes síntomas quiere decir que su angina de pecho es muy grave y que debe ir al hospital de inmediato:

- dolor o molestias muy severos, que empeoran, y que duran por más de 20 minutos
- dolor o molestias acompañados por una sensación de malestar del estómago, o desmayo
- dolor o molestias que no desaparecen incluso después de tomar tres tabletas de nitroglicerina
- dolor o molestias peores que los que ha tenido en el pasado

*continúa*

continuación

Si vive en un área en donde no existe un servicio de ambulancia de emergencia, haga que alguien lo lleve al hospital. Si se siente enfermo, no trate de guiar un automóvil para llegar al hospital.

También es importante hablar con familiares y amigos sobre su condición del corazón y dejar que lean esta publicación. Así ellos podrán reconocer los síntomas serios que indican la necesidad de ir al hospital. También dígales cuáles medicamentos tiene que tomar y el lugar en donde pueden encontrarlos en caso necesario.

## ¿QUÉ SUCEDERÁ EN LA SALA DE EMERGENCIAS DEL HOSPITAL?

En la sala de emergencias del hospital, el médico determinará si usted tiene un ataque de angina de pecho. Si éste es el caso, le darán medicamentos a través de la vena del brazo (intravenosos) para aliviar el dolor y prevenir que haya daño al corazón. Estos medicamentos ayudarán a prevenir coágulos de sangre, permitiendo que su corazón pueda latir con menor esfuerzo. Probablemente también le darán a respirar oxígeno para mejorar la oxigenación de su sangre.

Frecuentemente, los médicos y las enfermeras le preguntarán cómo se siente y si los medicamentos han aliviado el dolor y las molestias. Es importante que les diga exactamente cómo se siente, ya que si los medicamentos no alivian las molestias, hay otras alternativas para ayudarle a sentirse mejor.

Las acciones en la sala de emergencias se tienen que realizar rápidamente y puede ser que los médicos y las enfermeras no tengan tiempo de explicarle lo que está sucediendo paso por paso. Habrá más tiempo para hablar y hacer todas sus preguntas una vez que el médico determine la seriedad de su condición.

### ¿Qué es un electrocardiograma?

En la sala de emergencias le harán un electrocardiograma (conocido también como "ECG"). El electrocardiograma muestra la actividad eléctrica del latido de su corazón. Esta información mostrará si el músculo del corazón está recibiendo suficiente sangre oxigenada.

### ¿Me tendré que quedar en el hospital?

Sus antecedentes (historial) médico, el electrocardiograma y el tipo de molestias que presente le indicarán al médico la seriedad de su condición.

*continúa*

continuación

Si el médico considera que su condición no es lo suficientemente seria para internarle en el hospital, le dará una cita para verlo de nuevo y para realizar más exámenes médicos. Si las molestias en su pecho se vuelven a presentar antes de esa cita (o son como se describe en la sección "La angina de pecho puede ser una emergencia médica"), debe regresar inmediatamente al hospital.

Diagnosticar la angina de pecho no es sencillo y es posible que el médico le tenga que ver varias veces para asegurarse del diagnóstico.

Si el médico decide internarlo en el hospital, puede ser que le den una cama en una sala regular o en la sala de cuidado intensivo. De cualquier manera, el tratamiento continuará mientras que se realizan más exámenes o estudios de evaluación.

Los exámenes médicos dependerán de la seriedad de su condición y la eficacia de los medicamentos en el control de sus molestias de angina de pecho.

## ¿CUÁLES EXÁMENES MÉDICOS REALIZARÁN?

Existe más de un examen de evaluación que se necesitará para determinar la seriedad de la obstrucción de sus coronarias. Algunos de estos exámenes se realizan mientras que está internado en el hospital. Otros exámenes se pueden realizar en el hospital, pero no tiene que pasar la noche ahí. Finalmente, algunos de los exámenes se pueden realizar en el consultorio del médico.

### Exámenes de tolerancia al esfuerzo ("stress tests")

Probablemente realizarán un examen de tolerancia al esfuerzo. En este examen, le conectarán a una máquina de electrocardiograma mientras que realiza ejercicio en una bicicleta fija o en una banda deslizante. Puede ser que el médico también le inyecte una sustancia contrastante (tinte) radioactiva que permita ver sus vasos sanguíneos con unas cámaras especiales. El examen proporciona imágenes de los movimientos del músculo de su corazón y la manera en la que fluye la sangre.

El examen permite observar las alteraciones que suceden en el corazón mientras que su cuerpo realiza ejercicio. Durante el examen, el personal médico especializado vigilará su condición preguntándole cómo se siente. Asegúrese de seguir sus instrucciones cuidadosamente y decirles exactamente cómo se siente, (Si usted no habla inglés y no hay un médico o enfermera que hable español mientras realizan el examen, asegúrese que un familiar o amigo que hable ambos idiomas le acompañe.)

*continúa*

continuación

Si usted padece de otros problemas de la salud que impidan que realice ejercicio, le harán otro tipo de examen de tolerancia. Para realizar este examen, se le da un medicamento especial que hace que su corazón lata más rápidamente y que abre las arterias coronarias. El electrocardiograma que se toma durante este tipo de examen proporciona la misma información que se obtendría con el otro examen.

Los exámenes de tolerancia al esfuerzo con o sin ejercicio permiten determinar qué tan bien funciona su corazón. A pesar de que estos exámenes son útiles, el médico no puede obtener información precisa en cuanto al lugar o el grado de obstrucción de las coronarias. El grado de precisión de estos exámenes es de 90 por ciento. Por esta razón, es posible que también sea necesario realizar un cateterismo (angiograma) cardíaco.

## Cateterismo cardíaco

El angiograma (coronariografía) o cateterismo cardíaco permite que el médico observe las arterias coronarias directamente. Se introduce un tubo delgado conocido como catéter a través de una arteria en el brazo o la pierna. Viendo a través de una pantalla, el médico pasa el tubo por las arterias hasta llegar al corazón.

Con el catéter se mide la presión y circulación de la sangre en las arterias del corazón. Después se inyecta un líquido a través del catéter para tomar radiografías. Estas radiografías permiten ver el grado y ubicación de las obstrucciones de las coronarias.

El angiograma es un examen de evaluación no un tratamiento para la angina de pecho. El tratamiento para la angina de pecho que es parecido al angiograma se conoce como angioplastia.

## ¿QUÉ MUESTRAN ESTOS EXÁMENES?

Los exámenes de tolerancia al esfuerzo muestran el grado de peligro que existe al corazón como resultado de las obstrucciones de las coronarias. El angiograma muestra la severidad y ubicación de las obstrucciones. El médico le informará que tiene enfermedad en una, dos o tres de las coronarias principales y el porcentaje de la obstrucción.

El número y porcentaje de la obstrucción de las coronarias se usan para medir la gravedad de su enfermedad. Por lo general, el mayor número de obstrucciones en las coronarias y la mayor deficiencia en la función cardíaca indican una enfermedad más severa.

*continúa*

continuación

Estos exámenes dan mucha información sobre su condición. Es entonces que el médico le podrá dar más información en cuanto a la gravedad de su enfermedad y en cuanto a los tratamientos disponibles en su caso.

## TRATAMIENTOS PARA LA ANGINA DE PECHO INESTABLE

Usted y el médico pueden decidir el tratamiento más adecuado en su caso. Las recomendaciones de tratamiento dependen de los resultados de sus exámenes médicos, si sigue teniendo molestias, y de sus propias preferencias. Por lo general, los tres principales tipos de tratamiento disponibles son la terapia con medicamentos, la angioplastia, o la cirugía de puente coronario ("bypass").

### La terapia con medicamentos

Probablemente le dieron medicamentos durante su estadía en el hospital o la sala de emergencias. Algunos de estos medicamentos sólo se administran en el hopsital, como el medicamento que se usa para evitar coágulos sanguíneos (heparina).

Muchos otros medicamentos que se usan en el tratamiento de la angina de pecho inestable se pueden tomar en casa. Estos incluyen pastillas (tabletas) o cremas que usted mismo puede administrar.

El sólo uso de medicamentos logra controlar la condición en muchos pacientes. Recuerde que si los medicamentos no le brindan el alivio necesario, la angioplastia y la cirugía de puente coronario siempre siguen siendo opciones futuras.

Casi todos los pacientes de angina de pecho inestable recibirán algún tipo de medicamento. El médico o la enfermera le explicará exactamente cómo y cuándo tomarlos.

Existen varios tipos de medicamentos que se usan para aliviar las molestias de la angina de pecho inestable. Muchos de ellos también ayudan a reducir el esfuerzo del corazón para bombear sangre. Los medicamentos se pueden usar como tratamiento único o en combinación con los otros tratamientos que se describen más tarde.

El uso de medicamentos como tratamiento único probablemente es la opción adecuada para los pacientes que tienen otras enfermedades, o para los pacientes que no quieren someterse a la cirugía u otros tratamientos.

*continúa*

continuación

---

### El uso de medicamentos como tratamiento único ayuda a los pacientes que

- tienen una o varias obstrucciones pero sólo en una de las coronarias
- tienen obstrucciones menos severas
- no padecen molestias severas de angina de pecho
- se han estabilizado durante su estadía en el hospital

---

Probablemente deseará hacer las siguientes preguntas sobre el tratamiento a su médico:

- ¿Cuáles son los efectos secundarios (molestias) que tendré como resultado del uso de los medicamentos?
- ¿Tendré que tomar medicamentos toda mi vida?

Algunos pacientes presentan efectos secundarios molestos provocados por los medicamentos, pero la mayoría de ellos notan mejoría de sus síntomas de angina de pecho. Si tiene una reacción negativa a los medicamentos, asegúrese de llamar al médico. Frecuentemente, la reacción negativa desaparece o disminuye con el tiempo; o se pueden hacer cambios en el uso de los medicamentos que permitirán ayudarle a sentirse mejor.

Recuerde, ninguno de los medicamentos elimina las obstrucciones en sus coronarias. Estos solamente disminuyen las molestias de la angina de pecho porque permiten que su corazón tenga mejor irrigación de sangre o que funcione con menos dificultad.

Algunos de los medicamentos de uso común en el tratamiento de la angina de pecho inestable incluyen la aspirina, los nitratos y los betabloqueantes.

### *Aspirina*

**Cómo funciona:** La mayoría de las personas piensan en la aspirina como un medicamento para aliviar los dolores de cabeza o la fiebre. Pero la aspirina también evita la formación de coágulos sanguíneos y estos coágulos son los que pueden obstruir las coronarias y causar un ataque cardíaco.

La investigación científica de los pacientes con angina de pecho inestable demuestra que una aspirina al día reduce el riesgo de ataques cardíacos y muerte. El Tylenol® (acetaminofén) y el Advil® (ibuprofén) no son lo mismo que la aspirina y, en el caso de la angina de pecho, no se deben usar en lugar de ésta.

*continúa*

continuación

**Efectos secundarios.** A la mayoría de los pacientes con angina de pecho inestable se les recomendará el uso diario de aspirina. Cuando se usa la aspirina recubierta se presentan menos efectos secundarios. Se debe evitar el uso de aspirina si usted es alérgico a ella o si ha tenido úlceras u otros problemas de sangrados (hemorragias).

*Nitratos*

**Cómo funcionan.** Los nitratos (por lo general la nitroglicerina o el isosorbide) se usan para abrir las coronarias. Hacen menos difícil el funcionamiento del músculo del corazón y las coronarias porque aumentan la irrigación sanguínea. Los nitratos pueden aliviar las molestias de angina de pecho muy rápidamente.

Los nitratos vienen en varias formas de administración: Hay algunos que son unas pastillas (tabletas) que se colocan debajo de la lengua, otras tabletas que se tragan, parches que se colocan en la piel, o cremas que también se untan en la piel.

Las pastillas, las cremas y los parches tienen uso por un tiempo limitado y, después de este período ya no funcionan. Es importante que hable con el farmacéutico acerca de las fechas límite de uso de estos medicamentos y cuándo se deben reemplazar por nuevos.

Las cremas y parches de nitrato únicamente se usan como terapia de mantenimiento. Si los usa, también tendrá que tomar las pastillas para aliviar las molestias de la angina de pecho.

Tome una pastilla de nitroglicerina en cuanto sienta las molestias. Si las molestias no desaparecen en 5 minutos, tome otra pastilla. Si las molestias no desaparecen en otros 5 minutos, tome una tercera pastilla.

**Si las molestias no han desaparecido despues de tomar tres pastillas en un período de 20 minutos, vaya al hospital de inmediato. ¡Vaya de inmediato!**

Las molestias persistentes (que no desaparecen) pueden ser señales que está sufriendo un ataque cardíaco y tiene que recibir atención médica inmediata.

*continúa*

continuación

**Efectos secundarios.** Probablemente sentirá mareo inmediatamente después de tomar los nitratos, así es que por lo general le dirán que los tome mientras se encuentra sentado. A algunos pacientes les dan dolores de cabeza.

*Betabloqueantes*

**Cómo funcionan.** Estos medicamentos disminuyen el esfuerzo y la cantidad de oxígeno que necesita el corazón para funcionar.

**Efectos secundarios.** Estos medicamentos son fuertes y pueden provocar muchos efectos secundarios. Aproximadamente el 10 por ciento de los pacientes que toman betabloqueantes se sienten cansados o mareados. El 5 por ciento de los pacientes pueden presentar depresión emocional, diarrea, o irritaciones de la piel. La confusión mental, los dolores de cabeza, agruras (acidez estomacal) o dolor de estómago y la falta de aliento (aire) son efectos secundarios mucho menos comunes.

## La angioplastia

Este procedimiento es similar al angiograma. Se introduce un catéter (tubo delgado) en una arteria de la ingle y se dirige directamente hacia la coronaria con la obstrucción. El catéter tiene un pequeño globo (balón) en la punta. Cuando el catéter llega al área de la obstrucción, el médico infla el globo lo suficiente para abrir el estrechamiento de la coronaria y permitir el flujo libre de la sangre, deteniendo así las molestias de la angina de pecho.

Estas son preguntas sobre la angioplastia que probablemente deseará hacer al médico:

- ¿Necesitaré más angioplastias o cirugías de puente coronario en el futuro?
- ¿Qué se siente al tener una angioplastia?
- ¿Cuál es la probabilidad de que muera durante la angioplastia, y cuál es la probabilidad de tener otros problemas?

*continúa*

continuación

**Imagen longitudinal de una arteria coronaria mostrando la manera en la que la angioplastia abre la obstrucción**

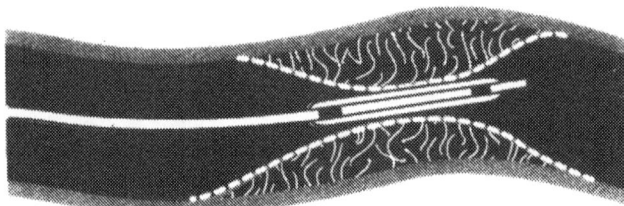

Se coloca el catéter con el globo en la obstrucción de la coronaria

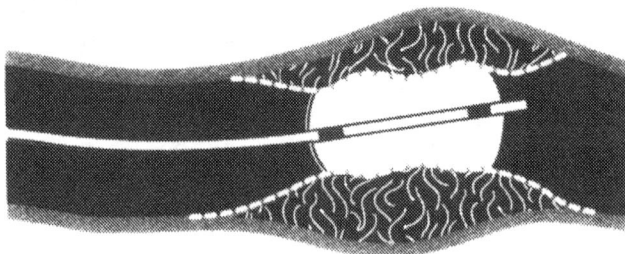

Se infla el globo

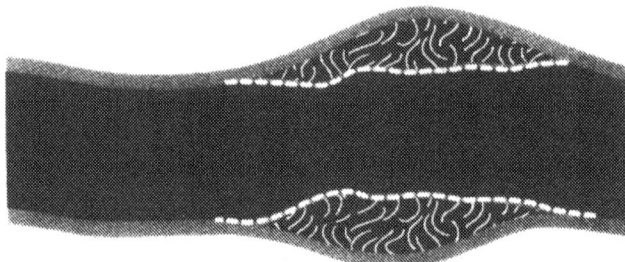

Se retira el catéter dejando la arteria abierta

*continúa*

continuación

---

**Beneficios y desventajas de la angioplastia**

*Posibles beneficios*

- Aliviar el dolor causado por la angina de pecho
- Poder aumentar el nivel de actividad o ejercicio del paciente
- Permitir que el paciente realice actividades que había tenido que suspender debido a la condición
- Reducir las cantidades de medicamento necesarias
- Reducir el nivel de ansiedad/temor

*Posibles desventajas*

- Empeorar la angina de pecho
- Necesidad de realizar una cirugía de puente coronario ("bypass") de emergencia
- Ataque cardíaco
- Daño a la coronaria
- Que la coronaria se vuelva a obstruir (bloquear)
- Muerte

---

### Cirugía de puente coronario ("bypass")

La cirugía se recomienda cuando el paciente tiene obstrucción severa en la coronaria principal izquierda o enfermedad en varias de las coronarias. La cirugía también es una opción cuando los medicamentos no controlan las molestias provocadas por la angina de pecho.

La cirugía de puente coronario puede ser muy eficaz en aumentar la cantidad de sangre que recibe el corazón y en aliviar las molestias de la angina de pecho.

Como puede ver en la siguiente ilustración, en la cirugía se corta un segmento (injerto) de vena de la pierna o de una arteria del pecho, para crear un puente (bypass) que permita el paso a través del área de la coronaria que tiene la obstrucción más severa. Uno de los extremos del segmento se liga a la aorta, que es la arteria por donde pasa toda la sangre desde su corazón al resto del cuerpo. El otro extremo del segmento se liga con la coronaria por debajo de donde está la sección obstruida para así crear un puente de paso para la irrigación de la sangre.

*continúa*

continuación

Estas son algunas preguntas sobre la cirugía de puente coronario que le deseará hacer al médico:

- ¿Cómo se siente el tener una cirugía de puente coronario?
- ¿Es normal sentir temor de someterse a esta cirugía?
- ¿Cuál es la probabilidad de que muera durante la cirugía, y cuál es la probabilidad de tener otros problemas?
- ¿Necesitaré más cirugías en el futuro?

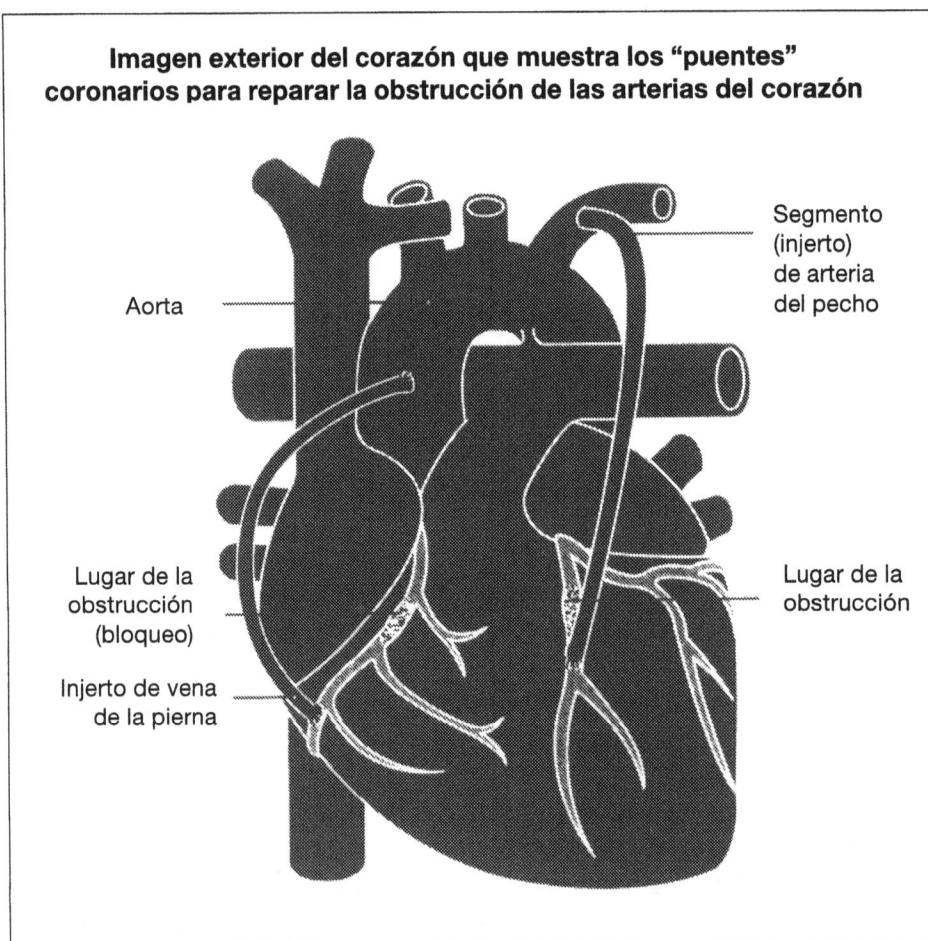

**Imagen exterior del corazón que muestra los "puentes" coronarios para reparar la obstrucción de las arterias del corazón**

continúa

continuación

---

**Beneficios y desventajas de la cirugía de puente (bypass) coronario**

*Posibles beneficios*

- Prolongar la vida
- Aliviar el dolor causado por la angina de pecho
- Aumentar el nivel de actividad o ejercicio del paciente
- Permitir que el paciente realice actividades que había tenido que suspender debido a la angina de pecho
- Reducir la necesidad de uso de medicamentos
- Reducir los niveles de ansiedad/temor

*Posibles desventajas*

- Sangrado (hemorragia) que requiera más cirugía
- Infección de la herida de la cirugía '
- Derrame (ataque) cerebral
- Coágulos sanguíneos
- Insuficiencia hepática (hígado), renal (riñón), o pulmonar
- Ataque cardíaco
- Muerte

---

**¿Angioplastia o cirugía de puente coronario?**

La cirugía y la angioplastia cumplen el mismo propósito, es decir, aumentar la irrigación de sangre al músculo del corazón. Su opción entre estos procedimientos depende de la gravedad de su condición.

¿Cómo sabrá cuál es la mejor opción en su caso? El médico le recomendará el procedimiento más indicado y le ayudará a tomar una decisión. Pero, generalmente, la angioplastia:

- No es una cirugía mayor, como lo es la operación de puente coronario.
- Le mantendrá en el hospital por menos tiempo.
- Le permitirá reanudar sus actividades de la vida diaria más rápidamente.

*continúa*

continuación

También es importante saber lo siguiente antes de tomar una decisión:

- En aproximadamente el 2 al 5 por ciento de los casos, la angioplastia no funciona, y el paciente tiene que someterse a la cirugía de puente coronario de emergencia.
- En aproximadamente 40 por ciento de los casos, las arterias se vuelven a bloquear dentro de los primeros 6 meses después de la angioplastia. Cuando ésto sucede, el paciente tiene que volver a someterse a la angioplastia, o a una cirugía de puente coronario.

## HABLAR CON EL PERSONAL MÉDICO A CARGO DE SU CUIDADO

Muchos pacientes piensan que los médicos están demasiado ocupados para tomarse el tiempo para responder a sus preguntas, y otras personas no saben cómo hacer las preguntas para obtener información. En todos los casos de problemas de la salud, sin embargo, el hablar con el médico, las enfermeras y otras pesonas a cargo de su cuidado es muy importante.

Sus preguntas son importantes y las personas a cargo de su cuidado médico tienen que tomarse el tiempo para responder a sus inquietudes y dudas. Su opinión en cuanto a los tratamientos que preferiría recibir es muy importante en el proceso de tomar decisiones.

Probablemente le ayudará el ir a sus citas médicas acompañado de un familiar o amigo (especialmente alguien bilingüe en caso que el médico no hable español). Esta persona se puede asegurar que usted entienda toda la información, le puede ayudar a hacer preguntas y a hablar con el médico sobre los asuntos que le inquietan y sus preferencias en cuanto a las opciones de cuidado.

A continuación, algunas de las preguntas que puede hacer al médico antes de tomar la decisión en cuanto a su tratamiento:

- ¿Qué es más recomendable en mi caso, el tratamiento con medicamentos, la angioplastia, o la cirugía de puente coronario?
- ¿Cuál es la probabilidad que mis arterias se vuelvan a obstruir después de la angioplastia o la cirugía de puente coronario? ¿Qué tan pronto puede suceder esto?
- ¿Tendré que cambiar de trabajo o jubilarme?
- ¿Cuándo puedo volver a realizar mis actividades de la vida diaria? ¿Cuándo puedo volver a tener relaciones sexuales?
- ¿Cuál es el costo de estos tratamientos médicos?
- ¿Tengo que iniciar una dieta baja en sodio (sal) o grasas? Si es así ¿Por cuánto tiempo?
- ¿Sufriré un ataque cardíaco? ¿Siempre tendré dolor de angina de pecho?

*continúa*

continuación

## ¿SE PUEDEN VOLVER A OBSTRUIR LAS CORONARIAS?

Ni la angioplastia ni la cirugía curan la angina de pecho. Los depósitos de grasa que pueden volver a obstruir las coronarias continúan produciéndose incluso después de estos tratamientos.

Ambos procedimientos se pueden volver a realizar si es necesario, pero la única manera de detener la enfermedad de las coronarias es prevenir las obstrucciones de las arterias.

Los médicos no han descubierto la razón por la que se forman las obstrucciones. Lo que sí saben, a través de estudios con números extensos de pacientes, es que existen algunas personas que tienen mayor riesgo de tener este problema.

Probablemente el médico recomendará que vaya a un programa de rehabilitación cardíaca. Generalmente los hospitales locales ofrecen estos programas y los seguros médicos pagan por los costos. En estos programas, los médicos, enfermeras, especialistas en actividad física y otros le ayudarán a cambiar las actividades y conducta de la vida diaria que hasta la fecha le han puesto en alto riesgo para esta condición. Le enseñarán a hacer ejercicio físico sin riesgo a su condición cardíaca y a adaptar su vida a su enfermedad.

---

### La prevención de las obstrucciones

Las mejores formas de prevenir que se depositen grasas en las paredes de las coronarias son:

- tomar aspirina diariamente
- dejar de fumar
- comer alimentos con bajo contenido de grasas
- aumentar la actividad física (ejercicio)
- controlar la presión arterial, si ésta es alta
- mantener un buen peso
- menores niveles de tensión emocional

---

## LA VIDA DIARIA PARA LAS PERSONAS CON ENFERMEDADES CARDÍACAS

Es normal que se preocupe debido a su condición de salud y su futuro. Es importante que sepa que la mayoría de las personas que tienen angina de pecho no sufren de ataques cardíacos. Por lo general, la angina de pecho se estabiliza en aproximadamente ocho semanas. De hecho, las personas que reciben tratamiento para esta condición pueden vivir productivamente por muchos años.

*continúa*

continuación

La enfermedad de las coronarias no desaparece y sus hábitos de vida influyen su condición de salud. Por eso es tan importante seguir los consejos del médico y el resto del personal a cargo de su cuidado.

Cada año se les dice a miles de personas que tienen enfermedades de las coronarias. Esto puede sorprenderles, especialmente si hasta la fecha nunca se han sentido enfermos. Por ésto, es común que la persona sienta temor, se preocupe por su futuro y su capacidad de cuidar a su familia. Esto hace que sienta que no tiene control sobre su vida.

Muchos médicos, enfermeras, miembros del clero (iglesia), los consejeros y otros saben cómo ayudar a los pacientes con enfermedades de las coronarias. Ellos pueden ayudar a usted y su familia, y es importante hablar con ellos sobre su condición fisica y mental.

La mejor forma de volver a tomar control sobre su vida es aprender todo lo posible sobre las enfermedades de las coronarias y sus tratamientos. Hable sobre todas sus preguntas con el médico o la enfermera.

**NOTAS:**

Source: "La Angina de Pecho Inestable," Agency for Health Care Policy and Research, U.S. Department of Health and Human Services, AHCPR Publication No. 94-0605, July 1994.

# Heart Attack

## DEFINITION OF HEART ATTACK

- It is damage to the heart muscle that cannot be fixed. Health care professionals call a heart attack a "myocardial infarction."
- A narrowing of the coronary artery interrupts blood and oxygen flow to the heart.
- A lack of blood and oxygen to the heart causes damage to the heart muscle.

## FACTORS THAT MAY INCREASE RISK

- Smoking
- Stress
- Obesity
- Sedentary lifestyle
- Diet high in saturated fats
- Age (typically affects men age 50–60 and women age 60–70)
- History of heart disease, high blood pressure, or diabetes

## SIGNS AND SYMPTOMS

- Hard to breath
- Palpitations
- Nausea or vomiting
- Weakness
- Sweating
- Anxiety

- Chest pain
  - can vary from mild discomfort to very severe, crushing pain
  - may radiate to neck, arms, shoulders, or jaw
  - unrelieved by rest or nitroglycerin

## MEASURES TO PREVENT ANOTHER HEART ATTACK

- Reach ideal weight to decrease workload of the heart.
- Eat diet low in saturated fat, cholesterol, and sodium.
- Exercise regularly:
  - Begin with a cardiac rehabilitation program under the guidance of a health professional.
  - Stop exercise immediately if any pain, shortness of breath, or dizziness is noted.
  - Progress exercise gradually.
  - Do not exercise for one to two hours after eating.
- Check and control blood pressure.
- Learn stress management techniques.
- Don't use tobacco and alcohol.
- Avoid constipation to decrease strain on the heart.
- Take medications as ordered, and have regular medical checkups.

Source: Donna Meyers, *Client Teaching Guides for Home Health Care,* Aspen Publishers, Inc., © 1989.

# Nitroglycerin

### ACTIONS

- Relaxes blood vessels
- Widens coronary arteries
- Increases supply of blood and oxygen to the heart

### USES

- Used to relieve angina (chest pain)
- Use to prevent pain before strenuous exercise
- Used to relieve smooth muscle pain that is not heart related

### ADVERSE REACTIONS

- Headache
- Dizziness
- Lowered blood pressure
- Fast heart rate
- Hot, flushed feeling

Note: These will generally only last a few minutes.

### STORAGE

- Keep in brown glass bottle.
- Refill prescription every 3 to 6 months.
- Do not store other medications in the same bottle.
- Do not keep cotton in the bottle; it absorbs the nitroglycerin.
- Freshness is decreased with time, heat, air, and moisture.

### SIGNS TO USE NITROGLYCERIN

- Jaw, neck, shoulders, arm/hand discomfort
- Chest pain/pressure
- Cold sweats, nausea
- Shortness of breath
- Anytime you are in doubt, treat discomfort

### HOW TO TAKE NITROGLYCERIN

Sit or lie down upon the first indication of chest pain. Often, chest pain will disappear with rest. If after 5 minutes, pain persists and you have:

#### Tablets

- Place 1 nitroglycerin tablet under tongue.
- Wait 3 to 5 minutes.
- Repeat if pain/pressure is not completely relieved, taking 1 tablet every 3 to 5 minutes for a total of three tablets.
- If not completely relieved of pain, seek help. You can continue taking 1 tablet every 3 to 5 minutes until you get to an emergency room, or until you can contact your doctor.
- Relax 15–20 minutes after taking nitroglycerin to prevent dizziness or faintness.

#### Spray

- Do not shake the drug container. Hold it upright with the opening of the mechanism as close as possible to your mouth.
- Press the spray mechanism with your forefinger to release the spray onto or under your tongue, close your mouth immediately. Do not inhale or swallow the spray.
- Follow the same directions as for tablet administration.

Courtesy of Lynette Bennett, RN, Educator, Northwest Health Systems, Springdale, Arkansas.

# What Is Heart Failure?

## YOUR HEART

The human heart is a remarkable organ that continuously pumps blood to nourish and provide energy to the body. As big as a fist, this powerful muscle uses its own electrical system to pump blood. It pumps 5 to 6 quarts of blood a minute during rest, but more than 20 quarts a minute during exercise.

Normally, the heart automatically adjusts to changing demands. As the body needs more nourishment and energy (for example, when climbing stairs), the heart responds. It should beat faster and more forcefully, causing more blood to circulate through the body. The blood will carry more oxygen and nourishment to muscles and organs and then return to the heart to begin the process again.

If you have heart failure, your heart is weak and its pumping power is reduced. Although it still beats normally, your heart cannot pump as much blood with each beat. Your symptoms will depend on how severe your heart failure is.

### What Heart Failure Means

"Heart failure" simply means that your heart's pumping power is weaker than normal. Although it still beats, a weakened heart pumps too little blood rich with oxygen and nutrients to meet the body's needs. Walking, carrying groceries, or climbing stairs can be difficult. You may feel short of breath; the body is not getting all the oxygen it needs.

For most patients, heart failure is a chronic condition, which means it can be treated and managed, but not cured. If it is a complication of other medical conditions such as blocked coronary arteries or heart valve disease, surgery may help.

### Causes of Heart Failure

The most common causes are:

- Coronary artery disease, usually with previous heart attack (myocardial infarction [MI])
- Heart muscle disorder (cardiomyopathy)
- High blood pressure (hypertension)
- Heart valve disease

*continues*

continued

Sometimes the exact cause of heart failure is not found. However, the actual cause is not as important as your heart's reduced pumping power and what can be done about it.

## Symptoms

Check (✔) your symptoms:

☐ Difficulty breathing, especially with exertion or when lying flat in bed
☐ Waking up breathless at night
☐ Frequent dry, hacking cough, especially when lying down
☐ Fatigue, weakness
☐ Dizziness or fainting
☐ Swollen feet, ankles, and legs (edema)
☐ Nausea, with abdominal swelling, pain, and tenderness

Other medical problems can cause the same symptoms. A thorough physical exam and a complete health history, plus certain tests, are needed to diagnose heart failure and find its possible causes.

## Causes of Symptoms

A healthy heart can increase how much oxygen-rich blood is pumped to vital organs and muscles as it is needed.

When a heart pumps with less power and force than normal, it cannot pump enough blood to organs and muscles. As a result, your body cannot do as much. Blood and fluids may collect or "pool" in the lungs. This can cause breathing problems when you lie down. Fluids can also collect in other parts of the body, swelling the feet, ankles, legs, and abdomen.

## HOW YOUR HEART'S CHAMBERS AND VALVES WORK

Understanding how your heart works will help you understand the reasons behind the treatment plan your heart care team designs for you. The more you know, the more you can be involved.

Blood moves through four chambers (two atriums and two ventricles) in the heart before circulating through the body (below). With each heartbeat, blood returns from the body through the veins, enters one of the chambers—the right atrium—and moves through the valve into the

*continues*

continued

right ventricle below it. At the same time, blood from the lungs that is rich in oxygen enters the left atrium on the other side of the heart. From the left atrium, the blood passes through a valve into the left ventricle.

## Blood Flow to Heart Chambers

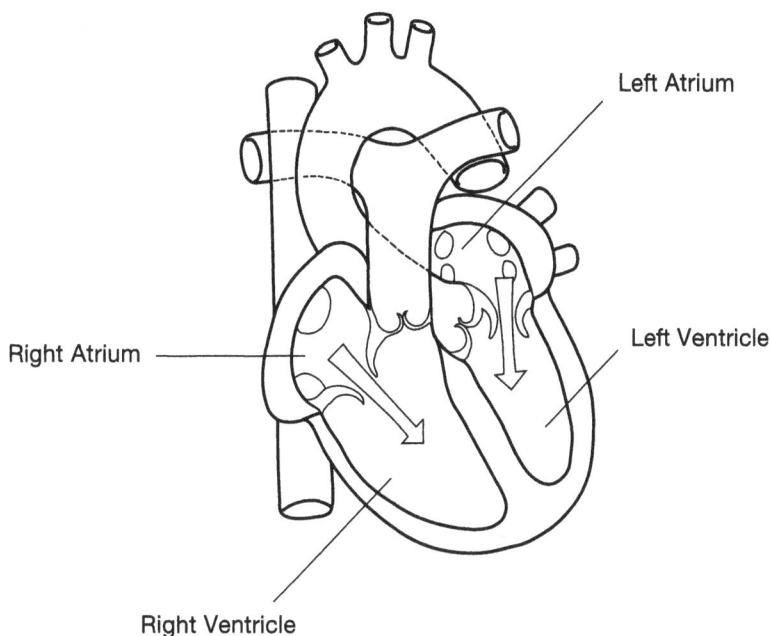

Next, the right ventricle contracts after getting blood from the right atrium, sending blood to the lungs to get oxygen (below). At the same time, the left ventricle contracts after getting blood from the left atrium. When the left ventricle contracts, it pumps blood through the aorta to arteries in all parts of the body.

The heart has four valves. Two prevent blood from flowing back between the atriums and ventricles. The other two valves prevent blood from flowing backward from the arteries and into the ventricles.

Normally, the left ventricle pumps one-half or more of the blood in it with each beat. With heart failure, the left ventricle cannot contract strongly enough, pumping two-fifths or less of the blood in it with each beat.

*continues*

continued

## Blood Flow from Heart Chambers

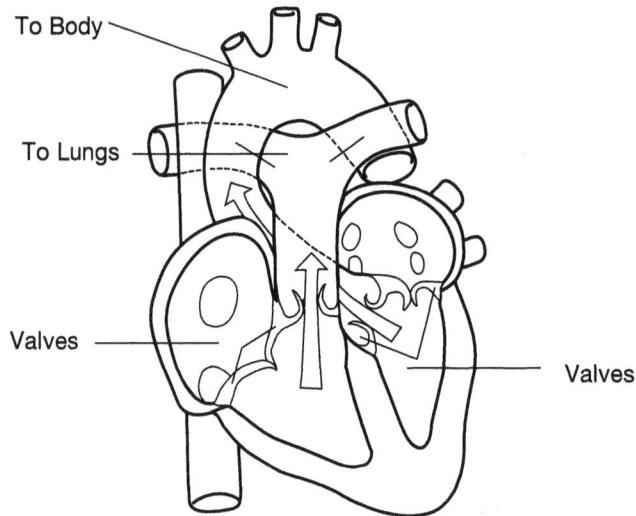

To Body

To Lungs

Valves

Valves

## YOUR HEALTH CARE TEAM

Because heart failure is complex, a team of health care professionals is needed for special skills and expertise.

By working with your health care team in learning how to treat your condition, you may live longer and also improve the quality of your life.

Health care providers on the team may include:

- Your **primary care doctor**—the doctor you normally see for health problems. General internists or family physicians normally provide primary care.
- A **cardiologist,** if your primary care doctor believes a heart specialist is needed.
- Other **doctors,** such as surgeons and other specialists, if needed and recommended by your primary care doctor or cardiologist.
- **Clinical nurse specialists** and **nurse practitioners,** who care for you and are sources of information, education, and counsel.
- **Other health care professionals,** including physician's assistants, nurses, dietitians, physical and occupational therapists, pharmacists, case managers, social workers, and other mental health professionals.

*continues*

continued

You and your family are important parts of this health care team. Before seeing other members of the health care team, write down your questions. Mark anything in this handout you don't understand or would like to know more about. Using the list and this handout, ask your health care provider questions. Tell him or her how you feel about your care.

**Be involved in management of your condition. The health care team is there to serve you.**

## DIAGNOSIS AND EVALUATION

Your health care team will want to know:

- What are your symptoms and how long have you had them?
- Have you ever had a heart attack, a heart murmur, or other heart problems? If so, how are these problems being treated?
- What is your general health history and status? What other health problems do you have, and how are they being treated? Are your diet, activities, or exercise restricted? Have family members had heart problems?
- What is your lifestyle and what are your health habits? What is your daily life like? What do you do to prevent health problems?
- Do you use tobacco, alcohol, or illegal drugs? How often?

Be honest and candid. Information you share with health care providers is confidential. Evaluating, treating, and managing heart failure depends on accurate information, including facts that only you and your family can provide.

A health history, physical exam, chest x-ray, and electrocardiogram (called ECG or EKG) help diagnose heart failure.

A normal heart pumps one-half (50 percent) or more of the blood in the left ventricle with each heartbeat. With heart failure, the weakened heart may pump two-fifths (40 percent) or less, and less blood is pumped with less force to all parts of your body.

Based on your symptoms and first test results, your health care team may want to measure the amount of blood pumped from the heart with each beat (the ejection fraction). Tests to measure the ejection fraction include **echocardiography** and **radionuclide ventriculography.**

**Echocardiography** uses sound waves to make images of the heart and its chambers. The procedure is safe and does not require entering the body with any instruments or devices.

*continues*

continued

**Radionuclide ventriculography** is a special test that tracks very low doses of a radioactive substance as it travels through the heart. The radioactive substance is safe and completely leaves the body.

## MANAGING HEART FAILURE

To manage heart failure, follow the instructions of your health care team. If you take medicines as prescribed and change how you live, you may reduce symptoms and improve how you feel.

Work with your health care team to make the best choices and set goals to keep your life interesting and enjoyable.

Your management plan consists of:

- Medicines
- Diet
- Daily activities
- Exercise
- Lifestyle and health habits
- Family support

Work with your health care team to learn how to treat your condition.

If you do not want to change how you live or take medicines as prescribed, tell your health care provider and explain your reasons.

Source: "Living with Heart Disease: Is It Heart Failure?" Agency for Health Care Policy and Research, U.S. Department of Health and Human Services, AHCPR Publication No. 94–0614, June 1994.

# Managing Heart Failure

## MONITORING YOUR PROGRESS

Managing heart failure requires keeping track of symptoms and monitoring how well you follow instructions of your health care team. Report changes in your health to your health care provider.

### Your Responsibilities

As part of your health care team, you should:

- Monitor your general health and report any changes in how you feel.
- Report changes in your symptoms.
- Take medicines as prescribed and report any side effects.
- Follow your guidelines for activities and exercise, and report when you are not able to do an activity or exercise easily.
- Follow a prescribed diet.
- Report any sudden weight changes.

### Family Responsibilities

Your family is part of your health care team. Ask family members for help in monitoring your condition. They should know when to report new symptoms, or a change in symptoms, to your health care provider if you do not.

When calling the health care provider's office, your family should:

- Say you are being treated for heart failure
- Describe your symptoms
- Describe what has already been done to bring relief or comfort
- Give the names and amounts of medicines you take

## THE FUTURE

Ask your primary care doctor to explain how heart failure is likely to affect your life. Many people adjust to limits imposed by heart failure and still lead active lives.

Although a sudden change in symptoms is not expected, certain activities may become harder because you are tired and short of breath. If your symptoms do change suddenly, call your health care provider right away.

## EMERGENCIES

In an emergency, such as if your heart or breathing stops, acceptance of medical care and treatment is assumed. However, you have a right to accept or refuse any medical care and

*continues*

continued

treatment in advance. You can direct that you do not want emergency medical workers to restore your heartbeat or use special equipment to breathe for you.

Specific instructions for family members and others may be needed so they will know how to react in a medical emergency. A legal document called an advance directive lets others know what to do in a medical emergency. This document states what lifesaving measures you want taken if you cannot think clearly or speak for yourself.

Advance directives include these legal documents:

- living wills
- medical durable power of attorney
- "No cardiopulmonary resuscitation" (CPR) instructions
- substitute decisionmakers (medical proxies)

If you do not have an advance directive, discuss your medical care and treatment wishes with your family and health care team before preparing one. Ask your health care team or attorney for more information about advance directives. These decisions may be difficult. Your health care team will help you understand how these decisions may affect you. Each state has different laws which govern the content and use of advance directives.

## SUPPORT GROUPS AND COUNSELING

Diagnosis of heart failure can generate a wide range of feelings. You and your family should talk about these feelings with your health care team. Seek help in dealing with feelings that cause problems.

In addition to professional counseling, local support groups can be a source of help. These groups offer the chance for you to talk about your feelings with other heart patients and families during regular meetings. Support groups may also offer educational programs about heart problems.

Ask your health care team about support groups where you live. If no support group exists, your health care team may help you start one.

For more information about support groups for heart patients and their families, contact:

**The Mended Hearts, Inc.**
7272 Greenville Avenue
Dallas, TX 75231
(214) 706-1442

**The Coronary Club, Inc.**
9500 Euclid Avenue, E-37
Cleveland, OH 44195
(216) 444-3690

Source: "Living with Heart Disease: Is It Heart Failure?" Agency for Health Care Policy and Research, U.S. Department of Health and Human Services, AHCPR Publication No. 94–0614, June 1994.

# Medicines for Heart Failure

## IMPORTANCE

Taking medicine every day is vital to treating heart failure. Depending on your symptoms and diagnosis, your doctor may start treatment by prescribing one medicine and then adding others later. Sometimes, treatment will begin with two or more medicines.

It may take several days or weeks to find the right doses of prescribed medicines. Be patient as you and your health care provider work together to find:

- the right medicines for you
- the right amount of each one
- the best time of day to take each medicine

The benefits of these medicines will be lost or reduced if you do not take your medicines as prescribed. Skipping doses or not refilling a medicine's prescription can cause serious problems. Do not take more than the prescribed dose of any medicine.

**Be sure to tell your health care provider about other health conditions you have and other medicines you take.** These medicines include nonprescription medicines such as aspirin, antacids, and cold remedies.

## SIDE EFFECTS

Any medicine can have unplanned results. If you have any side effects, tell your health care provider right away. He or she can work with you to lessen bothersome effects. If the first medicines prescribed do not work as expected, others are available.

Ask your health care team about side effects caused by taking prescribed medicines with:

- other prescribed medicines
- medicines you can buy without a doctor's prescription (such as aspirin, antacids, and cold remedies)
- certain foods

**Always report side effects to your health care provider. He or she will know what to do about side effects.**

*continues*

continued

## COMMON KINDS OF MEDICINES

Medicines commonly prescribed for treating heart failure include:

- **ACE inhibitors** (angiotensin-converting enzyme inhibitors) to make it easier for the heart to pump
- **Diuretics** or "water pills," to help remove excess fluid and salt from the body
- **Digitalis** to strengthen each heartbeat, allowing more blood to be pumped

When other heart or health problems exist with heart failure, your doctor may prescribe additional medicines, such as drugs to lower blood pressure.

## ACE Inhibitors

ACE inhibitors have been shown to help heart failure patients live longer and feel better. The drugs relax blood vessels and make it easier for the heart to pump. For some people, it may take weeks before they feel better from taking the medicine.

Depending on your initial diagnosis and evaluation, an ACE inhibitor may be the first medicine prescribed. Based on your symptoms, a diuretic and digitalis may be prescribed with the ACE inhibitor or added later.

Captopril, enalapril, lisinopril, and quinapril are generic names for ACE inhibitors now being used for heart failure. Others may be used in the future.

Although most patients take an ACE inhibitor without problems, some patients have side effects. They include:

- Cough
- Dizziness
- Skin rash

Tell your health care provider if any of these symptoms occur.

ACE inhibitors may also produce high potassium levels and affect kidney function. Blood tests are needed to monitor these actions.

**If you have any side effects, tell your health care provider right away.**

*continues*

continued

## Diuretics

By making you urinate more often, diuretics keep fluid from collecting in your feet, ankles, legs, and abdomen. Skipping doses can cause swelling in these parts of the body and shortness of breath when lying down or during physical activity.

The most commonly used diuretics are hydrochlorothiazide and furosemide (Lasix).

Regular use of some diuretics can lead to the body losing too much potassium and to other imbalances. Blood tests are needed to monitor these levels.

To replace lost potassium, you *may* have to:

- Eat more foods rich in potassium, including bananas and raisins, and drink orange juice and other citrus juices
- Take a prescribed potassium supplement

Diuretics may also cause:

- Leg cramps
- Dizziness or lightheadedness
- Incontinence (accidental urine leakage)
- Gout (a type of arthritis)
- Skin rash

Tell your health care provider if you have any of these symptoms. (Urinating more often is not a side effect. It is caused by the diuretic.)

## Digitalis

Digitalis helps the heart pump more effectively and may improve your ability to exercise. Prescribed as Digoxin or Lanoxin, digitalis is taken daily by many heart patients.

Digitalis has been proven safe for most patients. If too much digitalis is in your body, you may have:

- Nausea, loss of appetite
- Mental confusion
- Blurred or yellow-colored vision
- Rapid, forceful heartbeat (palpitations)

Tell your health care provider right away if you have these side effects. Do not stop taking digitalis unless told to do so by your health care provider.

*continues*

continued

## KEEPING TRACK OF YOUR MEDICINES

Having a system can help tell you when to take medicines, especially if you take several each day. Use the Weekly Medicine Record below each day to remind you:

- which medicines to take each day
- what each pill looks like
- when to take them
- when each medicine was taken

Make copies of the blank form for future use.

**Always carry with you a list giving the doses of each medicine you take.** In an emergency, this information can help medical workers help you.

## COST OF MEDICINES

The retail cost of medicines varies greatly among different pharmacies. If cost is a problem, ask your health care provider or pharmacist if there is a lower-cost and acceptable generic form of your medicine. You can also compare prices of different pharmacies and mail-order prescription services.

If you need financial assistance, it may be available through social service agencies where you live. You also may qualify for help through programs established by drug companies.

Let your health care provider know if the cost of medicines is a problem. Your health care team can help you apply for assistance.

Source: "Living with Heart Disease: Is It Heart Failure?" Agency for Health Care Policy and Research, U.S. Department of Health and Human Services, AHCPR Publication No. 94–0614, June 1994.

# Medication Information for the Patient Who Has Heart Failure

*Instructions to the patient:* Take your medication exactly as ordered. Report side effects to your healthcare provider. Do not stop taking any medication unless told to do so by your healthcare provider.

| Type of Medication | How Does It Work? | Possible Side Effects | The Medicine I Am Taking Is: (name, dose, frequency, storage) |
|---|---|---|---|
| **ACE Inhibitors**<br><br>Examples: Captopril, Enalapril, Fosinopril | Relaxes blood vessels so heart doesn't have to work hard to pump blood. Decreases fluid retention. Lowers blood pressure. | Fast heart beat<br>Dizziness<br>Dry cough | |
| **Diuretics**<br><br>Examples: Lasix, Bumex, Hydrochlorothiazide (HCTZ), Metalozone | Helps you to urinate more. This removes excess fluid from your lungs and body. Less fluid makes it easier for your heart to work effectively. | Dehydration, thirst<br>Loss of certain substances like potassium and sodium may cause muscles cramps or irregular heart beat. | |
| **Digoxin** | Helps your heart to beat stronger and slower. | Heart rate could get too slow or irregular. Check your pulse daily and report a pulse less than _____ as well as any new irregular beats to your health care provider. | |
| **Calcium Channel Blockers**<br><br>Examples: Amlodipine, Diltiazem, Nifedipine, Verapamil | Helps to relax the heart and blood vessels. Makes it easier for the heart to pump blood. Reduces blood pressure. | Lightheadedness<br>Slow heart rate<br>Ankle swelling | |

*continues*

continued

| Type of Medication | How Does It Work? | Possible Side Effects | The Medicine I Am Taking Is: (name, dose, frequency, storage) |
|---|---|---|---|
| **Beta Blockers**<br><br>Examples: Esmolol, Metoprolol | Helps to relax the heart and blood vessels. Decreases blood pressure and heart rate. | Lightheadedness<br>Feeling tired<br>Wheezing<br>Ankle swelling | |
| **Nitrates**<br><br>Examples: Isordil, Nitrodur, Nitroglycerine, Nitropatch | Relaxes blood vessels. Decreases amount of blood returning to heart so heart doesn't have to work as hard to pump. | Headache<br>Dizziness when first getting up<br>Fast heart rate<br>Flushed feeling | |
| **Vasodilators**<br><br>Examples: Clonidine, Doxazosin, Hydralazine, Methyldopa, Prazosin | Relaxes blood vessels, thus reducing blood pressure. Decreases work of the heart. | Lightheadedness<br>Changes in heart rate—some may be faster and some may be slower. | |

**NOTES:**

Courtesy of VA Medical Center, San Diego, California.

# Weekly Medicine Record

Your Name _____

Week of _____

| Name of Medicine and Dose | Size, Shape, and Color of Pill | When to Take | Place an ⊠ after each medicine when taken | | | | | | |
|---|---|---|---|---|---|---|---|---|---|
| | | | Sun | Mon | Tues | Wed | Thur | Fri | Sat |
| 1 | | | | | | | | | |
| 2 | | | | | | | | | |
| 3 | | | | | | | | | |
| 4 | | | | | | | | | |

## HOW TO USE YOUR WEEKLY MEDICINE RECORD

Use the weekly medicine record to keep track of what medicines to take every day, when to take them, and when you took them.

Write your name and the date, starting on Sunday, at the top of the record.

Each numbered row is for one medicine. Write the name and dose (amount) of each medicine under the first column. For example: **Lanoxin .25 mg.** The medicine's name and dose appear on the label of the medicine container.

In the second column, write the size, shape, and color of the pill. For example: **Small, round, white pill.**

In the third column, write when to take the medicine. For example: **Before breakfast.**

When you take a medicine, place an X in the column for the day of the week. If you take a medicine more than once a day, mark it each time.

Make copies of the form. Use it every day.

Source: "Living with Heart Disease: Is It Heart Failure?" Agency for Health Care Policy and Research, U.S. Department of Health and Human Services, AHCPR Publication No. 94–0614, June 1994.

# Diet and Heart Failure

In addition to taking medicines for heart failure, you must change and then monitor your diet.

## SALT

Because salt (sodium) causes fluid to build up in the body, you must restrict salt intake. If you do not, your feet, ankles, legs, and abdomen may swell, and you may find it hard to breathe. If these symptoms become severe, you may require hospital treatment.

Your health care provider will tell you how much salt, if any, can be in your diet. You and your family may be asked to see a dietitian, nurse specialist, or other health educator for special diet instructions and counseling. They may also suggest new ways to prepare foods and how to modify family recipes. For example, lemon juice and many spices and herbs can add flavor to unsalted foods.

Be especially aware of foods with "hidden" salt such as frozen or canned foods, cheeses, and processed meats. Foods such as hot dogs, salami, and canned soups often contain a lot of salt. Check the nutrition labels for salt content.

## ALCOHOL

If you drink alcoholic beverages, you may have to stop or have only one drink per day. One drink means a glass of beer or wine, or a mixed drink or cocktail containing no more than 1 ounce of alcohol.

## CHANGING YOUR DIET

Changing your diet can be complicated and confusing. The goal is to reduce salt, and possibly fat, in your food without sacrificing the pleasure of eating. If you have trouble changing your diet, ask your health care team for help.

## WATCHING YOUR WEIGHT

Watch your weight. Obtain an accurate scale and weigh yourself each morning after urinating, but before eating breakfast or dressing.

If you have gained 3 to 5 pounds since last visiting your health care provider, tell him or her promptly. The weight gain may mean your body is retaining fluid.

Source: "Living with Heart Disease: Is It Heart Failure?" Agency for Health Care Policy and Research, U.S. Department of Health and Human Services, AHCPR Publication No. 94–0614, June 1994.

# Lifestyle and Heart Failure

## DAILY ACTIVITIES

How heart failure affects you depends on how severe it is. Mild heart failure may have little effect on work or recreation. Severe heart failure may restrict activities that used to be easy. Talk to your health care team about:

- **Work.** Can you still work? Full time or part time?
- **Recreation.** Can you go hiking, play golf, swim, and attend sporting events?
- **Leisure.** Can you travel, work in the garden, and do volunteer work?
- **Sex.** Can you have sexual intercourse?

Involve your family members in discussions about activities. They need to know how to support and help you. This is especially true when what you can do changes over time. Some activities (such as work or recreation) may become more difficult while others do not change.

Do not be afraid of discussing private aspects of your life. Your health care team must rely on what you say to help reduce symptoms and improve the quality of your life.

As you learn to live with heart failure and change your lifestyle, you may discover new satisfactions and pleasures. Changes to daily life can be positive and rewarding. Work restrictions may lead to interesting and enjoyable leisure activities. Recreation may become a valuable part of daily life. Sexual relations can be very enjoyable as you and your partner discover less demanding ways to express and share affection.

## EXERCISE

Exercise regularly within your doctor's guidelines. Many people with heart failure say they feel better when they exercise regularly. Usually you can exercise safely at home or in a supervised rehabilitation setting such as a hospital, health club, recreation center, YMCA, or YWCA.

Exercise includes:

- Walking
- Cycling
- Swimming
- Low-impact aerobic routines

Your health care provider will advise you about the right kind and amount of exercise. Find out before starting. You may be asked to see a cardiac rehabilitation specialist to help plan and monitor an exercise program. Also, you may need an exercise stress test to see how much you can do safely.

*continues*

continued

## LIFESTYLE AND HEALTH HABITS

Your lifestyle reflects attitudes and values. Health habits involve what you do to reduce chances of illness or injury. Heart failure means you may have to change your lifestyle and health habits.

Examine your lifestyle and health habits. The following changes can reduce the symptoms of heart failure and improve the quality of your life:

- Lose weight if you are overweight.
- Do not smoke or chew tobacco.
- Eliminate or reduce alcohol.
- Do not use illegal drugs.

You should also:

- Avoid exercise that exceeds your exercise guidelines.
- Avoid coming in contact with people who have colds.
- Get a flu and pneumonia shot.

You may want to make other changes too, such as learning how to reduce stress. Work with your health care team to decide which choices are best.

## FAMILY SUPPORT

Your family can be a great source of support and encouragement. As much as possible, include family members in all decisions that affect you. These decisions involve your lifestyle and your ability to work and earn a living. Support from family members can be especially important as you adjust to lifestyle changes and if you face emotional difficulties. Let family members know how they can help.

Family members can help you to

- keep track of medicines
- prepare special meals
- exercise
- find more information on treating heart failure
- join a support group

The diagnosis of heart failure may affect your family as much as you. Family support can help you change your lifestyle and health habits.

Source: "Living with Heart Disease: Is It Heart Failure?" Agency for Health Care Policy and Research, U.S. Department of Health and Human Services, AHCPR Publication No. 94–0614, June 1994.

# Chest Pain and Heart Failure

Some people have chest pain (angina) in addition to heart failure symptoms. Angina is caused by blockage in the coronary arteries. When angina is a symptom, a test called **cardiac angiography** (heart catheterization with angiography) may be needed.

In this diagnostic procedure, fluid is injected into the coronary arteries through a long, thin tube called a catheter. Special x-rays show where and how much arteries are blocked. Ask your health care provider about expected benefits and risks of the procedure before agreeing to it.

The results of cardiac angiography are usually used to help health care providers plan your care. Treatment may include surgery. Cardiac angiography may not be needed if you do not want heart surgery. Ask your health care provider how information from the procedure will affect your care.

**NOTES:**

Source: "Living with Heart Disease: Is It Heart Failure?" Agency for Health Care Policy and Research, U.S. Department of Health and Human Services, AHCPR Publication No. 94–0614, June 1994.

# Chest Pain Chart

Name:

| ??? Time: | | | | | | | | | | |
|---|---|---|---|---|---|---|---|---|---|---|
| 1. How severe was the pain? 1–10 (severe) | | | | | | | | | | |
| 2. How long did it last? | | | | | | | | | | |
| 3. What was I doing? | | | | | | | | | | |
| 4. Did I take any nitroglycerin? How many? | | | | | | | | | | |
| 5. Was the pain relieved? | | | | | | | | | | |
| 6. Did I call the nurse? | | | | | | | | | | |

Courtesy of VA Medical Center, San Diego, California.

# Surgery for Heart Failure

If a heart valve problem or coronary artery disease is suspected as the cause of your heart failure, you may be asked to consider heart surgery. Detailed information should be provided. You should know what may result from heart surgery. You should know its:

- benefits
- risks, including the risks of doing nothing
- alternatives, including their benefits and risks
- total cost and how much is paid by insurance

Before deciding to have surgery, ask for a second opinion from another health care provider. Health insurance often requires a second opinion before surgery.

If heart surgery is a realistic choice for you, seek an experienced surgeon and hospital for the surgery. Ask for information about their success rates and costs before selecting a surgeon and hospital.

## HEART VALVE SURGERY

Repairing or replacing one or more heart valves may be needed if heart failure is caused by heart valve problems. This surgery is common and has proven to be successful in many cases.

## CORONARY ARTERY BYPASS GRAFT SURGERY AND ANGIOPLASTY

Coronary artery bypass graft (CABG) surgery is major surgery. In it, veins or arteries from other parts of the body are used to bypass blocked coronary arteries on the heart to restore more normal blood flow to the heart. As a muscle, the heart needs its own blood supply for nourishment so it can pump blood throughout the body.

An alternative to CABG surgery is angioplasty (or PTCA, percutaneous transluminal coronary angioplasty). In this major procedure, a catheter (long, thin tube) is inserted into the arteries on the heart. Inflating a small balloon on the catheter's tip expands the coronary artery and crushes the blockage, restoring blood flow.

Current research indicates that CABG surgery may benefit many people with angina (chest pain) and worsening heart failure resulting from coronary artery disease. The long-term benefits of angioplasty for such patients have not been established by research.

After heart surgery, you must follow a plan for managing and monitoring your heart health.

*continues*

continued

## HEART TRANSPLANT SURGERY

Heart transplantation is considered only in cases of very severe heart failure. Heart transplants are only performed in specialized centers.

## NOTES:

Source: "Living with Heart Disease: Is It Heart Failure?" Agency for Health Care Policy and Research, U.S. Department of Health and Human Services, AHCPR Publication No. 94–0614, June 1994.

# Post Coronary Artery Bypass Graft (CABG)

## ACTIVITY RESTRICTIONS

You must be careful with some motions to avoid placing too much pressure on your healing breastbone.

### Do Not

- Pull or push anything until approved by your surgeon.
- Lift anything greater than five pounds until instructed by your surgeon.
- Rise from a chair by placing your arms out to your side on the arms of the chair and pushing your body up.
- Overdo your exercise program.
- Walk more than one flight of steps more than two times per day.

## DIET RESTRICTIONS

A heart-healthy diet is suggested to reduce further heart-related problems. A diet that is healthy for your heart is restricted in fat. Saturated fats raise your blood cholesterol level, which is a precursor to cardiac disease. Saturated fats, such as lard, shortening, and butter, are generally solid at room temperature. Unsaturated fats, such as oils, are generally liquid at room temperature. As fats become more saturated, higher temperatures are required to melt them. For example, butter requires a higher temperature to melt than margarine does. Your nurse or dietitian can provide you with a detailed heart-healthy diet.

A diet containing a limited amount of salt will reduce the amount of fluid you retain and consequently will reduce your blood pressure. Salt comes in many forms. You are most familiar with table salt. Some salt is hidden. Read content labels carefully and avoid foods that list "salt" or "sodium" as one of the first three ingredients. Some general guidelines to decrease salt intake are:

- Use *minimal* amounts of salt while cooking.
- Do not add salt to any foods once prepared.
- Avoid
  - luncheon meats
  - processed cheese (American, cheese spreads)
  - cured meats such as ham, bacon, and sausage
  - salted pretzels, potato chips, and other crunchy salted snacks
  - anything that is pickled, such as pickles, olives, or hot peppers
  - frozen vegetables and meals
  - canned soups and meat

*continues*

continued

These guidelines often make you wonder what you can eat. There are many foods that you may eat. Use common sense and remember that if you cheat by adding more salt than usual while you're cooking, your blood pressure will rise. You may safely eat:

- freshly prepared meats
- fresh vegetables
- fresh, frozen, or canned fruits
- unsalted snack foods—boxes are marked "salt free" or "unsalted"
- low-sodium cheeses
- unsalted margarine or spreads (again, read those labels!)

## DAILY WEIGHTS

It is important to check your weight every day, especially in the presence of fluid retention. You should weigh yourself:

- at the same time of the day (preferably in the morning)
- unclothed (or with the same clothing on, such as underwear)
- on the same hard, flat surface

Report a weight gain of three pounds in a 24-hour period or a gradual weight gain over days to your doctor immediately.

## WHAT AND WHEN TO NOTIFY YOUR DOCTOR

Report immediately:

- heart pain not relieved by your prescribed medication (This pain may be felt as sharp, dull pressure or tightness. Heart pain is most commonly in the chest and may move into the arm(s) or jaw. Don't be confused—some people never feel anything in their chest but have other symptoms. When in doubt, it is best to check it out.)

**You should expect to have some itching, redness, and a little soreness from your incisions.**

- persistent nausea, vomiting, or heartburn
- cold skin that is moist
- pale or gray color to skin—blue tint to lips
- increased shortness of breath or difficulty with breathing
- weight gains, as specified previously, or increased fluid retention
- temperature above 101°F orally (or 100°F rectally)
- onset or increased drainage from incision

*continues*

continued

- change in color of drainage
- increase in discomfort level of incision
- unusual feelings or problems
- unpleasant side effects from your medications

## MEDICAL APPOINTMENT FOLLOW-THROUGH

It is very important that you schedule and keep your doctor appointments. Your doctor has ordered home care to **supplement** his or her care, not to replace it. Your doctor is the only person who can make changes in your medication and order tests that may be indicated. Discuss any transportation problems you may have with your nurse—there may be ways to help you.

## WHAT IS CORONARY ARTERY DISEASE?

Coronary artery disease (CAD) is a disease affecting the arteries that supply blood to the heart muscle. As a result, the heart muscle is deprived of food and oxygen, which may lead to death if extensive deprivation occurs.

## WHAT IS A CORONARY ARTERY BYPASS GRAFT?

A coronary artery bypass graft, sometimes called a CABG, is a type of surgery. The surgeon takes a healthy artery from the leg or the chest area and transplants it to the heart muscle. The transplanted artery takes on the work of the clogged arteries, allowing food and oxygen to reach the heart muscle. If the surgeon used an artery from your chest (internal mammary), you may have numb or sensitive areas on your chest for up to six months.

## SIGNS AND SYMPTOMS OF CORONARY ARTERY DISEASE

Signs and symptoms of coronary artery disease include

- chest pain (Pain is any sensation from mild pressure to burning, tingling, and being extremely uncomfortable. This pain may radiate down the arm(s) or up into the jaw, neck, or between the shoulder blades.)
- pain associated with activity that usually lasts less than 15 minutes and is relieved by rest and prescribed nitroglycerin products
- restlessness (Feelings of anxiety are common.)
- pain attacks characterized by:
  - profuse sweating
  - cold, moist skin
  - faintness and weakness
  - nausea and vomiting, sometimes indigestion

*continues*

continued

## STRESSORS AND RISK FACTORS LEADING TO CORONARY ARTERY DISEASE

Some of the stressors and risk factors that can lead to coronary artery disease include

- family history of cardiac disease
- gender—men are more prone
- tobacco use
- high blood cholesterol
- high blood pressure
- excessive weight
- physical inactivity
- increased stress
- type A personality—personality characteristics are commonly described as competitive, demonstrating urgency in requests of others, always busy, and lacking patience or tolerance with others
- diabetes mellitus
- oral contraceptive use

## HOW TO GET RELIEF FROM STRESSORS

There are three steps you can take to get relief from stressors

1. Understand your stressors:
   - What causes you stress?
   - What is your reaction to each stressor?
     – Is it physical? Do you feel your stomach jump or do you clench your teeth?
     – Is it emotional? Do you yell or hold back your thoughts?
2. Devise new responses to your stressors. This step may include asking your daughter not to visit you with her children for more than an hour at a time, or it may include concentrating on relaxation techniques.
3. Use stress reduction methods:
   - Listen to relaxing music.
   - Focus on a peaceful scene or place. Use all of your senses—see the place, listen to its sounds, feel and smell the air, and taste what may be there to taste.
   - Consider how you perceive and think about stressors, and climb out of your thoughts and into another dimension. Change the way you think.
   - Obtain professional help with significant stressors. You may want to consider biofeed-back (measuring the muscle activity as you work with stress-reduction methods) or hypnosis.
   - Learn the process of meditation. Kick off your shoes; get comfortable; close your eyes; take slow, deep breaths; and concentrate on relaxing your body from your toes up to your head. Continued practice makes meditation easier.

*continues*

continued

## CARDIAC REHABILITATION

Exercise is an important part of getting better. It is very important that you follow your doctor's specific instruction. Until your heart "grows more circulation" or compensates for its lost circulation, it is important that you limit activity. For this reason you were placed on strict bedrest for a short period of time. Next, your doctor allowed you to get out of bed in a chair and then take short walks. Once approved by your physician, the goal of cardiac rehabilitation is to increase the strength of your heart to accommodate a normal lifestyle. Gradually you will increase your exercise to a goal of tolerating moderately intense exercise from 15 to 30 minutes, three times per week. If you have not heard about a structured cardiac rehabilitation program yet, ask your doctor on your next visit.

**NOTES:**

Source: Barbara Stover Gingerich and Deborah Anne Ondeck, *Clinical Pathways for the Multidisciplinary Home Care Team,* Aspen Publishers, Inc., © 1995.

# La insuficiencia cardíaca

## EL PROPÓSITO DE ESTA GUÍA

Esta guía le ayudará si usted o alguien en su familia padece de insuficiencia cardíaca debido a que el corazón tiene menor capacidad de bombear sangre (disfunción ventricular sistólica izquierda). El aprender acerca de esta condición y seguir algunas recomendaciones sencillas pueden ayudar a mejorar la calidad de vida del paciente.

La guía le ayudará al paciente y su familia a participar en su cuidado médico, trabajando en cooperación con el grupo de cuidado de salud (médicos, enfermeras y otros profesionales). Esta guía le ayudará a mejorar su vida a pesar de la condición; así que probablemente deseará compartirla con sus familiares y otras personas a cargo de su cuidado.

Leer esta guía le ayudará a entender cómo y por qué la insuficiencia cardíaca afecta a su cuerpo. También le dará información sobre cómo responder a los síntomas y lo que puede esperar de los tratamientos disponibles. El aprender sobre la condición y participar activamente en su atención médica le permitirá mejorar su calidad de vida.

## EL CORAZÓN

El corazón es un órgano importante del cuerpo que se encarga de bombear contínuamente la sangre que le proporciona al cuerpo nutrientes y oxígeno. Es del tamaño de un puño y es un poderoso músculo que utiliza su propio sistema "eléctrico" para funcionar como una bomba y circular la sangre. Durante el descanso, el corazón irriga entre 5 a 6 litros ("quarts") de sangre al cuerpo cada minuto; pero esta cantidad de sangre puede aumentar hasta 20 litros por minuto cuando la persona está haciendo ejercicio o esfuerzo físico.

Normalmente el corazón responde automáticamente a las necesidades del cuerpo. Es decir, cuando el cuerpo necesita más nutrientes y oxígeno porque está haciendo esfuerzo físico (como subir escaleras), el corazón responde latiendo más rápido y más fuerte. Al latir más rápidamente, el corazón distribuye más sangre rica en nutrientes y oxígeno a todos los músculos y órganos del cuerpo. A su vez, la sangre que necesita más nutrientes y oxígeno, regresa al corazón para volver a circular a través del cuerpo.

Cuando una persona padece de insuficiencia cardíaca, su corazón se encuentra débil y tiene menor capacidad para bombear sangre. A pesar que puede continuar latiendo normalmente el corazón no distribuye la misma cantidad de sangre con cada latido. Los síntomas de cada paciente varían de acuerdo a la severidad de la condición.

*continúa*

continuación

# ¿QUÉ ES LA INSUFICIENCIA CARDÍACA?

La insuficiencia cardíaca quiere decir que su corazón tiene una menor capacidad para bombear sangre. Resulta en que el cuerpo recibe menos nutrientes y oxígeno de los que necesita. El paciente tendrá dificultad para caminar, cargar cosas o subir escaleras. Probablemente sentirá que le falta el aliento (aire) porque el cuerpo no tiene suficiente oxígeno para funcionar normalmente.

Para la mayoría de los pacientes, la insuficiencía cardíaca es una condición crónica. Es decir que pueden recibir tratamiento para controlarla, pero no existe una curación. Si la condición es el resultado de otros problemas médicos como la obstrucción de las arterias coronarias, o problemas de las válvulas cardíacas, la cirugía del corazón puede ayudar al paciente.

## Las causas de la insuficiencia cardíaca

Las causas más comunes de la insuficiencia cardíaca son las siguientes:

- enfermedades de las arterias coronarias, por lo general con un ataque cardíaco previo (infarto miocárdico)
- defecto muscular cardíaco (cardiomiopatía)
- alta presión sanguínea (hipertensión)
- enfermedades de las válvulas cardíacas

A veces no se puede identificar la causa de la insuficiencia cardíaca. Sin embago, la causa de la condición no es tan importante como lo que se puede hacer para ayudarle en caso que su corazón tenga menos capacidad para bombear sangre.

## Síntomas

Marque (✔) los síntomas que usted presente:

- ☐ Dificultad para respirar, especialmente cuando hace un esfuerzo físico, o cuando se encuentra descansando (acostado)
- ☐ Despertar del sueño y sentir que le falta el aliento (aire)
- ☐ Tos seca y frecuente, especialmente cuando se encuentra acostado
- ☐ Sentirse cansado o débil
- ☐ Mareos o desmayos
- ☐ Hinchazón de los pies, los tobillos, y las piernas (edema)
- ☐ Náuseas, con inflamación abdominal, dolor, o dolor al contacto

*continúa*

continuación

Existen otros problemas que pueden producir los mismos síntomas, así es que es necesario que se le realice un examen médico completo. Para diagnosticar e identificar la causa probable de la insuficiencia cardíaca, es necesario obtener un historial médico y ciertos exámenes de evaluación.

### Las causas de los Síntomas

Cuando el corazón está sano, puede responder a las necesidades del cuerpo y aumentar el flujo de sangre oxigenada a los órganos vitales y los músculos.

Cuando el corazón no está sano y tiene menos capacidad y menos fuerza, no puede bombear suficiente sangre para responder a las necesidades de los músculos y órganos. Por esto, su cuerpo no puede realizar las mismas actividades que antes.

Otro síntoma es que se acumulan o retienen sangre y líquidos en los pulmones, causando problemas para respirar cuando el paciente se encuentra acostado. Los líquidos también se pueden acumular en otras partes del cuerpo causando hinchazón de los pies, los tobillos, las piernas o el abdomen (estómago).

## EL FUNCIONAMIENTO DE LAS CAVIDADES Y VÁLVULAS CARDÍACAS

Aprender sobre el funcionamiento de su corazón le ayudará a entender su plan de tratamiento y le permitirá desempeñar un papel activo en las decisiones sobre éste.

### La sangre en el corazón

Antes de circular en el cuerpo, la sangre pasa por las cavidades cardíacas que incluyen dos aurículas y dos ventrículos. Como podrá ver en el dibujo 1, la sangre del cuerpo regresa al corazón a través de las venas y entra a la aurícula derecha (a). De ahí, la sangre baja al ventrículo derecho (b). Mientras tanto, la sangre oxigenada de los pulmones entra a la aurícula izquierda (c) en el otro lado del corazón. Entonces, la sangre pasa por una válvula para llegar al ventrículo izquierdo (d).

*continúa*

continuación

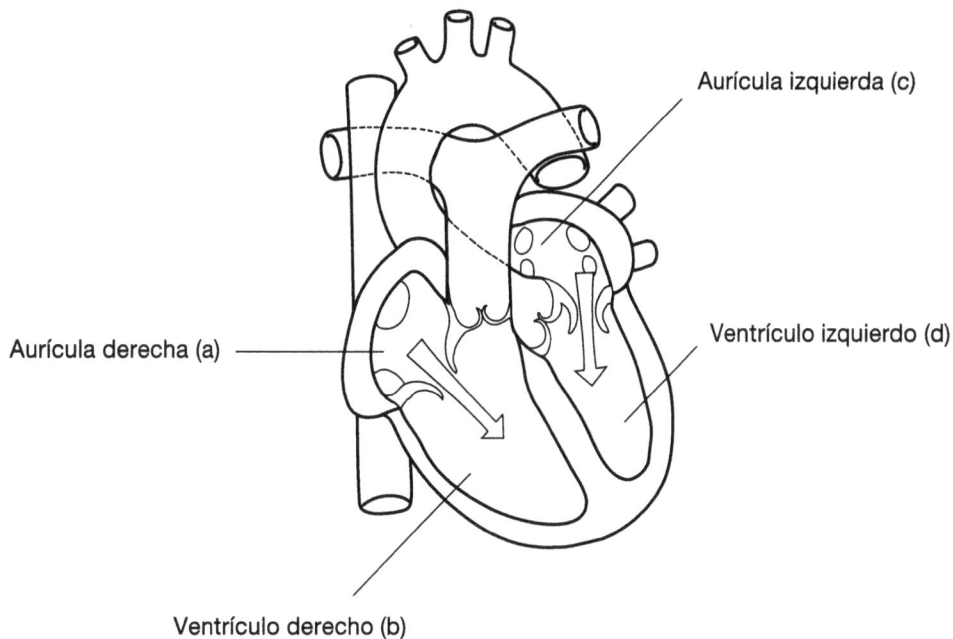

**Dibujo 1**

Aurícula izquierda (c)

Ventrículo izquierdo (d)

Aurícula derecha (a)

Ventrículo derecho (b)

En el dibujo 2, puede ver el ventrículo derecho, éste se contrae después de recibir la sangre de la aurícula derecha y envía la sangre a los pulmones para que reciba oxígeno (a). Al mismo tiempo, el ventrículo izquierdo se contrae después de recibir sangre oxigenada y la envía al resto del cuerpo (b).

El corazón también tiene cuatro válvulas. Dos de ellas se encargan de impedir que la sangre retroceda entre las aurículas y los ventrículos. De la misma manera, las otras dos válvulas se encargan de evitar que el flujo sanguíneo retroceda de las arterias hacia los ventrículos.

Normalmente, en cada latido del corazón el ventrículo izquierdo se encarga de bombear más de la mitad de la sangre que irriga al cuerpo. Cuando existe insuficiencia cardíaca, el ventrículo izquierdo no se puede contraer con la suficiente fuerza y sólo puede bombear el 40 por ciento de la sangre que debería impulsar con cada latido del corazón.

*continúa*

continuación

## La sangre saliendo del corazón

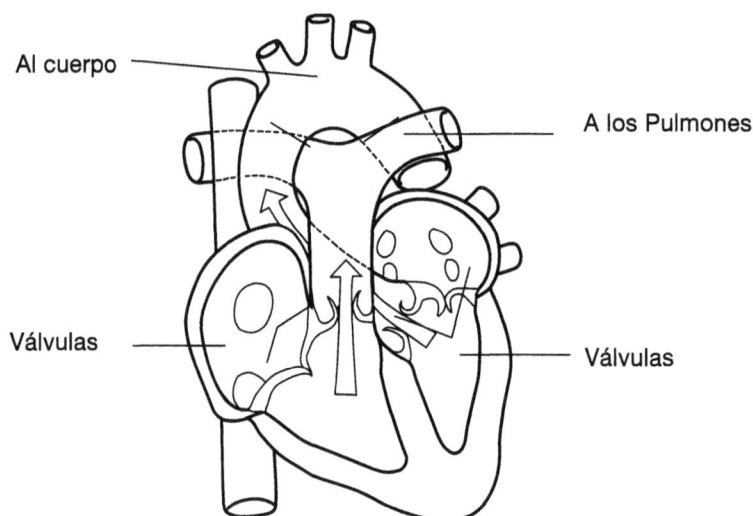

**Dibujo 2**

## EL GRUPO DE CUIDADO MÉDICO

Debido a que la insuficiencia cardíaca es una condición complicada, es necesario que reciba atención de varios tipos de profesionales de la salud especializados en diferentes capacidades.

El cooperar con este grupo de cuidado para aprender más sobre su condición le permitirá vivir mejor y por más tiempo.

Los profesionales a cargo de su cuidado pueden incluir a:

- El **médico de cabecera** (internista, "primary care doctor") es el médico que generalmente le da todo su cuidado de salud. Los internistas o médicos de familia son los encargados de proporcionar el cuidado básico de salud.
- Un **cardiólogo** es un especialista en enfermedades del corazón a quien le enviará su médico de cabecera si así lo cree necesario.
- **Otros médicos** incluyen los cirujanos y otros especialistas que pueden participar en su cuidado si así lo creen necesario el médico de cabecera o el cardiólogo.
- **Enfermeras clínicas y otras enfermeras** a cargo de su cuidado médico en diferentes momentos pueden ser una fuente de información y de educación en cuanto a su condición.
- **Otros profesionales de la salud** incluyen asistentes médicos (profesionales capacitados para tratar ciertas enfermedades y condiciones sin ser médicos titulados), enfermeras, especialistas en dietética (alimentación), especialistas en terapias física y ocupacional, farmacéuticos, especialistas en el manejo de cada caso ("case managers"), trabajadores sociales, y otros especialistas en salud mental.

*continúa*

continuación

Usted y su familia son parte importante del grupo de cuidado médico. Antes de visitar al médico o cualquier otro de los miembros de su grupo de atención de la salud, escriba todas sus preguntas. Si así lo desea, marque las partes que no entienda de esta guía para que se las expliquen, y pídales cualquier otra información necesaria. Con la ayuda de la lista de preguntas que se presenta al final de esta guía, converse con el médico o la enfermera sobre sus dudas y otros asuntos que considere importantes sobre su atención médica.

Participe en las decisiones de su tratamiento.

## EL DIAGNÓSTICO Y LA EVALUACIÓN

La siguiente información es importante para su evaluación médica:

- ¿Cuáles son sus síntomas y por cuánto tiempo los ha tenido?
- ¿Ha tenido usted anteriormente un ataque cardíaco, un soplo cardíaco ("murmur"), u otros problemas? Si este es el caso ¿cuáles tratamientos ha recibido para estos problemas?
- ¿Cuáles son sus antecedentes de salud y su estado general de salud? ¿Qué otros problemas de salud tiene? ¿Qué tratamientos está recibiendo para estos problemas? ¿Tiene restricciones en su alimentación, actividades o programa de ejercicios? ¿Existen otros miembros de su familia que tienen problemas del corazón?
- ¿Cuáles son los detalles sobre su estilo de vida, y sus rutinas diarias? ¿Qué hace para prevenir problemas de la salud?
- ¿Bebe alcohol (licor), fuma, o consume drogas ilegales?

Trate de ser honesto al proporcionar esta información a su médico o enfermera. Recuerde que esta información es confidencial y no se le dará a nadie más. La evaluación, tratamiento y control de la condición dependen de esta información. Existen ciertos detalles que sólo usted y sus familiares le pueden proporcioner al médico.

Una cuidadosa entrevista para obtener el historial médico de familias, una radiografía de pecho, un examen físico y un electrocardiograma también ayudarán a diagnosticar correctamente la insuficiencia cardíaca.

Además de la información obtenida de los síntomas específicos y los resultados de los exámenes de evaluación iniciales, también será necesario realizar otro examen que mide la cantidad de sangre que bombea el corazón con cada latido (conocido como examen de fracción de eyección). Cuando se cree que el paciente tiene insuficiencia cardíaca, también se realizará una ecocardiografía o una ventriculografía radionúclida para medir la fracción de eyección.

*continúa*

continuación

- **Ecocardiografía.** Se usan ondas de sonido (sonograma) para producir imágenes de las cavidades cardíacas. El examen no tiene peligros y no es necesario introducir instrumentos al cuerpo.
- **Ventriculografía radionúclida.** En este examen, se introduce una sustancia de contraste (tinte) radioactiva para obtener imágenes del corazón conforme ésta circula en las diversas cavidades cardíacas. La sustancia radioactiva no es peligrosa y se elimina completamente después del examen.

Como ya dijimos, con cada latido el corazón sano bombea el 50 por ciento o más de la sangre que se encuentra en el ventrículo izquierdo. Cuando existe insuficiencia cardíaca, el corazón debilitado sólo puede bombear el 40 por ciento, o menos, de la sangre al resto del cuerpo.

## EL CONTROL DE LA INSUFICIENCIA CARDÍACA

Para controlar la insuficiencia cardíaca, el paciente tiene que seguir cuidadosamente las instrucciones y recomendaciones de su médico. Se pueden aliviar los síntomas y mejorar la calidad de vida con el uso de medicamentos y ciertos cambios en la rutina de vida.

Coopere con su médico y enfermera para tomar las decisiones más adecuadas en cuanto a su tratamiento y para definir ciertas metas que le puedan ayudar a mantener una vida plena.

El plan de control de su condición incluye

- medicamentos
- dieta
- actividades diarias
- ejercicio
- hábitos y estilo de vida
- apoyo de familiares

Si usted no está de acuerdo con las recomendaciones de tratamiento o los medicamentos, tiene que hablar con el médico sobre sus razones y cooperar con él para encontrar alternativas.

Coopere con el médico para aprender a controlar su condión.

### Medicamentos

*Su importancia*

Tomar los medicamentos indicados es una parte importante del tratamiento de la insuficiencia cardíaca. Dependiendo de sus síntomas y diagnóstico, es probable que el médico inicie el

*continúa*

continuación

tratamiento con un medicamento y que agregue otros con el tiempo. A veces, el tratamiento se iniciará con el uso de dos o más medicamentos.

Pueden pasar varios días o semanas antes de encontrar medicamentos o dosis (cantidades) adecuados en su caso. Sea paciente y coopere con su médico para encontrar

- los medicamentos adecuados
- las dosis adecuadas de cada medicamento
- la mejor hora del día para tomar cada medicamento

Los beneficios de cada medicamento se perderán o serán menores si usted no los toma exactamente como lo indique el médico. No tomar una de las dosis, o no comprar más medicamentos cuando se acaben, puede resultar en problemas muy serios. También es importante que no tome mayores dosis de las que le indiquen.

Asegúrese de informar al médico sobre otros problemas de salud y los medicamentos que toma para éstos.

Informe al médico si toma medicamentos sin receta, tales como la aspirina, los antiácidos y los medicamentos para el resfrío. También infórmele de otros remedios que tome, para asegurarse que no hay problemas con el uso combinado de éstos y sus nuevos medicamentos.

### *Efectos secundarios*

Cualquier medicamento puede tener efectos no deseados. Si los medicamentos que toma para su condición le causan cualquier efecto secundario, es importante que se lo diga al médico o la enfermera de inmediato. Ellos le pueden ayudar a evitar o aliviar los efectos molestos. Si los medicamentos que le recetan inicialmente no son eficaces, existen otras alternativas.

Pregunte al médico o a la enfermera sobre los efectos secundarios que pueden resultar al consumir sus medicamentos y

- tomar medicamentos recetados por un médico para otras enfermedades o problemas de salud
- tomar medicamento que compra sin receta médica, tales como la aspirina, los antiácidos, los medicamentos para el resfrió y otros remedios
- comer ciertos alimentos

Siempre informe de inmediato al médico o a la enfermera sobre los efectos secundarios.

*continúa*

continuación

## *Los medicamentos comunes en el tratamiento de la condición*

Los medicamentos más comunes en el tratamiento de la insuficiencia cardíaca incluyen los siguientes:

- **Inhibidores de la enzima convertidora ("ACE inhibitors")** se usan para permitir que el corazón lata con menor dificultad.
- **Diuréticos** se usan para desechar el exceso de líquidos y sales que se acumulan en el cuerpo.
- **Digitales ("digitalis")** se usan para fortalecer los latidos del corazón y permitir un mayor flujo de sangre.

Cuando existen otros problemas de salud o del corazón además de la insuficiencia cardíaca, es probable que su médico le recete otros medicamentos tales como aquellos para controlar la alta presión sanguínea.

**Inhibidores de la enzima convertidora.** Se ha comprobado que estos medicamentos permiten que los pacientes que padecen de insuficiencia cardíaca vivan mejor y por más tiempo. Los inhibidores relajan los vasos sanguíneos y ayudan a mejorar el latido del corazón. Algunos pacientes tienen que esperar varias semanas antes de sentir los beneficios.

Dependiendo de su diagnóstico y evaluación iniciales, es posible que estos medicamentos sean los primeros que se le receten. Dependiendo de sus síntomas, es posible que le receten diuréticos y digitales al mismo tiempo, o que se agreguen más tarde.

Los inhibidores de la enzima convertidora que se usan en el tratamiento de la insuficiencia cardíaca son el captopril, enalapril, lisinopril y quinapril. Probablemente en el futuro se usarán otros medicamentos de este tipo para la insuficiencia cardíaca.

La mayoría de los pacientes no sufren problemas cuando toman estos medicamentos. Cuando se presentan problemas, los más comunes incluyen

- tos
- mareo
- irritaciones de la piel

Si presenta cualquiera de estos síntomas, repórtelo a su médico o enfermera.

Estos medicamentos también pueden producir altos niveles de potasio y afectar la función renal (de los riñones). Para vigilar estos problemas, es necesario realizar exámenes de la sangre.

*continúa*

continuación

**Diuréticos.** Al hacer que orine con más frecuencia, los diuréticos ayudan a eliminar los líquidos que se pueden acumular en los pies, tobillos, piernas o abdomen (estómago). El olvidar tomar una de las dosis de estos medicamentos puede causar hinchazón de estas partes del cuerpo o falta de aliento cuando se acueste o realice actividades físicas.

Los diuréticos de uso más común son la hidroclorotiazida y la furosemida (Lasix).

El uso prolongado de diuréticos puede resultar en que el cuerpo pierda potasio y causar otros problemas. Para vigilar los niveles de estas sustancias es necesario realizar análisis de sangre.

Para reemplazar el potasio en el cuerpo es probable que le recomienden:

- Comer más alimentos ricos en potasio, como los plátanos (guineos), las pasas, el jugo de naranja y otros cítricos.
- Tomar suplementos de potasio.

Los diuréticos también pueden causar:

- calambres (contracciones) en las piernas
- mareos
- incontinencia urinaria (perder orina involuntariamente)
- gota (un tipo de artritis)
- irritaciones de la piel

Hable con su médico o enfermera si presenta cualquiera de estos síntomas. El orinar más frecuentemente es el efecto deseado, así es que no tiene que reportarlo al médico.

**Digitales.** Los digitales mejoran el latido del corazón y pueden ayudarle a realizar mayor esfuerzo físico y ejercicio. Muchos pacientes con condiciones cardíacas toman digitales diariamente, recetados bajo los nombres comerciales de Digoxina o Lanoxina.

Los digitales generalmente no son peligrosos, pero si un paciente tiene demasiado en su sangre, puede presentar

- náusea, pérdida del apetito
- confusión mental
- visión nublada o amarillenta
- latidos del corazón fuertes o acelerados (palpitaciones)

Hable con su médico inmediatamente si presenta cualquiera de estos efectos secundarios, pero no deje de tomarlos a menos que así lo indique el médico.

*continúa*

continuación

### Vigilar el uso de sus medicamentos

Si toma varios medicamentos a diferentes horas del día, el mantener una lista de su uso puede ayudarle a seguir su tratamiento. Use la tabla al final de esta guía para recordarle

- cuáles medicamentos tomar diariamente
- la apariencia de cada pastilla o píldora que debe tomar
- cuándo tomar cada medicamento
- los medicamentos que ya ha tomado

Saque copias de la tabla para poder usarla muchas veces.

Siempre lleve consigo una lista de la dosis y los medicamentos que toma.

En caso de emergencia, esta información puede ayudar mucho a los médicos a cargo de su cuidado.

### Costo de los medicamentos

El costo de los medicamentos varía significativamente de una farmacia a otra. Si el costo de sus medicamentos es demasiado para usted, pida a su médico o farmacéutico que le ayude a encontrar medicamentos de marca genérica adecuados y a menor costo. También puede comparar los precios entre farmacias e incluso ordenar sus medicamentos a través del correo.

Si es necesario, puede obtener ayuda financiera a través de las agencias de servicios sociales en su comunidad. Probablemente, también podría reunir los requisitos necesarios para obtener ayuda a través de los programas de las compañías farmacéuticas.

Hable con el médico o la enfermera si tiene problemas para cubrir el costo de sus medicamentos. Ellos le pueden ayudar a solicitar la ayuda necesaria.

### Dieta

Además de tomar medicamentos, deberá hacer cambios y vigilar su alimentación. Debido a que la sal (sodio) causa acumulación de líquidos en el cuerpo, deberá de reducir el consumo de ésta. Si no lo hace, los líquidos se acumularán y causarán hinchazón en sus pies, tobillos, piernas y abdomen. También le pueden causar problemas para respirar. Si estos síntomas llegan a ser severos, es probable que necesite recibir atención médica en el hospital.

*continúa*

continuación

El médico le dirá cuál es la cantidad adecuada de sal que puede consumir, o si no puede consumirla. Probablemente le enviarían a consultar a un especialista en dietética (alimentación), una enfermera, u otro especialista que le dará las instrucciones necesarias en cuanto a su dieta. Probablemente le ayudarán a encontrar nuevas formas de cocinar los alimentos o a modificar las recetas de la familia. Por ejemplo, el uso del jugo de limón y otros condimentos y hierbas de olor puede reemplazar la sal en muchos alimentos.

Tiene que prestar atención especial a aquellos alimentos que tienen altos contenidos de sodio o sal, tales como las comidas de lata o congeladas, los quesos, y las carnes frías (embutidos). Ejemplos específicos de este tipo de alimentos son los embutidos como las salchichas y los chorizos, las sopas de lata y las papas y tortillas fritas. Lea las etiquetas de los ingredientes de los alimentos y busque el contenido de sal o sodio.

Si consume bebidas alcohólicas, es probable que tenga que dejar de hacerlo, o que sólo pueda tomar una ración al día. Una ración al día quiere decir un vaso de vino o cerveza, o sólo un trago de una bebida mixta con un contenido de alcohol no mayor de una onza.

Cambiar sus hábitos alimenticios puede ser complicado. La meta es reducir el contenido de sodio o sal y grasas en su alimentación, y al mismo tiempo tratar de mantener el mejor sabor. Si encuentra difícil cambiar su alimentación, hable con el médico o la especialista en dietética.

Vigile su peso. Para hacer esto debe comprar una báscula precisa y usarla al despertar después de orinar pero antes de desayunar o vestirse.

Si sube entre tres y cinco libras (uno kilo y medio a cuatro kilos) desde su última visita al médico, repórtelo de inmediato. Este aumento de peso puede indicar que su cuerpo está reteniendo líquidos.

### Actividades diarias

Puede ser que tenga que cambiar su estilo de vida y sus hábitos para mantener la salud.

La insuficiencia cardíaca afectará su vida diaria dependiendo de su severidad. La insuficiencia le puede afectar poco su trabajo y sus actividades recreativas. La insuficiencia severa, por otra parte, puede hacer que el paciente tenga que cambiar actividades diarias que antes le eran sencillas. Hable con el médico y la enfermera sobre:

- **Trabajo.** ¿Puede seguir trabajando de tiempo completo o de medio tiempo?
- **Actividades recreativas.** ¿Puede seguir haciendo ejercicio, caminar, o practicar deportes?
- **Pasatiempos.** ¿Puede viajar, trabajar en su jardín, o realizar actividades voluntarias para su iglesia?
- **Sexo.** ¿Puede tener relaciones sexuales?

*continúa*

continuación

Hable sobre sus actividades diarias con sus familiares ya que ellos le pueden dar apoyo y ayuda. Esto es de importancia especial cuando sus actividades tienen que cambiar con el tiempo. Ciertas actividades (como el trabajo y las actividades recreativas) pueden hacerse más difíciles conforme pasa el tiempo, mientras que la dificultad de otras actividades no cambia.

No tema hablar sobre aspectos privados de su vida. Es importante que el médico y la enfermera sepan lo más posible de su rutina diaria, para ayudarle a aliviar o reducir los síntomas y mejorar su calidad de vida.

Conforme aprenda más sobre su condición, probablemente encontrará nuevas satisfacciones y placeres en su vida. Los cambios a las rutinas de la vida diaria pueden ser positivos e interesantes. Al tener que reducir su carga de trabajo, probablemente encontrará nuevas actividades recreativas. Probablemente los pasatiempos se convertirán en una parte importante de su vida diaria. Las relaciones sexuales también pueden ser muy satisfactorias al explorar nuevas, y menos difíciles, formas de compartir el amor físico.

### Ejercicio

Realice ejercicio físico de acuerdo a las recomendaciones y limitaciones que le indique el médico. Muchos pacientes que padecen de insuficiencia cardíaca afirman que se sienten mejor cuando realizan ejercicio físico regularmente. Puede realizar ejercicio sin peligro en casa, en un centro de rehabilitación como el hospital, o en un club de ejercicio, un centro recreativo, la YMCA, o la YWCA.

Los ejercicios físicos incluyen

- caminar
- andar en bicicleta
- nadar
- ejercicios aeróbicos de bajo impacto

El médico le indicará el tipo y cantidad de ejercicio adecuado en su caso. Es importante consultarle antes de iniciar el programa de ejercicio. Probablemente le enviarán a visitar a un especialista en rehabilitación cardíaca, quien le ayudará a diseñar un plan de ejercicio y a vigilar sus resultados y efectos. Probablemente también será necesario que le realicen un examen de tolerancia al esfuerzo ("stress test") para determinar los límites de ejercicio físico que puede realizar sin correr peligro.

*continúa*

continuación

## Estilo de vida y los hábitos para mantener la salud

Su estilo de vida es el resultado de sus valores y sus creencias. Los hábitos para mantener la salud son aquellos que le ayudan a prevenir las probabilidades de padecer de enfermedades o de sufrir lesiones. Cuando una persona padece de insuficiencia cardíaca, probablemente tendrá que cambiar su estilo de vida y modificar sus hábitos para mantener la salud.

Los siguientes cambios le pueden ayudar a reducir los síntomas de la insuficiencia cardíaca y a mejorar su calidad de vida:

- Si pesa demasiado, tiene que reducir su peso.
- No fume o mastique tabaco.
- Elimine o reduzca su consumo de bebidas alcohólicas.
- No consuma drogas ilegales.

También:

- Evite realizar ejercicio que exceda las recomendaciones de su médico.
- Evite estar en contacto con personas que tienen resfriados.
- Vacúnese regularmente contra la pulmonía y la influenza ("flu").

Probablemente también le ayudará el hacer ciertos cambios como el reducir el nivel de tensión emocional. Hable con su médico y enfermera sobre otros cambios que le pueden ayudar a mejorar su calidad de vida.

## Apoyo de su familia

Su familia puede ser una fuente de apoyo. En cuanto sea posible, inclúyalos en todas las decisiones que afectarán su vida. Estas decisiones probablemente tendrán impacto en su estilo de vida y en su capacidad de trabajar y ganar dinero. El apoyo de la familia puede ser de importancia especial cuando se tienen que realizar cambios y el paciente enfrenta dificultades emocionales. Dígale a sus familiares cómo le pueden ayudar, por ejemplo:

- a administrar y vigilar el uso de los medicamentos
- a preparar alimentos especiales
- a realizar ejercicio
- a obtener información útil en cuanto al tratamiento y control de la insuficiencia cardíaca (especialmente si usted no habla inglés)
- a participar en grupos de apoyo

*continúa*

continuación

El diagnóstico de insuficiencia cardíaca tiene un impacto fuerte en el paciente y su familia. El apoyo de sus familiares es una parte importante para ayudar al paciente a realizar los cambios necesarios en su estilo de vida y modificar sus hábitos para mantener la salud.

## ANGINA (DOLOR) DE PECHO

Además de tener síntomas de insuficiencia cardíaca algunos pacientes también sienten dolor o angina de pecho. La angina de pecho causa dolor debido a obstrucciones o estrechamientos de las arterias coronarias. Cuando éste es el caso, es probable que sea necesario realizar un examen médico conocido como angiografía cardíaca (se introduce un catéter o tubo hasta el corazón para observarlo).

Durante la angiografía se introduce una sustancia a través del catéter y se toman rayos-x que muestran el grado de obstrucción de las coronarias. Antes de someterse a este examen, hable con el médico o la enfermera sobre sus beneficios y posibles desventajas.

Los resultados de la angiografía ayudan al médico y otros especialistas a diseñar un plan de tratamiento que puede incluir una operación. Si el paciente no quiere someterse a la cirugía, la angiografía no es necesaria. Nuevamente, es importante que hable con el médico sobre las posibles alternativas de tratamiento disponibles, de acuerdo a los resultados de los exámenes de evaluación.

## CIRUGÍA DEL CORAZÓN

Si el médico cree que su insuficiencia cardíaca es el resultado de algún problema con las válvulas o arterias del corazón, es probable que recomiende una cirugía. Antes de aceptar esta alternativa, tiene que considerar toda la información disponible y los resultados posibles. Debe hablar con el médico sobre los siguientes aspectos:

- beneficios
- desventajas, incluyendo la posibilidad que no dé resultados
- otras alternativas, y los beneficios y desventajas de éstas
- el costo total, y cuánto pagará su compañía de seguro de salud

Antes de decidir someterse a la cirugía, busque una segunda opinión de otro médico. Por lo general, las compañías de seguro de la salud exigen que el paciente tenga una segunda opinión médica antes de aceptar cubrir los costos de este procedimiento.

*continúa*

continuación

Si la cirugía del corazón es una opción adecuada en su caso, es importante que busque un cirujano y hospital con amplia experiencia en este tipo de cirugía. Pregunte en cuanto a sus índices de éxito al realizar estas cirugías y hable de los costos antes de elegir el hospital y al cirujano.

### Cirugía valvular cardíaca

Cuando existen problemas valvulares, puede ser necesario reparar o reemplazar una o varias válvulas del corazón. Este tipo de cirugía es bastante común y es eficaz en la mayoría de los casos.

### Cirugía de puente coronario ("bypass") y angioplastia

La cirugía de puente coronario es una cirugía mayor. Durante esta operación se utilizan trozos (injertos) de otras venas o arterias del cuerpo para crear un "puente" de paso para que la sangre pueda irrigar al músculo del corazón. La cirugía corrige obstruccions en las arterias que proveen de sangre al corazón que, como cualquier otro músculo, necesita oxígeno para funcionar y bombear sangre.

La angioplastia es una alternativa a la cirugía de puente coronario ("percutaneous transluminal coronary angioplasty"). Durante este procedimiento, se inserta un catéter (tubo delgado) a través de una arteria y hasta el corazón. Al llegar al área de la obstrucción, se infla un globo en la punta del catéter. El globo expande la arteria coronaria y, al retirarlo, permite una mejor circulación de la sangre.

La investigación científica reciente indica que la cirugía de puente coronario puede ayudar a los pacientes que han empeorado y tienen insuficiencia cardíaca y angina de pecho causada por enfermedades de las coronarias. Sin embargo, aún no se han comprobado los beneficios a largo plazo del uso de la angioplastia.

Después de someterse a la cirugía, el paciente tiene que seguir un cuidadoso programa para vigilar y controlar su condición cardíaca.

### Cirugía de transplante de corazón

Los transplantes de corazón sólo se consideran en los casos en los que la insuficiencia cardíaca es muy grave. Los transplantes de corazón sólo se realizan en centros especializados en este tipo de cirugía.

continuación

## VIGILAR SU PROGRESO

Para controlar la insuficiencia cardíaca es necesaria una cuidadosa observación de los síntomas y los efectos de los tratamientos. Seguir las instrucciones del médico y otros especialistas también permite proveer el mejor cuidado. Reporte cualquier cambio en su condición a su médico o enfermera.

### Las responsabilidades del paciente

Como un miembro del grupo a cargo de su atención médica, tiene que hacer lo siguiente:

- vigilar su estado de salud en general y reportar al médico cualquier cambio
- reportar cualquier cambio en sus síntomas
- tomar los medicamentos siguiendo las indicaciones, y reportar cualquier efecto secundario
- seguir las recomendaciones de los especialistas en ejercicio y reportar cuando tenga dificultad para hacer cualquier actividad o ejercicio
- seguir las recomendaciones en cuanto a su alimentación (dieta)
- reportar al médico cuando tenga cambios súbitos de peso

### Las responsabilidades de la familia

La familia puede ayudar al paciente a seguir las recomendaciones para controlar y vigilar su condición. Ellos también deben saber y ayudarle a reportar al médico los cambios en los síntomas o cuando se presentan nuevos síntomas. Esto es especialmente importante si usted no habla inglés y alguien en su familia le ayuda en sus conversaciones con los médicos y las enfermeras.

Al llamar al médico u otro especialista, sus familiares deben

- indicar que está recibiendo tratamiento para la insuficiencia cardíaca
- describir sus síntomas
- describir lo que ya se ha hecho para brindarle alivio
- dar los nombres y las dosis de los medicamentos que está tomando

## EL FUTURO

Hable con su médico de cabecera sobre la manera en la que la insuficiencia cardíaca afectará su vida. Muchos pacientes aprenden a disfrutar de la vida a pesar de las limitaciones que impone el padecer de esta condición.

continúa

continuación

A pesar que no es común que el paciente presente cambios súbitos en sus síntomas, existen ciertas actividades que ya no podrá realizar debido a que se cansa o le falta el aliento (aire). Si nota un cambio súbito en sus síntomas, es importante que lo reporte al médico de inmediato.

## Emergencias

En caso que se presente una emergencia médica, tal como que deje de respirar o que haya un paro del corazón, se asume que el paciente acepta el tratamiento médico. En los Estados Unidos existen ciertas alternativas legales en cuanto al tratamiento médico. Estas decisiones son derechos de cada individuo. Si usted siente que necesita ayuda para tomarlas, puede hablar con un familiar, un sacerdote, un miembro del clero o un consejero. Recuerde, ésta es una decisión solamente suya; lo puede hacer o no hacer. Usted tiene el derecho de rehusar o aceptar los tratamientos médicos antes de que éstos sean necesarios debido a una emergencia. Puede aclarar en un documento legal que usted no quiere que los técnicos de emergencia traten de volver a hacer que lata el corazón o que le coloquen una máquina especial que restaure la respiración.

Puede ser necesario que dé instrucciones específicas a sus familiares y otras personas para que sepan por adelantado cuáles son sus deseos en el caso de una emergencia. En los Estados Unidos existe un documento legal conocido como "instrucciones de cuidado médico" ("advance directive") que especifica sus deseos en caso de una emergencia. El documento especifica las medidas y tratamientos que usted aprueba y no aprueba en caso que durante la emergencia usted no pueda pensar o hablar claramente.

Las instrucciones de cuidado médico incluyen varios documentos:

- "testamento en vida" ("living will"), que especifica sus deseos en caso de una emergencia médica, incapacitación severa, o enfermedad crónica
- agente de poder en caso de emergencia médica ("medical durable power of attorney"), que da poder legal a un pariente o amigo a que se encargue de ejecutar y autorizar sus deseos en cuanto a su cuidado médico

Antes de preparar este tipo de documento, si usted decide que lo quiere hacer, debe hablar con sus familiares y profesionales a cargo de su cuidado médico. Estas son decisiones serias y su grupo de cuidado médico le podrá ayudar a entender las consecuencias de estas decisiones. Hable con ellos y sus abogados en cuanto a estos documentos y las variaciones que existen de acuerdo a las leyes de su estado o comunidad (en los Estados Unidos).

*continúa*

continuación

## Grupos de apoyo y consejería

El diagnóstico de una enfermedad crónica como la insuficiencia cardíaca tiene un efecto emocional tanto en el paciente como en su familia. Es importante que discuta estas reacciones con su médico y otros profesionales a cargo de su cuidado de salud. Si es necesario, debe buscar ayuda para poder controlar estas emociones.

Además de los servicios profesionales de consejería, los grupos de apoyo en su localidad pueden ser de ayuda. El hablar en reuniones regulares con las familias y pacientes que tienen esta condición le será útil. Los grupos de apoyo probablemente también ofrecen programas educativos sobre las condiciones cardíacas.

Hable con su médico o enfermera sobre los grupos de apoyo, los servicios disponibles en español y otras fuentes de ayuda. Con la ayuda de su médico o enfermera usted mismo puede iniciar un grupo de apoyo.

Para obtener más información, consulte a:

**The Mended Hearts, Inc.**
7272 Greenville Avenue
Dallas, TX 75231
(214) 706-1442

**The Coronary Club, Inc.**
9500 Euclid Avenue, E-37
Cleveland, OH 44195
(216) 444-3690

Recuerde preguntar si cuentan con servicios en español.

## CÓMO USAR LA TABLA PARA ANOTAR EL USO DE MEDICAMENTOS

Use la siguiente tabla para anotar y vigilar el uso de medicamentos. Anote los medicamentos que toma cada día, la hora a la que los toma, y cuándo los ha tomado.

En la parte superior de la hoja, escriba su nombre y la fecha, empezando con el domingo.

Cada línea numerada es para un medicamento. En la primera columna, escriba el nombre y la dosis (cantidad) de cada medicamento, por ejemplo: **Lanoxin .25 mg.** Puede encontrar el nombre y dosis del medicamento en la etiqueta del frasco que le dan en la farmacia.

En la segunda columna, escriba el tamaño, forma y color de la pastilla (píldora), por ejemplo: **Antes de desayunar.**

Cuando ha tomado el medicamento, marque una × en la columna que corresponde al día de la semana. Si toma un medicamento varias veces al día, marque cada vez que lo haya tomado.

Haga copias de esta tabla para que la pueda usar cada semana.

*continúa*

continuación

# Tabla semanal de uso de medicamentos

Su nombre _____

Semana del _____

| Nombre y dosis del medicamento | Tamaño, forma y color del medicamento | Cuándo tomarlo | Marque con una ☒ en el día correspondiente cada vez que tome el medicamento | | | | | | |
|---|---|---|---|---|---|---|---|---|---|
| | | | Dom | Lun | Mar | Miér | Jue | Vier | Sáb |
| 1 | | | | | | | | | |
| 2 | | | | | | | | | |
| 3 | | | | | | | | | |
| 4 | | | | | | | | | |

Source: "La Insuficiencia Cardiaca," Agency for Health Care Policy and Research, U.S. Department of Health and Human Services, AHCPR Publication No. 94-0615, June 1994.

# Pulmonary Edema

## WHAT IS PULMONARY EDEMA?

- It is abnormal accumulation of fluid that results when the heart cannot pump enough blood from the lungs to the rest of the body.
- Fluid from the small blood vessels of the lungs rapidly oozes from the vessels into the lungs.
- It typically occurs at night, after lying down for several hours.

## POSSIBLE CAUSES

- Heart failure (most common)
- Kidney failure
- Intravenous fluid overload
- Intravenous drug overdose
- Drowning

## SIGNS AND SYMPTOMS

Symptoms usually begin after lying down for a few hours.

### First Stage

- Persistent cough
- Slight shortness of breath
- Restlessness
- Anxiety

### Later Stage

- Extreme shortness of breath
- Noisy, moist respirations
- Cough with frothy, pink-tinged sputum
- Profuse perspiration
- Rapid heart rate
- Gray complexion
- Extreme anxiety

### Acute Stage

- Decreased level of consciousness
- Shock (blood pressure drops, and person may lose consciousness)

## PREVENTING PULMONARY EDEMA

- Follow activity as ordered, with planned rest periods.
- Restrict sodium.
- Weigh yourself daily for early detection of fluid retention.
- Sleep with head of bed elevated (place head of bed on ten-inch blocks).
- Avoid people with upper respiratory infections.
- Notify doctor if the following symptoms occur:
  - change in sputum characteristics
  - decreased activity tolerance
  - increased cough or chest fullness
  - noisy, moist breathing
  - swelling of lower extremities

## IF PULMONARY EDEMA OCCURS

- Call an ambulance and notify physician. (Have the emergency numbers next to the phone.)
- Sit with head and shoulders up and feet down to favor pooling of the blood to lower dependent portions of the body.
- Do not panic. (Family members should provide emotional support to decrease anxiety.)

## POSSIBLE COMPLICATIONS

- Respiratory failure
- Cardiac arrest

Source: Donna Meyers, *Client Teaching Guides for Home Health Care,* Aspen Publishers, Inc., © 1989.

# Thrombophlebitis

## WHAT IS THROMBOPHLEBITIS?

- It is an inflammation of the vein with a clot formation.
- It occurs most often in the veins of the legs but may also occur in other areas of the body.

## RISK FACTORS

- Long periods of immobility or lack of position changes
- Oral contraceptives
- Trauma
- Varicose veins or other vascular problems
- Intravenous therapy
- Advancing age
- Cardiac disease
- Cigarette smoking
- Obesity
- Surgery

## SIGNS AND SYMPTOMS

### Superficial Thrombophlebitis

- Increased firmness of the vein
- Redness and warmth along the vein
- Tenderness
- Fever
- Swelling

### Deep Vein Thrombosis

(NOTE: may not have any symptoms)

- Cramping leg pain aggravated by movement
- Increased warmth of the skin
- Fever
- Tenderness
- Edema
- Pain upon straightening or extending toes

## PREVENTING AND MANAGING THROMBOPHLEBITIS

- Promote good circulation
  - Avoid constrictive clothing (garters, girdles, etc.).
  - Avoid smoking (constricts blood vessels).
  - Avoid crossing legs and sitting for long periods.
  - Exercise regularly.
  - Wear support hose when standing for long periods.
  - Elevate legs periodically.
- Avoid oral contraceptives.
- Eat a well-balanced diet (calcium, vitamin E, and vitamin K all affect the clotting mechanism).
- Achieve and maintain ideal weight.
- Follow postoperative teaching
  - early ambulation
  - passive and active exercise
  - deep breathing exercise

## TREATMENTS

- Pain relief
  - warm, moist heat to affected area as ordered
  - analgesics as ordered
- Anticoagulant medications to thin the blood as ordered
- Bed rest or activity as instructed
- Prevention of emboli
  - fluids increased to at least six to eight glasses per day
  - massaging of affected part avoided
- Anti-embolism stockings

## POSSIBLE COMPLICATIONS

- Pulmonary embolism (blood clot to the lung)
- Stroke (blood clot to the brain)

Source: Donna Meyers, *Client Teaching Guides for Home Health Care,* Aspen Publishers, Inc., © 1989.

# Pulmonary Embolism

## WHAT IS A PULMONARY EMBOLISM?

- It is a blood clot lodged in the artery of a lung.
- The blood clot blocks blood flow to a portion of the lung.
- Without adequate blood supply, the lung cannot function properly, and lung tissue may be destroyed.

## RISK FACTORS

- Immobility
- Fractures and injury
- Advanced age
- Obesity
- Pregnancy
- Recent surgery
- Vascular disease
- Estrogen therapy
- Certain diseases (for example, diabetes, chronic obstructive pulmonary disease, and heart disease)

## SIGNS AND SYMPTOMS

### Medium-Size

- Chest pain
- Shortness of breath
- Cough with blood-tinged sputum
- Rapid heart rate
- Slight fever
- Perspiration
- Apprehension

### Massive

- Pallor
- Severe shortness of breath
- Crushing chest pain
- Shock (blood pressure drops, and client may lose consciousness)

## MEASURES TO PREVENT PULMONARY EMBOLISM

- Promote good circulation:
  - Exercise regularly, especially leg exercises.
  - Elevate legs 30 degrees or more when sitting.
  - Wear anti-embolism stockings.
  - Avoid crossing legs or sitting for long periods of time.
  - Avoid constrictive clothing.
  - Stop smoking (constricts blood vessels).
- Increase fluid intake to at least six to eight glasses per day.
- Take medication as prescribed.
- Follow general safety precautions to prevent injury (good lighting, handrails, etc.).
- Avoid laxatives because they affect vitamin K absorption.

## POSSIBLE COMPLICATIONS

- Pulmonary infarction (death of lung tissue)
- Pulmonary hypertension
- Heart failure
- Collapse of a lung

Source: Donna Meyers, *Client Teaching Guides for Home Health Care,* Aspen Publishers, Inc., © 1989.

# Recovering from Heart Problems through Cardiac Rehabilitation

## THE KEYS TO HEART HEALTH

**Exercise:** Regular physical activity that is tailored to your abilities, needs, and interests.

**Education:** Learning about your heart problem, its causes and treatments, and how you can manage it.

**Counseling:** Advice on why and how to change your lifestyle to lower your risk of further heart problems.

**Behavior change:** Learning specific skills to enable you to stop unhealthy behaviors such as smoking or to begin healthy behaviors such as eating a heart-healthy diet.

## PURPOSE OF CARDIAC REHABILITATION

Cardiac rehabilitation (rehab) services are designed to help patients with heart disease recover faster and return to full and productive lives. Cardiac rehab includes exercise, education, counseling, and learning ways to live a healthier life. Together with medical and surgical treatments, cardiac rehab can help you feel better and live a healthier life.

You can benefit from cardiac rehab if you:

- have heart disease, such as angina or heart failure, or have had a heart attack
- have had coronary bypass surgery or a balloon catheter (PTCA) procedure on your heart
- have had a heart transplant

Cardiac rehab can make a difference. It is a safe and effective way to help you:

- feel better faster
- get stronger
- reduce stress
- reduce the risks of future heart problems
- live longer

Almost everyone with heart disease can benefit from some type of cardiac rehab. No one is too old or too young. Women benefit from cardiac rehab as much as men. This handout can help you learn how to lower your risk for future heart problems. You will also learn tips for finding a cardiac rehab plan that is right for you. Most important, you will learn what you can do to be healthier.

*continues*

continued

When you have heart disease, breaking old habits and learning new ones can be stressful. Wondering about your future health can be stressful, too. But the support of family and friends, as well as health care providers, can make a big difference in how well you adjust to these changes. Share this handout with others so they will learn about cardiac rehab and how they can help you.

## RISK FACTORS FOR CORONARY DISEASE

The controllable risk factors for coronary disease are shown below. There are some risk factors that you cannot change, such as older age or a family history of heart disease. But you can change or control the ones shown below. Cardiac rehab can help you do this.

### Coronary Disease Risk Factors You Can Control

- Smoking
- High blood pressure
- High blood cholesterol
- Sedentary lifestyle
- Overweight
- Diabetes
- Stress

## THE CARDIAC REHAB TEAM

Cardiac rehab services can involve many health care providers. Your team may include:

- Doctors (your family doctor, a heart specialist, perhaps a surgeon)
- Nurses
- Exercise specialists
- Physical and occupational therapists
- Dietitians
- Psychologists or other behavior therapists

Sometimes a primary care provider, such as your family doctor or nurse practitioner, works alone playing many roles or refers you to other health care specialists as needed. But the most important member of your cardiac rehab team is you. No one else can make you exercise. Or quit smoking. Or eat a more healthful diet.

*continues*

continued

To be an active member of your cardiac rehab team

- Learn about your heart condition.
- Learn what you can do to help your heart.
- Follow the treatment plan.
- Feel free to ask questions.
- Report symptoms or problems.

## Support Networks

A support network can help you. Your support network may be family, friends, or a group of other people with heart problems.

Family members and friends can make a difference. They may want to learn more about heart problems so their help can be even more valuable. For example, family members may have to learn to let you do things for yourself. Or they may want to learn about preparing heart-healthy meals. Your family and friends can give you emotional support as you adjust to a new, healthier lifestyle.

You may also want the support of other people who have heart disease. Ask your cardiac rehab team if they know of a support group you can join.

## HOW DO I GET STARTED?

Cardiac rehab often begins in the hospital after a heart attack, heart surgery, or other heart treatment. It continues in an outpatient setting after you leave the hospital. Once you learn the habits of heart-healthy living, stick with them for life.

Outpatient rehab may be located at the hospital, in a medical or professional center, in a community facility such as the YMCA, or at your place of work. You may even have cardiac rehab at home. You will be advised to increase the amount of exercise you do. You will also receive education and encouragement to control your risk factors. After you have learned the skills of heart-healthy living, you should continue to use them for life.

You need your doctor's approval to get started in cardiac rehab. Tell your doctor or nurse that you're interested in cardiac rehab and ask which rehab services or plans are best for you.

*continues*

continued

## HOW DOES CARDIAC REHAB WORK?

Cardiac rehab has two major parts:

1. **Exercise training** to help you learn how to exercise safely, strengthen your muscles, and improve your stamina. Your exercise plan will be based on your individual ability, needs, and interests.
2. **Education, counseling, and training** to help you understand your heart condition and find ways to reduce your risk of future heart problems. The cardiac rehab team will help you learn how to cope with the stress of adjusting to a new lifestyle and to deal with your fears about the future.

Cardiac rehab often takes place in groups. However, each patient's plan is based on his or her specific risk factors and special needs. Cardiac rehab helps you recognize and change unhealthy habits you may have and establish new, more healthy ones. Your rehab may last 6 weeks, 6 months, or even longer. It is important that you complete the recommended rehab plan.

No matter how difficult it seems, your hard work in cardiac rehab will have lifetime benefits.

## IS IT SAFE FOR ME?

Cardiac rehab is safe. Studies show that serious health problems caused by cardiac rehab exercise are rare. The cardiac rehab team is trained to handle emergencies. Your health care provider can help you choose a plan that is safe for you. Many patients can safely exercise without supervision once they learn their own exercise plan.

Checking how your heart reacts and adapts to exercise is an important part of cardiac rehab. You may be connected to an EKG transmitter while you exercise. If your cardiac rehab is done at home, you may be connected to an EKG machine by telephone, or you may phone the cardiac rehab team to let them know how you are doing. In some settings, you check your own pulse rate or estimate how hard you are exercising.

## WHAT'S IN IT FOR ME?

The goals of cardiac rehab are different for each patient. In helping set your personal goals, your health care team will look at your general health, your personal heart problem, your risks for future heart problems, your doctor's recommendations, and, of course, your own preferences.

Cardiac rehab can reduce your symptoms and your chances of having more heart problems. And it has many other benefits:

*continues*

continued

- Exercise tones your muscles and improves your energy level and spirits. It helps both your heart and your body get stronger and work better. Exercise also can get you back to work and other activities faster.
- A healthy diet can lower blood cholesterol, control weight, and help prevent or control high blood pressure and other problems such as diabetes. Plus, you will feel better and have more energy.
- Cardiac rehab can help you quit smoking. Kicking the habit means less risk of lung cancer, emphysema, and bronchitis, as well as less risk of heart attack, stroke, and other heart and blood vessel problems. It means more energy, and it means better health for your loved ones.
- You can learn to manage stress instead of letting it manage you. You will feel better and improve your heart health.

Aerobic exercise raises your pulse rate and makes you perspire. It helps improve the flow of oxygen-rich blood throughout your body. Strength training, such as using weights, improves your muscle strength and your stamina. Both types of exercise in the right amount are safe and important for your heart health.

**Make a habit of the heart-healthy lifestyle you learn in cardiac rehab. Your life depends on it!**

## HOW DO I FIND A PLAN THAT'S RIGHT FOR ME?

Your doctor or nurse may recommend a cardiac rehab plan or help you to arrange for exercise training, education, counseling, and other services. Many hospitals and outpatient health care centers offer cardiac rehab—so do some local schools and community centers. You can also check the Yellow Pages of your telephone book.

When choosing a cardiac rehab plan, ask about:

- **Time.** Is it offered when you can get there without causing added stress? Cardiac rehab services offered at the workplace are sometimes an option.
- **Place.** Is it easy to get to? Keep in mind that traffic problems can add to your stress. Is there parking? Public transportation?
- **Setting.** Is it an individual or group plan? Is it home-based or in a facility? Think about whether you want to be in a group with professional supervision.
- **Services.** Does it offer a wide range of services? More importantly, does it include the areas you need help with, such as quitting smoking?
- **Cost.** Is it affordable? Is it covered by insurance? Your insurance may cover all or part of the cost of some cardiac rehab services but not others. Find out what will be covered and for how long. Consider what you can afford and for how long.

*continues*

continued

Cardiac rehab has life-long favorable effects, so choose a plan that will serve your needs. For example, if you smoke, look for a plan that will help you quit. Choose a plan that includes activities you enjoy, such as regular walking in a shopping mall or park. Before you sign up, visit and ask any questions you may have.

## HOW CAN I GET THE MOST OUT OF CARDIAC REHAB?

Studies show that controlling your risk factors for heart disease can help you lead a healthier life. So make sure your cardiac rehab plan works for you. Here's how:

- Plan. Work with your health care team to design or change your services to meet your needs.
- Communicate.
- Ask questions. If you don't understand the answers, keep asking until you do. Report changes in your feelings or symptoms.
- Take charge of your recovery. No one else can do it for you. Your new lifestyle is healthy for your heart, so stick with it—for life.

To gain more control over your cardiac rehab, remember your goals and keep important information where you can find it. You may want to have a special calendar just for your rehab activities or keep a notebook like the one shown below.

Sometimes people who have big changes in their lives feel depressed. Some people with heart problems feel depressed when they find out about their disease, or after surgery. Cardiac rehab may help you feel better, but if you are seriously depressed you will need additional help. When you are depressed, it is hard to do things to help yourself get better, such as going to cardiac rehab or getting back to your usual activities. If you are depressed, tell your doctor. Depression can be treated.

*continues*

continued

# SAMPLE NOTEBOOK

Schedule of Activities:

Activity: _____

When: _____

Where: _____

Activity: _____

When: _____

Where: _____

Activity: _____

When: _____

Where: _____

----------------------------------------------------------------

The name, phone number, and job of each person on the rehab team:

_____

_____

_____

_____

_____

_____

continued

## Questions and concerns to talk about with the program staff:

_____

_____

_____

_____

_____

_____

_____

## Goals for the week (include check marks showing which plans have been carried out and which goals have been reached):

[   ] _____

[   ] _____

[   ] _____

[   ] _____

[   ] _____

[   ] _____

[   ] _____

## Smaller successes (little steps I've taken to reach my larger goals):

[   ] _____

[   ] _____

[   ] _____

[   ] _____

[   ] _____

[   ] _____

[   ] _____

Source: "Recovering from Heart Problems through Cardiac Rehabilitation," Agency for Health Care Policy and Research, U.S. Department of Health and Human Services, AHCPR Publication No. 96–0674, October 1995.

# How To Take Your Pulse—Determining Heart Rate

Pulse (heart rate) is the number of times your heart beats per minute. A normal resting heart beats approximately 60 to 100 times per minute.

## FACTORS AFFECTING THE HEART RATE

- Women average five to ten beats per minute faster than men.
- Emotions, humidity, and exercise increase heart rate.
- The heart rate decreases with increasing age.
- The heart rate increases during and after eating.
- The heart rate increases as body temperature increases.
- A change from a lying position to a sitting position raises the heart rate.
- Do not become alarmed if the pulse goes above 100 beats per minute when affected by the above factors.
- The beating effect that you feel against the artery every time the heart forces blood into it is a pulse, which tells how fast or slow the heart is beating.

### The Radial Artery (on the thumb side of the wrist)

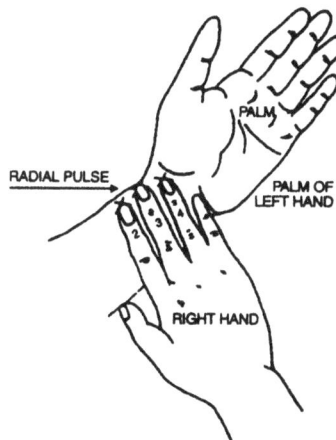

### TO TAKE YOUR RADIAL PULSE

1. Sit down and relax for five minutes before taking a resting pulse.
2. Gently place your second, third, and fourth fingers over the radial artery (on the thumb side) to feel a pulsation in your wrist. Never use your thumb to feel a pulse.
3. After locating the beat, count the number of beats for six seconds and then add a zero. Record your pulse rate.

Source: Annette R. Karnash, ed., *Focus on Geriatric Care and Rehabilitation,* 5:1, Aspen Publishers, Inc., © 1991.

# Target Zone Heart Rate

A target zone for your heart rate is one in which there is sufficient activity to condition the muscles and cardiovascular system to achieve fitness but not so much activity as to exceed safe limits.

- Determine the amount of exercise necessary to place you in the target zone by counting the heart rate **immediately** upon stopping the exercise (the rate changes very quickly when exercise slows up or stops).
- Each individual's target zone is between 60 percent and 80 percent of their own maximal aerobic power. Below 60 percent there is little benefit, and above 80 percent there is little added benefit. There is a point at which the heart and the circulation are no longer able to deliver more oxygen to the tissues and are unable to exercise longer or harder without becoming exhausted; the heart cannot beat any faster and the oxygen cannot be carried by the blood to the muscles fast enough to create energy for exercise. The 35 to 40 minutes of regular aerobic activity while the heart is in the target zone provide significant cardiovascular conditioning.

To obtain your range of target heart rates, first find your maximal heart rate by subtracting your age from 220 (male) or 226 (female). Subtract from the result your resting heart rate; then multiply by 60 percent to 70 percent, and add to that result your resting heart rate.

To find your minimum target heart rate for cardiovascular conditioning, fill in the blanks, subtract, multiply, and add as shown.

Your age: _____

Your resting heart rate: _____

Find your maximal heart rate:

220 (male) or 226 (female) – _____ = _____
                                            age       maximal
                                                  heart rate

Find your target rate:

_____ – _____ = _____ × .60 = _____ + _____ = _____
maximal      resting                                       resting      your
heart       heart                                         heart     target
rate        rate                                         rate      rate

*continues*

continued

## TARGET ZONE RANGE (using 60 as resting heart rate)

| | 60% | | 70% | |
|---|---|---|---|---|
| *Age* | *Male* | *Female* | *Male* | *Female* |
| 20 | 144 | 148 | 158 | 162 |
| 25 | 141 | 145 | 155 | 159 |
| 30 | 138 | 142 | 151 | 155 |
| 35 | 135 | 139 | 148 | 152 |
| 40 | 132 | 136 | 144 | 148 |
| 45 | 129 | 133 | 141 | 145 |
| 50 | 126 | 130 | 137 | 141 |
| 55 | 123 | 127 | 134 | 138 |
| 60 | 120 | 124 | 130 | 134 |
| 65 | 117 | 121 | 127 | 131 |
| 70 | 114 | 118 | 123 | 127 |
| 75 | 111 | 115 | 120 | 124 |
| 80 | 108 | 112 | 116 | 120 |
| 85 | 105 | 109 | 113 | 117 |

Source: Annette R. Karnash, ed., *Focus on Geriatric Care and Rehabilitation,* 5:1, Aspen Publishers, Inc., © 1991.

# Walking for Heart Health

The American way of life has changed the American way of fitness. Today, few jobs require regular or vigorous physical activity. Many Americans:

- Ride rather than walk.

- Use elevators instead of stairs.

- Sit at home rather than being physically active during free time.

Evidence suggests that even low- to moderate-intensity activities can have both short- and long-term benefits. If performed daily, they help lower your risk of heart disease. For inactive people, the trick is to get started.

Walking is an easy way to begin a physical activity program because it does not require special facilities or equipment other than well-made, comfortable shoes and a safe place to walk.

Below is a sample walking program. If you find a particular week's pattern tiring, repeat it before going on to the next pattern. You do not have to complete the walking program in 15 weeks. Use the walking log below to chart your progress.

*continues*

continued

| Sample Walking Program (3 sessions per week) | | | |
|---|---|---|---|
| | Warm Up | Exercise Period | Cool Down | Total |
| Week 1 | Walk slowly 5 minutes | Walk briskly 5 minutes | Walk slowly 5 minutes | 15 minutes |
| Week 2 | Walk slowly 5 minutes | Walk briskly 7 minutes | Walk slowly 5 minutes | 17 minutes |
| Week 3 | Walk slowly 5 minutes | Walk briskly 9 minutes | Walk slowly 5 minutes | 19 minutes |
| Week 4 | Walk slowly 5 minutes | Walk briskly 11 minutes | Walk slowly 5 minutes | 21 minutes |
| Week 5 | Walk slowly 5 minutes | Walk briskly 13 minutes | Walk slowly 5 minutes | 23 minutes |
| Week 6 | Walk slowly 5 minutes | Walk briskly 15 minutes | Walk slowly 5 minutes | 25 minutes |
| Week 7 | Walk slowly 5 minutes | Walk briskly 18 minutes | Walk slowly 5 minutes | 28 minutes |
| Week 8 | Walk slowly 5 minutes | Walk briskly 20 minutes | Walk slowly 5 minutes | 30 minutes |
| Week 9 | Walk slowly 5 minutes | Walk briskly 23 minutes | Walk slowly 5 minutes | 33 minutes |
| Week 10 | Walk slowly 5 minutes | Walk briskly 26 minutes | Walk slowly 5 minutes | 36 minutes |
| Week 11 | Walk slowly 5 minutes | Walk briskly 28 minutes | Walk slowly 5 minutes | 38 minutes |
| Week 12 | Walk slowly 5 minutes | Walk briskly 30 minutes | Walk slowly 5 minutes | 40 minutes |

After week 12, continue with at least three exercise sessions per week. Gradually increase your brisk walking time to 30–60 minutes, three or four times per week.

*continues*

continued

# Walking Log

Use the Walking Log to keep track of how many minutes you walk per day.

| Week | Monday | Tuesday | Wednesday | Thursday | Friday | Saturday | Sunday |
|---|---|---|---|---|---|---|---|
| Week 1 | | | | | | | |
| Week 2 | | | | | | | |
| Week 3 | | | | | | | |
| Week 4 | | | | | | | |
| Week 5 | | | | | | | |
| Week 6 | | | | | | | |
| Week 7 | | | | | | | |
| Week 8 | | | | | | | |
| Week 9 | | | | | | | |
| Week 10 | | | | | | | |
| Week 11 | | | | | | | |
| Week 12 | | | | | | | |

Source: "The Sports Guide: NHLBI Planning Guide for Cardiovascular Risk Reduction Projects at Sporting Events," Office of Prevention, Educating, and Control, National Heart, Lung, and Blood Institute, NIH Publication No. 95–3802, October 1995.

# Calories Burned during Physical Activities

| Activity | Calories Burned Per Hour |
|---|---|
| Bicycling, 6 mph | 240 |
| Bicycling, 12 mph | 410 |
| Cross-country skiing | 700 |
| Jogging, 5 ½ mph | 740 |
| Jogging, 7 mph | 920 |
| Jumping rope | 750 |
| Running in place | 650 |
| Running, 10 mph | 1,280 |
| Swimming, 25 yds/min. | 275 |
| Swimming, 50 yds/min. | 500 |
| Tennis-singles | 400 |
| Walking, 2 mph | 240 |
| Walking, 3 mph | 320 |
| Walking, 4 ½ mph | 440 |

**Note:** These figures are for a 150-pound person. The amount of calories you burn up depends on how much you weigh. The more you weigh, the more calories you burn. For example, a 100-pound person burns only 0.67 times the calories of a 150-pound person (100/150=0.67). So, to find the number of calories a 100-pound person burns in an activity, multiply the number of calories in the chart by 0.67. For a 200-pound person, multiply by 1.3. To find the number of calories you burn up in any activity, divide your weight by 150 and multiply the number of calories in the chart by that number.

min. = minutes
yds. = yards
mph = miles per hour

Source: *Exercise and Your Heart—A Guide to Physical Activity*, National Heart, Lung, and Blood Institute/American Heart Association, DHHS, PHS, NIH Publication No. 93-1677.

# What Makes Blood Cholesterol High or Low

Why do some people have too much cholesterol in their blood? Many factors help determine whether your blood cholesterol level is high or low. The following factors are the most important.

## HEREDITY

Your genes partly determine the amount of cholesterol your body makes. High blood cholesterol can run in families.

## DIET

Two nutrients in the foods you eat make your blood cholesterol level go up: *saturated fat,* a type of fat found mostly in foods that come from animals; and *cholesterol,* which comes from animal products. Saturated fat raises your cholesterol level more than anything else in your diet. Reducing the amounts of *saturated fat* and *cholesterol* you eat is an important step in reducing your blood cholesterol levels.

## WEIGHT

Excess weight tends to increase your blood cholesterol level. If you are overweight and have a high blood cholesterol level, losing weight may help you lower it.

## PHYSICAL ACTIVITY/EXERCISE

Regular physical activity may help to lower LDL-cholesterol and raise HDL-cholesterol levels.

## AGE AND SEX

Before menopause, women have total cholesterol levels that are lower than those of men the same age. Pregnancy raises blood cholesterol levels in many women, but blood cholesterol levels should return to normal about 20 weeks after delivery. As women and men get older, their blood cholesterol levels rise. In women, menopause often causes an increase in their LDL-cholesterol level. Some women may benefit from taking estrogen after menopause, because estrogen lowers LDLs and raises HDLs.

## ALCOHOL

Alcohol intake increases HDL-cholesterol. However, doctors don't know whether it also reduces the risk of heart disease. Drinking too much alcohol can certainly damage the liver and heart muscle and cause other health problems. Because of these risks, you should not drink alcoholic beverages to prevent heart disease.

*continues*

continued

## STRESS

Stress over the long term has not been shown to raise blood cholesterol levels. The real problem with stress may be how it affects your habits. For example, when some people are under stress, they console themselves by eating fatty foods. The saturated fat and cholesterol in these foods probably cause higher blood cholesterol, not the stress itself.

**NOTES:**

Source: "So You Have High Blood Cholesterol," National Heart, Lung, and Blood Institute, NIH Publication No. 93–2922, December 1993.

# Cholesterol and Your Risk of Heart Disease

Cholesterol is a waxy substance that occurs naturally in all parts of the body. Your body needs cholesterol, which it uses to make many hormones and vitamin D. Cholesterol is also involved in producing bile acids, which help the body process the fats you eat. Your body produces enough cholesterol to meet its needs.

## HOW HIGH BLOOD CHOLESTEROL LEADS TO HEART DISEASE

When there is too much cholesterol in your blood, the excess can become trapped in the walls of your arteries. By building up there, the cholesterol helps to cause "hardening of the arteries" or atherosclerosis. And atherosclerosis causes most heart attacks. How? The cholesterol buildup narrows the arteries that supply blood to the heart, slowing or even blocking the flow of blood to the heart. So, the heart gets less oxygen than it needs. This weakens the heart muscle, and chest pain (angina) may occur. If a blood clot forms in the narrow artery, a heart attack (myocardial infarction) or even death can result.

Cholesterol buildup happens very slowly—you are not even aware of it. If you lower your high blood cholesterol level, you can slow, stop, or even reverse the buildup—and lower your risk of illness or death from heart disease.

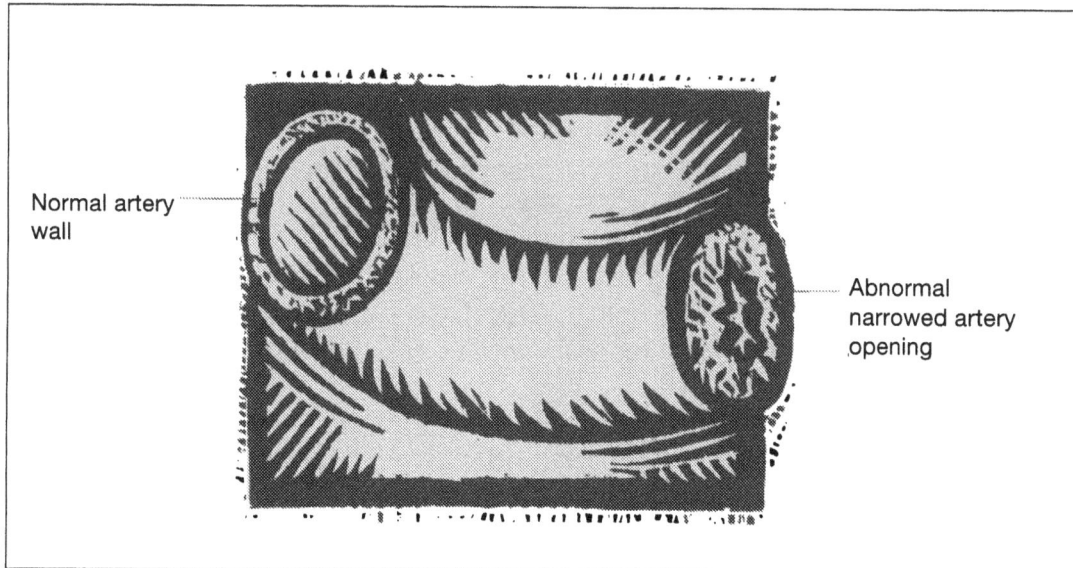

Normal artery wall

Abnormal narrowed artery opening

*continues*

continued

## "GOOD" AND "BAD" CHOLESTEROL: THE LIPOPROTEINS

Cholesterol travels in the blood in packages called lipoproteins. Just like oil and water, cholesterol and blood do not mix. So, in order to be able to travel in the bloodstream, the cholesterol made in the liver is also coated with a layer of protein, making a lipoprotein. This lipoprotein then carries the cholesterol through the bloodstream.

Two types of lipoproteins affect your risk of heart disease.

**Low-density lipoproteins (LDLs)**—the "bad" cholesterol. LDLs carry most of the cholesterol in the blood, and the cholesterol and fat from LDLs are the main source of dangerous buildup and blockage in the arteries. Thus, the more LDL-cholesterol you have in your blood, the greater your risk of heart disease.

**High-density lipoproteins (HDLs)**—the "good" cholesterol. HDLs carry some of the cholesterol in the blood, but this cholesterol goes back to the liver, which leads to its removal from the body. So HDLs help keep cholesterol from building up in the walls of the arteries. If your level of good cholesterol is low, your risk of heart disease is greater.

## OTHER RISK FACTORS FOR HEART DISEASE

In addition to a high LDL-cholesterol level and a low HDL-cholesterol level, other factors also increase your chance of heart disease. The chart below lists these risk factors. The more of them you have, the higher your chance of developing heart disease. If you have any of these risk factors in addition to your high blood cholesterol, your risk of heart disease is even greater.

In addition to the risk factors on the chart, another factor that influences your risk of heart disease is where your body stores excess fat. If you have an "apple-shaped" body with most of your fat around the stomach, you are at a greater risk of heart disease than if your body is "pear-shaped," with most of your fat around your hips. Generally, men carry their fat around the stomach, while women carry it on the hips and thighs.

Talk to your doctor about all of your risk factors and what you can do to reduce your chance of heart disease. Often, the actions you take to control one risk factor help reduce others as well. For example, losing weight helps to reduce blood cholesterol levels and high blood pressure, and helps to control diabetes. Regular physical activity can help you lose weight as well as improve the fitness of your heart and lungs, which also can help lower your risk of heart disease.

*continues*

continued

## Risk Factors for Heart Disease

- Cigarette smoking
- High blood cholesterol (high total cholesterol and high LDL-cholesterol)
- Low HDL-cholesterol
- High blood pressure
- Diabetes
- Obesity
- Physical inactivity

- Age
  - 45 years or older for men
  - 55 years or older for women
- Family history of early heart disease (heart attack or sudden death):
  - Father or brother stricken before the age of 55
  - Mother or sister stricken before the age of 65

## SIGNS OF CORONARY HEART DISEASE

- Have ever had a heart attack
- Suffer from chest pain which has been diagnosed as angina
- Have had heart surgery such as a bypass operation, balloon, or angioplasty procedure
- Have ever been told by your doctor that you have a buildup or blockage in any of your arteries

**NOTES:**

Source: "So You Have High Blood Cholesterol," National Heart, Lung, and Blood Institute, NIH Publication No. 93–2922, December 1993.

# What Your Blood Cholesterol Levels Mean If You *Do Not* Have Heart Disease

Even if you don't now have any signs of heart disease, it doesn't mean you never will. Now is the best time for prevention. Otherwise, a high blood cholesterol level, as well as other risk factors, can lead to problems in the future.

## YOUR BLOOD CHOLESTEROL TESTS

Blood cholesterol levels are measured in a small blood sample taken from your finger or your arm. The blood is tested for total cholesterol and, if accurate results can be obtained, HDL-cholesterol levels. You do not have to fast or do anything special before having this blood test. Depending on the results you may also need a second blood test, a lipoprotein profile, to determine your LDL-cholesterol level. You do have to fast for this test. An LDL-cholesterol level gives the doctor more information about your risk of heart disease and helps to guide any necessary treatment.

## TOTAL AND HDL-CHOLESTEROL

### Classification: Total and HDL-Cholesterol*

|  | Desirable | Borderline-High Risk | High Risk |
|---|---|---|---|
| *Total Cholesterol* | less than 200 mg/dL | 200–239 mg/dL | 240 mg/dL and above |
| *HDL-Cholesterol* |  |  | Less than 35 mg/dL |

*For anyone 20 years of age or older.

*continues*

continued

| **Your Next Steps** | | **If You *Do Not* Have Heart Disease** |
|---|---|---|
| *If Your Total and HDL Levels are . . .* | | *Then . . .* |
| *Total Cholesterol* | *HDL-Cholesterol* | |
| less than 200 mg/dL | 35 mg/dL or greater | You are doing well and should have your total and HDL-cholesterol levels checked again in about 5 years. In the meantime, take steps to keep your total cholesterol level down: eat foods low in saturated fat and cholesterol, maintain a healthy weight, and be physically active. The last two steps, along with not smoking, will also help keep your HDL level up. |
| less than 200 mg/dL or 200–239 mg/dL | less than 35 mg/dL | You will need a lipoprotein profile to find out your LDL-cholesterol level. For this test you need to fast for 9–12 hours before the test. Have nothing but water, or coffee or tea with no cream or sugar. |
| 200–239 mg/dL | 35 mg/dL or greater | Your doctor will see if you have other risk factors for heart disease and determine whether more tests (including a lipoprotein profile to find out your LDL-cholesterol) need to be done. No matter what your risk is, it is important to eat foods low in saturated fat and cholesterol, to maintain a healthy heart. |
| 240 mg/dL and above | any level | You will need a lipoprotein profile to find out your LDL-cholesterol level. Again, you need to fast for 9–12 hours before the test, having nothing but water, or coffee or tea with no cream or sugar. |

*continues*

continued

# LDL-CHOLESTEROL

## What Your LDL-Cholesterol Levels Mean

A high LDL-cholesterol level increases your risk for heart disease. Use the chart below to find out about your risks and your next steps.

### Classification: LDL-Cholesterol

| Desirable | Borderline-High Risk | High Risk |
|---|---|---|
| less than 130 mg/dL | 130–159 mg/dL | 160 mg/dL and above |

| Your Next Steps | If You *Do Not* Have Heart Disease |
|---|---|
| *If Your LDL Level is . . .* | *Then . . .* |
| less than 130 mg/dL | You have a desirable LDL-cholesterol level. You will need to have your total and HDL-cholesterol levels tested again in 5 years. You should follow an eating plan low in saturated fat and cholesterol, maintain a healthy weight, be physically active, and not smoke. |
| 130 mg/dL or above | Your doctor will look at your other heart disease risk factors and decide what you need to do to lower your LDL-cholesterol level. The higher your level and the more other risk factors you have, the more you need to follow a diet low in saturated fat and cholesterol. For example, if your LDL is 160 mg/dL or greater and you have fewer than two other risk factors, your LDL goal is a level below 160 mg/dL. If your LDL is 130 mg/dL or greater and you have two or more other risk factors, your goal is to reduce your LDL level to below 130 mg/dL. It is also important to lose weight if your are overweight, to be physically active, and to not smoke. Discuss your treatment plan with your doctor. |

Source: "So You Have High Blood Cholesterol," National Heart, Lung, and Blood Institute, NIH Publication No. 93–2922, December 1993.

# What Your Blood Cholesterol Levels Mean If You *Do* Have Heart Disease

It's not too late to help your heart. In fact, if you already have heart disease, you should pay even more attention to your cholesterol level. You have even more to gain. A person with coronary heart disease has a much greater risk of having a future heart attack than a person without heart disease. If you lower your blood cholesterol level, you can definitely reduce your risk of future heart attacks and may, in fact, prolong your life.

### YOUR BLOOD CHOLESTEROL TESTS

Since you have heart disease, you need to have a blood test called a lipoprotein profile. This test will determine not only your total and HDL-cholesterol levels, but also your LDL-cholesterol level—and levels of another fatty substance called triglyceride. In order to take the test, you must fast. That means you can have nothing to eat or drink but water, or coffee or tea with no cream or sugar for 9–12 hours beforehand.

### CHECK YOUR LEVELS

Since you have heart disease, your doctor will use your LDL-cholesterol level to decide on the last treatment. Your aim should be to have an LDL-cholesterol level lower than that of people who do not have heart disease. Compare your levels to those in the following chart to find out what your next steps should be.

| Your Next Steps | If You *Do* Have Heart Disease |
|---|---|
| *If Your LDL Level Is . . .* | *Then . . .* |
| 100 mg/dL or less | You do not need to take specific steps to lower your LDL, but you will need to have your level tested again in 1 year. In the meantime, you should closely follow a diet low in saturated fat and cholesterol, maintain a healthy weight, be physically active, and not smoke. |
| greater than 100 mg/dL | You need to have a complete physical examination done to see if you have a disease or a health condition that is raising your cholesterol levels. You will probably need a diet that is lower in saturated fat and cholesterol, i.e., the Step II diet. Since this diet will be more effective, your doctor will likely encourage you to start there as well as to be physically active, to lose weight if you are overweight, and to not smoke. If your LDL level does not come down, you may need to take medicine. |

Source: "So You Have High Blood Cholesterol," National Heart, Lung, and Blood Institute, NIH Publication No. 93–2922, December 1993.

# Questions You May Have about Your High Blood Cholesterol

### Since I'm a Woman, Why Should I Worry about Having a Heart Attack?

It's true that before menopause, women are unlikely to die from heart disease. But as they get older, especially after menopause, their chance of developing heart disease goes up. Women and men in their seventies have an equal likelihood of dying from heart disease. That's why at any age it is important for women as well as men to take steps to prevent high blood cholesterol.

### At 69, I'm Feeling Fine. Why Do I Need To Make Changes Now?

You have three very good reasons to change some of your health habits.

1. The risk of heart disease increases as you get older. Although you are feeling well, you may already have some buildup of fat and cholesterol in your arteries. Unless you try to stop or reverse the buildup, you may have a heart attack later on.
2. Adopting a healthy lifestyle helps reduce the risk of heart disease—even for people your age. People in their seventies can lower their blood cholesterol levels, and therefore deposit less fat in their arteries. Being more physically active is another important step that helps to protect older people against heart disease. A heart-healthy diet should also be a balanced diet. Most people will not have to make extreme changes to make their eating and activity habits healthy. These changes can fit in with your overall lifestyle.
3. You've got a lot of living yet to do. A man at 69 can expect on average to live another 15 years: a woman at 69 can expect to live another 19 years. The changes you make now can help make those years more healthy and enjoyable.

### Will Lowering My Blood Cholesterol Help Me Live Longer?

Many studies show that lowering cholesterol levels reduces the risk of illness or death from heart disease, which kills more men and women each year than any other illness. If you have heart disease, lowering your cholesterol level will probably help you to live longer. If you don't have heart disease, the studies so far do not show that you will live longer, but you will definitely reduce your risk of illness and death from heart attack.

*continues*

continued

### Since Heredity Can Cause High Blood Cholesterol, Do My High Levels Mean That My Family Is at Risk?

If you have high blood cholesterol, your family may also have high levels. This includes your children, parents, brothers, and sisters. They should all have their cholesterol levels tested to help protect them from heart disease.

### How Much Does My Cholesterol Level Change from Day to Day?

Your cholesterol level varies somewhat from day to day, sometimes by more than 15–20 mg/dL. Different laboratories also may use different methods of analyzing blood cholesterol levels which can give different results. This is why you need more than one cholesterol test before starting any treatment.

### What Is a Cholesterol Ratio?

Some laboratories may calculate a cholesterol ratio. The ratio is obtained by dividing either total cholesterol or LDL-cholesterol by the HDL-cholesterol. **The ratio is not recommended since it is more important to know each value separately.** Be sure to get separate total cholesterol, LDL, and HDL values.

### My Blood Test Showed I Also Have High Triglycerides. How Does that Affect My Risk of Heart Disease?

Triglycerides are a form of fat that is carried through the bloodstream. Most of your body's fat tissue is in the form of triglycerides. High blood triglyceride levels alone usually do not raise your risk of heart disease. But many people have a high triglyceride level along with high LDL- and low HDL-cholesterol levels. In these cases, the three are often treated together.

Borderline-high and high triglyceride levels are first treated with the same diet and lifestyle changes used for high blood cholesterol levels. These changes include:

- Weight loss (if you are overweight)
- A diet low in saturated fat and cholesterol
- Increased physical activity
- No smoking
- No alcoholic beverages (for some people)

Usually "very high" levels are due to heredity: They may be lowered with the changes above, along with medicines.

*continues*

continued

## Does Eating Foods High in Salt and Sodium Increase My Blood Cholesterol Level?

No. The amount of sodium in your diet has no effect on your cholesterol level. However, sodium can cause blood pressure to rise in some people. Further, many people with high blood cholesterol also have high blood pressure. If you have both, it's a good idea to reduce your sodium intake.

The National High Blood Pressure Education Program recommends no more than 2,400 mg per day (the amount in about 1 teaspoon of table salt). On average, Americans take in 4,000 to 6,000 milligrams of sodium each day: This sodium comes from many different foods. Foods high in sodium include some canned soups, vegetables, and meats; instant soups and cereals; ready-to-eat cereals; salty snacks and crackers; pickles and olives; and many frozen meals.

**NOTES:**

Source: "So You Have High Blood Cholesterol," National Heart, Lung, and Blood Institute, NIH Publication No. 93–2922, December 1993.

# Three Steps To Reducing High Blood Cholesterol Levels

### THREE STEPS CAN HELP YOU REDUCE YOUR HIGH BLOOD CHOLESTEROL

1. Follow the Step I or Step II diet. These diets are described in the boxes below. Your doctor will first recommend one or the other. The diets contain all the daily nutrients you need and emphasize eating foods that are low in saturated fat, total fat, and cholesterol, and high in starch and fiber. You will probably be asked to follow the Step I diet first to see if it brings your blood cholesterol levels down sufficiently. If not, you may have to move to the Step II diet. If you already have coronary heart disease or a very high LDL level, your doctor may recommend starting with the Step II diet.
2. Be more physically active.
3. Lose weight if you are overweight.

### THESE THREE STEPS WORK TOGETHER

Eating less fat, especially saturated fat, also may help you decrease the amount of cholesterol and calories you eat. Why? Foods high in fat and saturated fat are high in calories and often high in cholesterol. In fact, all fats, including both saturated and unsaturated fat, have more than twice as many calories as either carbohydrate or protein. They provide nine calories per gram and the other two provide four calories per gram.

Being more physically active helps burn more calories, which helps in weight loss. It may also help you lower your LDL-cholesterol and raise your HDL-cholesterol, as well as improve the health of your heart and lungs. Losing excess weight if you are overweight can help lower your LDL-cholesterol and increase your HDL-cholesterol.

### HOW LOW WILL YOU GO?

By closely following your diet, being more physically active, and watching your progress with regular checkups, you can lower your blood cholesterol level. How much your cholesterol levels change depends on:

- how much fat, especially saturated fat, and how much cholesterol you ate before you changed your diet
- how closely you follow the changes
- how your body responds to these changes. Usually the higher your blood cholesterol is to begin with, the more the levels go down. However, sometimes due to heredity, levels will not change enough no matter how well you change your habits.

*continues*

continued

For example: Your total blood cholesterol level is 240 mg/dL, and you are eating a diet high in saturated fat and cholesterol. By going on the Step I diet, you could reduce your cholesterol level by 5–35 mg/dL; and 5–15 mg/dL more, if you then go on Step II. Over time, you may reduce your cholesterol level by 10–50 mg/dL or even more. This drop will slow the fatty buildup in your arteries and reduce your risk of illness and death from heart attack. In fact, studies have shown that, in adults with high blood cholesterol levels, for each 1 percent reduction in total cholesterol levels, there is a 2 percent reduction in the risk of heart attack. So if you reduce your cholesterol level by 10 percent (for example, from 240 mg/dL to 216 mg/dL), your risk of heart disease could drop by 20 percent. And many people will get even more of a drop in their cholesterol level.

## 1.  LEARN ABOUT THE STEP I AND STEP II DIETS

---

### Step I Diet

On the Step I diet, you should eat:

- 8–10 percent of the day's total calories from saturated fat.
- 30 percent or less of the day's total calories from fat.
- Less than 300 milligrams of dietary cholesterol a day.
- Just enough calories to achieve and maintain a healthy weight. (You may want to ask your doctor or registered dietitian what is a reasonable calorie level for you.)

---

### Step II Diet

On the Step II diet, you should eat:

- Less than 7 percent of the day's total calories from saturated fat.
- 30 percent or less of the day's total calories from fat.
- Less than 200 milligrams of dietary cholesterol a day.
- Just enough calories to achieve and maintain a healthy weight. (You may want to ask your doctor or registered dietitian what is a reasonable calorie level for you.)

---

### Practical Ways To Change Your Diet

Here are some tips on how to choose foods for the Step I and Step II diets.

*continues*

continued

*To cut back on saturated fats, choose:*

- Poultry, fish, and lean cuts of meat more often. Remove the skin from chicken and trim the fat from meat.
- Skim or 1 percent milk, instead of 2 percent or whole milk
- Cheeses with no more than 3 grams of fat per ounce (these include low-fat cottage cheese or other low-fat cheeses). Cut down on full-fat processed, natural, and hard cheeses (like American, brie, and cheddar).
- Liquid vegetable oils that are high in unsaturated fat (these include canola, corn, olive, and safflower oil). Use tub or liquid margarines that list liquid vegetable oil as the first ingredient (instead of lard and hydrogenated vegetable shortening, which are high in saturated fat). Choose products that are lowest in saturated fat on the label.
- Fewer commercially prepared and processed foods made with saturated or hydrogenated fats or oils (like cakes, cookies, and crackers). Read food labels to choose products low in saturated fats.
- Foods high in starch and fiber, instead of foods high in saturated fats

*Cutting back on saturated fat helps you to control dietary cholesterol as well. Two additional points to remember when cutting back on dietary cholesterol are:*

- Eat less organ meat (such as liver, brain, and kidney).
- Eat fewer egg yolks as whole eggs or on prepared foods (try substituting two egg whites for each whole egg in recipes or using an egg substitute).

*To include more foods high in starch and fiber, choose:*

- More whole grain breads and cereals, pasta, rice, and dry peas and beans
- More vegetables and fruits

## 2. MAKE PHYSICAL ACTIVITY WORK FOR YOU

### Regular Physical Activity

- lowers LDL levels
- raises HDL levels
- lowers high blood pressure
- lowers triglyceride levels
- reduces excess weight
- improves the fitness of your heart and lungs

*continues*

continued

If you have been inactive for a long time, start with low- to moderate-level activities such as walking, taking the stairs instead of the elevator, gardening, housework, dancing, or exercising at home. Begin by doing the activity for a few minutes most days, then work up to a longer program—at least 30 minutes per day, 3 or 4 days a week. This can include regular aerobic activities such as brisk walking, jogging, swimming, bicycling, or playing tennis.

If you have heart disease or have had a heart attack, talk with your doctor before starting an activity to be sure you are following a safe program that works for you. Otherwise you may experience chest pain or further heart damage. If you have chest pain, feel faint or light-headed, or become extremely out of breath while exercising, stop the activity at once and tell your doctor as soon as possible.

### 3. LOSE WEIGHT IF YOU ARE OVERWEIGHT

Two action steps are key:

- Eat fewer calories (cutting back on the fat you eat will really help).
- Burn more calories by becoming more physically active.

**NOTES:**

Source: "So You Have High Blood Cholesterol," National Heart, Lung, and Blood Institute, NIH Publication No. 93–2922, December 1993.

# Proteja su corazón—Baje su colesterol

*"Yo sabía que tenía que hacer algo para bajar mi nivel de colesterol alto en la sangre. Poco a poco hice algunos cambios al comprar y preparar los alimentos. Cada día trato de mantenerme activa, camino durante mi hora del almuerzo o salto cuerda con mis hijos. Vale la pena hacer cambios.*

*¡En tres meses uso dos tallas menos en los vestidos!*
*Y poco a poco está bajando mi nivel de colesterol.*
*¡Me siento bien!"* —Pilar Crespo

## SIGA ESTOS CONSEJOS PARA DISMINUIR SU RIESGO DE TENER UN NIVEL ALTO DE COLESTEROL EN LA SANGRE.

### COMA ALIMENTOS SALUDABLES PARA EL CORAZÓN.

- leche descremada o con 1% de grasa
- helado de yogur bajo en grasa
- quesos bajos en grasa o sin grasa
- pescado
- pavo y pollo sin pellejo
- cortes de carne bajos en grasa
- cereales, pastas, lentejas y frijoles (habichuelas)
- tortillas de maíz, panes
- frutas y vegetales

### ESCOJA SÓLO DE VEZ EN CUANDO ESTOS ALIMENTOS.

- leche con un 2% de grasa
- aceites y margarina
- aguacates (paltas), aceitunas y coco
- nueces

### TRATE DE EVITAR ESTOS ALIMENTOS.

- leche entera o regular
- cremas y helados de leche (mantecados)
- quesos hechos de leche entera
- mantequilla
- cortes de carne con alto contenido de grasa y chicharrones
- chorizos, salchichas y mortadela
- hígado, riñones y otros órganos animales
- yemas de huevo
- manteca, aceite de coco, de palma o de pepita de palma

*continúa*

continuación

## MANTÉNGASE ACTIVO FÍSICAMENTE TODOS LOS DÍAS.

## ¡ESCOJA ACTIVIDADES QUE USTED Y SU FAMILIA PUEDAN DISFRUTAR!

- caminar
- hacer ejercicios aeróbicos
- trabajar en el jardín
- bailar
- practicar deportes
- saltar cuerda con sus hijos

## TRATE DE LOGRAR UN PESO SALUDABLE. SIGA ESTOS CONSEJOS PARA BAJAR DE PESO SI TIENE SOBREPESO. TRATE DE PERDER PESO LENTAMENTE.

- Evite las comidas con alto contenido de grasa y calorías.
- Sírvase porciones pequeñas de comida.
- Coma frutas y vegetales como bocadillos.
- Hornee, ase o hierva sus comidas.
- Manténgase activo todos los días.

## NOTAS:

Source: "Proteja su Corazón-Baje su Colesterol!" NIH Publication No. 96-4044, U.S. Department of Health and Human Services, National Institutes of Health.

# Ask Your Health Professionals about High Blood Cholesterol

*In addition to your doctor, other health professionals can help you control your blood cholesterol levels. These persons include:*

- **Registered Dietitian (R.D.) or qualified nutritionist,** who can explain food plans and show you how to make changes in what you eat. They can give you advice on shopping for and preparing foods, and eating out. They also can help you set goals for changing the way you eat, so you can successfully lower your high blood cholesterol without making big changes all at once in your eating habits or in your lifestyle.

  To find a registered dietitian, contact:

  - The National Center for Nutrition and Dietetics Consumer Nutrition Hotline 1-800-366-1655
  - Your local hospital or health department
  - Your doctor

- **The nurse in your doctor's office,** who also may be able to answer questions about your high blood cholesterol or your diet.
- **Lipid specialists,** who are doctors with expertise in treating high blood cholesterol and similar conditions. In special cases, you may be referred to a lipid specialist if the treatment your doctor is prescribing does not successfully lower your blood cholesterol levels.
- **Your doctor,** who can answer your questions about the medicines you are taking. Be sure to tell your doctor about everything you are taking and if you feel different after you take any of them.
- **Pharmacists,** who are aware of the best ways to take medicines to lessen side effects and of the latest research on drugs.

Source: "So You Have High Blood Cholesterol," National Heart, Lung, and Blood Institute, NIH Publication No. 93–2922, December 1993.

# High Blood Cholesterol Glossary

**Atherosclerosis:** A type of "hardening of the arteries" in which cholesterol, fat, and other substances in the blood build up in the walls of arteries. As the process continues, the arteries to the heart may narrow, cutting down the flow of oxygen-rich blood and nutrients to the heart.

**Bile Acid Sequestrants:** One type of cholesterol-lowering medication, including cholestyramine and colestipol. The sequestrants bind with cholesterol-containing bile acids in the intestines and remove them in bowel movements.

**Calories:** Units of measurement that represent the amount of energy the body is able to get from foods. Different nutrients in foods provide different amounts of calories. Carbohydrates and protein provide about 4 calories per gram, while fat (both saturated and unsaturated) yields about 9 calories per gram.

**Carbohydrate:** One of the nutrients that supply calories to the body. Carbohydrates may be simple or complex. Complex carbohydrates also are called starch and fiber. They come from plants and can be found in whole-grain breads, cereals, pasta, rice, dried peas and beans, corn, lima beans, fruits, and vegetables.

**Cholesterol:** A soft, waxy substance. The body makes enough cholesterol to meet its needs. Cholesterol is used in the manufacture of hormones, bile acid, and vitamin D. It is present in all parts of the body, including the nervous system, muscle, skin, liver, intestines, and heart.

- **Blood cholesterol**—Cholesterol circulating in the bloodstream. It is made in the liver and absorbed from the food you eat. The blood carries it for use by all parts of the body. A high level of blood cholesterol leads to atherosclerosis and an increased risk of heart disease.
- **Dietary cholesterol**—Cholesterol in the food you eat. It is present only in foods of animal origin, not those of plant origin. Dietary cholesterol, like dietary saturated fat, raises blood cholesterol, which increases the risk for heart disease.

**Estrogen Replacement Therapy (ERT).** Treatment with the hormone estrogen, which has many effects, one of which is cholesterol lowering. It includes different amounts of estrogen and progestin, two hormones produced normally by women who have menstrual periods. ERT is given only to women who have gone through menopause. ERT may help prevent heart disease by lowering blood cholesterol levels, especially LDL.

*continues*

continued

**Fat.** One of the nutrients that supplies calories to the body. The body needs only small amounts of fat. Foods contain different types of fat, which have different effects on blood cholesterol levels. These include:

- **Total fat**—The sum of the saturated, monounsaturated, and polyunsaturated fats present in food. All foods have a varying mix of these three types.
- **Saturated fat**—A type of fat found in greatest amounts in foods from animals, such as fatty cuts of meat, poultry with the skin, whole-milk dairy products, lard, and in some vegetable oils, including coconut, palm kernel, and palm oils. Saturated fat raises blood cholesterol more than anything else eaten.
- **Unsaturated fat**—A type of fat that is usually liquid at refrigerator temperature. Monounsaturated fat and polyunsaturated fat are two kinds of unsaturated fat. When used in place of saturated fat, monounsaturated and polyunsaturated fats help to lower blood cholesterol levels.
  - **Monounsaturated fat**—An unsaturated fat that is found in greatest amounts in foods from plants, including olive and canola oils.
  - **Polyunsaturated fat**—An unsaturated fat found in greatest amounts in foods from plants, including safflower, sunflower, corn, and soybean oils.

**Fibric Acid Derivatives:** One type of cholesterol-lowering drug. It includes gemfibrozil. The fibric acids lower triglycerides and raise HDLs.

**HMG CoA Reductase Inhibitors:** See "Statins."

**Lipids.** Fatty substances, including cholesterol and triglycerides, that are present in blood and body tissues.

**Lipoproteins.** Protein-coated packages that carry fat and cholesterol through the bloodstream. Lipoproteins are classified according to their density:

- **High-density lipoprotein (HDL)**—Lipoproteins that contain a small amount of cholesterol and carry cholesterol away from body cells and tissues to the liver for excretion from the body. A low level of HDL increases the risk of heart disease, so the higher the HDL level, the better. HDL is sometimes called the "good" cholesterol.
- **Low-density lipoprotein (LDL)**—Lipoproteins that contain most of the cholesterol in the blood. LDL, the "bad" cholesterol, carries cholesterol to the tissues of the body including the arteries. For this reason, a high level of LDL increases the risk of heart disease.

*continues*

continued

**Lipoprotein Profile:** A test that uses blood from the arm to measure your total HDL- and LDL-cholesterol, and triglyceride levels. The test requires a fast for 9–12 hours beforehand. Nothing can be consumed but water, or coffee or tea with no cream or sugar.

**Milligram (mg):** A unit of weight equal to one-thousandth of a gram. There are about 28,350 mg in 1 ounce. Dietary cholesterol is measured in milligrams.

**Milligrams/Deciliter (mg/dL):** The measure used to express cholesterol and triglyceride levels in the blood. It stands for the weight of cholesterol in milligrams in a deciliter of blood. A deciliter is one-tenth of a liter or about one-tenth of a quart.

**Nicotinic Acid:** A cholesterol-lowering medicine that reduces total and LDL-cholesterol and triglyceride levels and also raises HDL-cholesterol levels. This is the same substance as Niacin or vitamin $B_1$, but in doses that lower cholesterol, it should only be used with your doctor's supervision.

**Risk Factor:** A habit, trait, or condition in a person that is associated with an increased chance (or risk) for a disease.

**Statins:** One type of cholesterol-lowering drug that includes lovastatin, pravastatin, and simvastatin. These drugs lower LDL levels by limiting the amount of cholesterol the body can make.

**Triglycerides:** Lipids carried through the bloodstream to tissues. Most of the body's fat tissue is in the form of triglycerides, stored for use as energy. Triglycerides are obtained primarily from fat in foods.

Source: "So You Have High Blood Cholesterol," National Heart, Lung, and Blood Institute, NIH Publication No. 93–2922, December 1993.

# Know Your Cholesterol Level

Lowering your high blood cholesterol is an important step for reducing your chance of developing heart disease. Remember to ask your doctor for your total cholesterol, LDL-cholesterol, and HDL-cholesterol levels *each* time they are measured. Write the levels down on the chart below to keep track of your progress.

Date _____          Date _____

Total Cholesterol _____          Total Cholesterol _____

HDL-Cholesterol _____          HDL-Cholesterol _____

LDL-Cholesterol _____          LDL-Cholesterol _____

Date _____          Date _____

Total Cholesterol _____          Total Cholesterol _____

HDL-Cholesterol _____          HDL-Cholesterol _____

LDL-Cholesterol _____          LDL-Cholesterol _____

Date _____          Date _____

Total Cholesterol _____          Total Cholesterol _____

HDL-Cholesterol _____          HDL-Cholesterol _____

LDL-Cholesterol _____          LDL-Cholesterol _____

Source: "So You Have High Blood Cholesterol," National Heart, Lung, and Blood Institute, NIH Publication No. 93–2922, December 1993.

# ¡Conozca su nivel de colesterol!

*"¡Mi nivel de colesterol en la sangre estaba alto—arriba de 240! Yo pensaba que iba a tener que dejar las comidas sabrosas para comer alimentos saludables. Muy pronto aprendí el secreto de saber escoger alimentos saludables y es fácil. Las comidas saben muy sabrosas. ¡Mi nivel de colesterol en la sangre bajó a un número deseable en sólo 6 meses! Además perdí peso."*

*—Alma Graciela González*

## MANTENGA SU COLESTEROL A UN NIVEL MENOR DE 200.

Su cuerpo produce todo el colesterol que necesita para que usted esté saludable. Además, el colesterol llega a su cuerpo cuando come alimentos con alto contenido de grasa saturada y colesterol. A través de los años, el exceso de colesterol en la sangre puede taparle las arterias. Esto aumenta su riesgo de sufrir un ataque al corazón.

Si usted es mayor de 20 años, mida el nivel de colesterol en la sangre por lo menos cada cinco años. Las personas con números altos necesitan medirse el colesterol en la sangre como lo indica su médico.

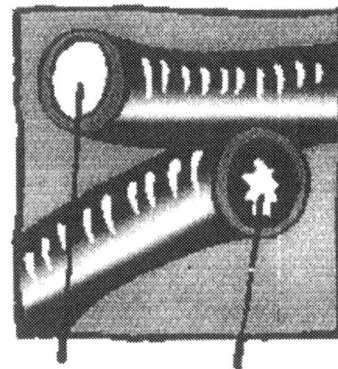

arteria normal

arteria obstruída con colesterol

## PROTEJA SU SALUD.

- Pídale a su médico que le haga el examen para medir su nivel de colesterol en la sangre. El médico le dirá su número.
- Conozca el significado de su número:

1. Un nivel de colesterol de menos de 200 es deseable. ¡Buena noticia! Manténgase activo. Coma alimentos con bajo contenido de grasa saturada y colesterol.
2. Si su número se encuentra entre 200 y 239, esté alerta. Usted está en riesgo de tener un ataque al corazón. Usted necesita aumentar su actividad física y hacer cambios en su alimentación. Disminuya el consumo de alimentos con alto contenido de grasa saturada y colesterol.
3. Si su número es 240 ó más, usted tiene un alto nivel de colesterol en la sangre. ¡Peligro! Usted tiene un alto riesgo de sufrir un ataque al corazón. Su médico puede indicarle cómo bajarlo.

*continúa*

continuación

## ¿CUÁL ES EL TIPO DE GRASA QUE MÁS AUMENTA SU NIVEL DE COLESTEROL EN LA SANGRE?

La grasa saturada aumenta su nivel de colesterol en la sangre. Esta se encuentra en alimentos que provienen de animales tales como:

- Leche entera (regular), mantequilla, crema, quesos con alto contenido de grasa
- Manteca de cerdo y manteca vegetal
- Carnes con alto contenido de grasa como las costillas, las salchichas, los chorizos y los chicharrones.

## ¿CUÁLES SON LOS ALIMENTOS CON MÁS ALTO CONTENIDO DE COLESTEROL?

- Yemas de huevo
- Carnes de vísceras tales como hígado, sesos y riñones

---

**Para la salud del corazón, estos pasos tomaré:**

☐ Medirme el nivel de colesterol en la sangre.
☐ Aprender el significado de mi número.
☐ Comer menos alimentos con alto contenido de grasa saturada y colesterol.
☐ Comer más frutas, vegetales y granos.
☐ Mantenerme activo físicamente.

---

Source: "Conozca su nivel de colesterol!" NIH Publication No. 96–4043, National Heart, Lung, and Blood Institute, National Institutes of Health, September 1996.

# Medicine for High Blood Cholesterol

If you have successfully changed your eating habits for at least 6–12 months, and your LDL-cholesterol level is still too high, you may need to take medicine. Some people will need to take medicine from the start of their treatment because of a very high LDL level or the presence of heart disease.

If your doctor prescribes medicine, you also will need to:

- Follow your cholesterol-lowering diet
- Lose weight if overweight
- Be more physically active
- Stop smoking

Taking all these steps together may lessen the amount of medicine you need, or make the medicine work better. And that reduces your risk of heart disease.

## MEDICINES YOUR DOCTOR MAY PRESCRIBE

Several types of medicine can help lower blood cholesterol levels. These include:

### Major Medicines

- Bile acid sequestrants (cholestyramine and colestipol)
- Nicotinic acid
- HMG CoA reductase inhibitors or "statins" (for example, lovastatin, pravastatin, and simvastatin)

### Other Medicines

- Fibric acid derivatives (gemfibrozil)
- Probucol

In addition, if you are a woman going through or past menopause, your doctor may talk with you about estrogens. Sometimes called Estrogen Replacement Therapy, this can lower blood cholesterol levels, and may make it unnecessary for you to take a cholesterol-lowering drug.

## TALKING TO YOUR DOCTOR ABOUT MEDICINES

Drugs that lower blood cholesterol work in different ways. Some may work for you while others may not. Before the doctor prescribes any medicine, be sure to state what other medicines you

*continues*

continued

are taking. And once a medicine is prescribed, take it exactly the way your doctor tells you to. If you have any side effects from a medicine, tell your doctor right away. The amount or type of drug can be changed to reduce or stop unwanted side effects.

Whatever medicine you take, continue to follow the Step I or Step II diet and to be more physically active. This will help keep the dose of medicine as low as possible.

**NOTES:**

Source: "So You Have High Blood Cholesterol," National Heart, Lung, and Blood Institute, NIH Publication No. 93–2922, December 1993.

**11. Nutrition for Heart Disease**

# Heart-Healthy Eating: The Step I and Step II Diets

## INTRODUCTION

All Americans should follow the general rules to lower blood cholesterol. In fact, this is a way that the whole family can eat (except infants under 2 years who need more calories from fat), because these guidelines are similar to those recommended for the general population. And if the whole family eats in this way, it will help **you** make your blood cholesterol-lowering diet your everyday way of eating.

If you have high blood cholesterol, you will have to pay attention to what you eat by following either the Step I diet or Step II diet, as advised by your doctor.

## STEP I DIET

### On the Step I diet eat

- 8–10 percent of the day's total calories from saturated fat
- 30 percent or less of the day's total calories from fat
- Less than 300 milligrams of dietary cholesterol a day
- Just enough calories to achieve and maintain a healthy weight (You may want to ask your doctor or registered dietitian what is a reasonable calorie level for you.)

If you do not lower your blood cholesterol enough on the Step I diet or if you are at high risk for heart disease, your doctor will ask you to follow the Step II diet. If you already have heart disease, you should start on the Step II diet right away. The Step II diet helps you cut down on saturated fat and cholesterol even more than the Step I diet. This helps lower your blood cholesterol even more.

## STEP II DIET

### On the Step II diet eat

- Less than 7 percent of the day's total calories from saturated fat
- 30 percent or less of the day's total calories from fat
- Less than 200 milligrams of dietary cholesterol a day
- Just enough calories to achieve and maintain a healthy weight (You may want to ask your doctor or registered dietitian what is a reasonable calorie level for you.)

*continues*

*continued*

To get the full benefits of the Step II diet, you should have help from a registered dietitian or other qualified nutritionist. If your levels do not go down enough, you may need to take medicine along with your diet.

The recommendations for saturated fat and total fat are based on a percentage of the calories you eat; the actual amount you should eat daily will vary depending on how many calories you eat. See the chart below to get an idea of the number of grams of saturated fat and total fat you should be eating.

## COUNTING SATURATED FAT AND TOTAL FAT ON THE STEP I AND STEP II DIETS

| If you eat this many calories . . . | | | | | |
|---|---|---|---|---|---|
| | 1,200 | 1,500 | 1,800 | 2,000 | 2,500 |

*This is the recommended amount of fat for each day:*

**Saturated Fat** *(grams)**

| | 1,200 | 1,500 | 1,800 | 2,000 | 2,500 |
|---|---|---|---|---|---|
| Step I | 12 | 15 | 18 | 20 | 25 |
| Step II | 8 | 10 | 12 | 13 | 17 |

**Total Fat** *(grams)***
Step I
and

| | 1,200 | 1,500 | 1,800 | 2,000 | 2,500 |
|---|---|---|---|---|---|
| Step II | 40 | 50 | 60 | 65 | 80 |

*Amounts are equal to 9 percent of total calories for Step I and 6 percent of total calories for Step II. Remember: 1 gram of fat equals 9 calories.

** Amounts are equal to 30 percent of total calories (rounded down to the nearest 5); your intake should be this much or less.

**Note:** On average, women consume about 1,800 calories and day and men consume about 2,500 calories a day.

*continues*

continued

## ABOUT SODIUM

If you have high blood pressure as well as high blood cholesterol (and many people do), your doctor may tell you to cut down on sodium or salt. As long as you are working on getting your blood cholesterol number down, this is a good time to work on your blood pressure, too. Try to limit your sodium intake to 2,400 milligrams a day.

## WHAT CAN YOU EXPECT?

Generally your blood cholesterol level should begin to drop a few weeks after you start on a cholesterol-lowering diet. How much your level drops depends on the amount of saturated fat and cholesterol you used to eat, how high your blood cholesterol is, how much weight you lose if you are overweight, and how your body responds to the changes you make. Over time, you may reduce your blood cholesterol level by 10–50 mg/dL or even more.


**NOTES:**

Source: "Step by Step: Eating to Lower Your High Blood Cholesterol," National Heart, Lung, and Blood Institute, NIH Publication No. 94–2920, August 1994.

# Sample Menus—Traditional American-Style Foods

## STEP I—2,500 CALORIES

**Breakfast**
1 medium bagel
  2 teaspoons low-fat cream cheese
1 1/2 cups shredded wheat cereal
1 small banana
1 cup 1 percent milk
3/4 cup orange juice
1 cup coffee
  2 tablespoons 1 percent milk

**Lunch**
1/2 cup minestrone soup, canned
1 lean roast beef sandwich
  2 slices whole wheat bread
  3 ounces lean roast beef, unseasoned
  3/4 ounce American cheese, low-fat
  1 leaf lettuce
  3 slices tomato
  2 teaspoons mayonnaise, low-fat
1 cup fresh mixed fruit salad
1 cup lemonade

**Snack**
1 fresh large apple

**Dinner**
3 ounces salmon
1 medium baked potato
  2 teaspoons tub margarine
1/2 cup green beans
  1/2 teaspoon tub margarine
1/2 cup carrots
  1/2 teaspoon tub margarine
1 medium white dinner roll
  1 teaspoon tub margarine
1 cup ice milk
1 cup iced tea, unsweetened

**Snack**
3 cups popcorn
  1 tablespoon tub margarine

*Note: No salt is used when making the food.*

## STEP II—2,500 CALORIES

**Breakfast**
1 medium bagel
  2 teaspoons jelly
1 1/2 cups shredded wheat cereal
1 small banana
1 cup skim milk
3/4 cup orange juice
1 cup coffee
  2 tablespoons skim milk

**Lunch**
1/2 cup minestrone soup, canned
1 lean roast beef sandwich
  2 slices whole wheat bread
  2 ounces lean roast beef, unseasoned
  3/4 ounce American cheese, low-fat
  1 leaf lettuce
  3 slices tomato
  2 teaspoons tub margarine
1 cup fresh mixed fruit salad
1 cup lemonade

**Snack**
1 fresh large apple

**Dinner**
3 ounces flounder
  1 teaspoon vegetable oil
1 medium baked potato
  2 teaspoons tub margarine
1/2 cup green beans
  1/2 teaspoon tub margarine
1/2 cup carrots
  1/2 teaspoon tub margarine
1 medium white dinner roll
  1 teaspoon tub margarine
1 cup frozen yogurt
1 cup iced tea, unsweetened

**Snack**
3 cups popcorn
  1 tablespoon tub margarine

| | | |
|---|---:|---:|
| Calories | 2,471 | 2,453 |
| Percent calories from fat | 29 | 28 |
| Percent calories from saturated fat | 8 | 7 |
| Cholesterol (milligrams) | 162 | 144 |
| Sodium (milligrams) | 2,400 | 2,426 |

*continues*

continued

## STEP I—1,800 CALORIES

**Breakfast**
1/2 medium bagel
1 teaspoon low-fat cream cheese
1 cup shredded wheat cereal
1 small banana
1 cup 1 percent milk
3/4 cup orange juice
1 cup coffee
    2 tablespoons 1 percent milk

**Lunch**
1/2 cup minestrone soup, canned
1 lean roast beef sandwich
    2 slices whole wheat bread
    3 ounces lean roast beef, unseasoned
    3/4 ounce American cheese, low-fat
    1 leaf lettuce
    3 slices tomato
    2 teaspoons mayonnaise, low-fat
1 medium apple
1 cup water

**Dinner**
3 ounces salmon
1 medium baked potato
    1 teaspoon tub margarine
1/2 cup green beans
    1/2 teaspoon tub margarine
1/2 cup carrots
    1/2 teaspoon tub margarine
1 medium white dinner roll
    1 teaspoon tub margarine
1/2 cup ice milk
1 cup iced tea, unsweetened

**Snack**
2 cups popcorn
    1 teaspoon tub margarine

*Note: No salt is used when making the food.*

## STEP II—1,800 CALORIES

**Breakfast**
1/2 medium bagel
1 teaspoon jelly
1 cup shredded wheat cereal
1 small banana
1 cup skim milk
1 cup orange juice
1 cup coffee
    2 tablespoons skim milk

**Lunch**
1/2 cup minestrone soup, canned
1 lean roast beef sandwich
    2 slices whole wheat bread
    2 ounces lean roast beef, unseasoned
    3/4 ounce American cheese, low-fat
    1 leaf lettuce
    3 slices tomato
    2 teaspoons tub margarine
1 medium apple
1 cup water

**Dinner**
3 ounces flounder
    1 teaspoon vegetable oil
1 medium baked potato
    1 teaspoon tub margarine
1/2 cup green beans
    1/2 teaspoon tub margarine
1/2 cup carrots
    1/2 teaspoon tub margarine
1 medium white dinner roll
    1 teaspoon tub margarine
1/2 cup low-fat frozen yogurt
1 cup iced tea, unsweetened

**Snack**
3 cups popcorn
    2 teaspoons tub margarine

| | | |
|---|---|---|
| Calories | 1,821 | 1,870 |
| Percent calories from fat | 30 | 29 |
| Percent calories from saturated fat | 9 | 7 |
| Cholesterol (milligrams) | 150 | 130 |
| Sodium (milligrams) | 2,046 | 2,148 |

Source: "Step by Step: Eating to Lower Your High Blood Cholesterol," National Heart, Lung, and Blood Institute, NIH Publication No. 94–2920, August 1994.

# Sample Menus—Southern-Style Foods

## STEP I—2,500 CALORIES

**Breakfast**
1 cup oatmeal, made with 1 percent milk
1 cup 1 percent milk
1 medium English muffin
   2 tablespoons low-fat cream cheese
1 cup orange juice
1 cup coffee
   2 tablespoons 1 percent milk

**Lunch**
3 ounces baked chicken, without the skin
   1 teaspoon vegetable oil
Salad
   1/2 cup lettuce
   1/2 cup tomato
   1/2 cup cucumber
   1 tablespoon regular oil and vinegar dressing
1 cup white rice
   1 teaspoon tub margarine
1 medium biscuit, made with vegetable oil
   2 teaspoons tub margarine
1 cup water

**Dinner**
3 ounces lean roast beef
1/4 cup onion
1 tablespoon beef gravy, made with 1 percent milk
1/2 cup turnip greens
   1/2 teaspoon tub margarine
1 medium sweet potato
   1 teaspoon brown sugar
1 medium slice cornbread, made with tub margarine
   1 teaspoon tub margarine
1/4 medium honeydew melon
2 medium pumpkin cookies, made with vegetable oil
1 cup iced tea, sweetened with sugar

**Snack**
8 saltine crackers, with unsalted tops
1 1/2 ounces part skim mozzarella cheese
2 medium dried prunes

*Note: No salt is used when making the food.*

## STEP II—2,500 CALORIES

**Breakfast**
1 cup oatmeal, made with skim milk
1 cup skim milk
1 medium English muffin
   2 teaspoons tub margarine
   2 teaspoons jelly
1 cup orange juice
1 cup coffee

**Lunch**
3 ounces baked chicken, without the skin
   1 teaspoon vegetable oil
Salad
   1/2 cup lettuce
   1/2 cup tomato
   1/2 cup cucumber
   1 tablespoon regular oil and vinegar dressing
1 1/4 cups white rice
   1 1/4 teaspoon tub margarine
1 medium biscuit, made with vegetable oil
   2 teaspoons tub margarine
1 cup water

**Dinner**
2 ounces roast beef
1/4 cup onion
1 tablespoon beef gravy, made with water
1/2 cup turnip greens
   1/2 teaspoon tub margarine
1 medium sweet potato
   1 teaspoon brown sugar
1 medium slice cornbread, made with tub margarine
   1 teaspoon tub margarine
1/4 medium honeydew melon
2 medium pumpkin cookies, made with vegetable oil
1 cup iced tea, sweetened with sugar

**Snack**
8 saltine crackers, with unsalted tops
3/4 ounce part-skim mozzarella cheese
2 medium dried prunes

| | STEP I | STEP II |
|---|---|---|
| Calories | 2,560 | 2,536 |
| Percent calories from fat | 30 | 29 |
| Percent calories from saturated fat | 10 | 7 |
| Cholesterol (milligrams) | 241 | 177 |
| Sodium (milligrams) | 2,174 | 2,035 |

*continues*

continued

## STEP I—1,800 CALORIES

**Breakfast**
3/4 cup oatmeal, made with 1 percent milk
3/4 cup 1 percent milk
1 medium English muffin
  2 tablespoons low-fat cream cheese
3/4 cup orange juice
1 cup coffee
  2 tablespoons 1 percent milk

**Lunch**
3 ounces baked chicken, without the skin
  1 teaspoon vegetable oil
Salad
  1/2 cup lettuce
  1/2 cup tomato
  1/2 cup cucumber
  2 teaspoons regular oil and vinegar dressing
1/2 cup white rice
  1/2 teaspoon tub margarine
1/2 medium biscuit, made with vegetable oil
  1 teaspoon tub margarine
1 cup water

**Dinner**
3 ounces lean roast beef
1/4 cup onion
1 tablespoon beef gravy, made with 1 percent milk
1/2 cup turnip greens
  1/2 teaspoon tub margarine
1 medium sweet potato
  1/2 teaspoon brown sugar
1/2 medium slice cornbread, made with tub margarine
1/2 teaspoon tub margarine
1/4 medium honeydew melon
1 medium pumpkin cookie, made with vegetable oil
1 cup iced tea, sweetened with sugar

**Snack**
4 saltine crackers, with unsalted tops
3/4 ounce part-skim mozzarella cheese
2 medium dried prunes

*Note: No salt is used when making the food.*

## STEP II—1,800 CALORIES

**Breakfast**
3/4 cup oatmeal, made with skim milk
1 cup skim milk
1 medium English muffin
  2 teaspoons tub margarine
  2 teaspoons jelly
3/4 cup orange juice
1 cup coffee
  2 tablespoons skim milk

**Lunch**
3 ounces baked chicken, without the skin
  1 teaspoon vegetable oil
Salad
  1/2 cup lettuce
  1/2 cup tomato
  1/2 cup cucumber
  2 teaspoons regular oil and vinegar dressing
1/2 cup white rice
  1/2 teaspoon tub margarine
1/2 medium biscuit, made with vegetable oil
  1 teaspoon tub margarine
1 cup water

**Dinner**
2 ounces lean roast beef
1/4 cup onion
  1 tablespoon beef gravy, made with water
1/2 cup turnip greens
  1/2 teaspoon tub margarine
1/2 medium mashed sweet potato
  1/2 teaspoon brown sugar
1/2 medium slice cornbread, made with tub margarine
  1/2 teaspoon tub margarine
1/4 medium honeydew melon
1 medium pumpkin cookie, made with vegetable oil
1 cup iced tea, sweetened with sugar

**Snack**
4 saltine crackers, with unsalted tops
1/2 ounce part-skim mozzarella cheese
2 medium dried prunes

| | | |
|---|---|---|
| Calories | 1,823 | 1,841 |
| Percent calories from fat | 30 | 29 |
| Percent calories from saturated fat | 9 | 7 |
| Cholesterol (milligrams) | 191 | 159 |
| Sodium (milligrams) | 1,471 | 1,492 |

Source: "Step by Step: Eating to Lower Your High Blood Cholesterol," National Heart, Lung, and Blood Institute, NIH Publication No. 94–2920, August 1994.

# Sample Menus—Mexican American-Style Foods

## STEP I—2,500 CALORIES

**Breakfast**
1/2 cup cantaloupe
1 cup farina, made with 1 percent milk
2 slices white bread
    2 teaspoons tub margarine
    2 teaspoons jelly
3/4 cup orange juice
1 cup hot cocoa, made with 1 percent milk

**Lunch**
Beef Enchilada
    2 corn tortillas
    3 ounces lean roast beef
    1 teaspoon vegetable oil
    1 ounce low fat cheddar cheese
    1/8 cup onion
    1/8 cup tomato
    1/4 cup lettuce
    2 teaspoons chili peppers
3/4 cup refried beans, made with vegetable oil
6 carrot sticks
6 celery sticks
1/2 cup 1 percent milk

**Dinner**
Chicken Taco
    2 corn tortillas
    3 ounces chicken breast without the skin
    1 teaspoon vegetable oil
    1 ounce low-fat cheddar cheese
    2 tablespoons guacamole
    2 tablespoons salsa
1/2 cup corn
    1/2 teaspoon tub margarine
1 cup Spanish rice, made with tub margarine
1 medium banana
1 cup coffee
    2 tablespoons 1 percent milk

**Snack**
3/4 cup ice milk

*Note: No salt is used when making the food.*

## STEP II—2,500 CALORIES

**Breakfast**
1/2 cup cantaloupe
1 cup farina, made with skim milk
2 slices white bread
    2 teaspoons tub margarine
    2 teaspoons jelly
3/4 cup orange juice
1 cup hot cocoa, made with skim milk

**Lunch**
Beef Enchilada
    2 corn tortillas
    2 ounces lean roast beef
    1/2 teaspoon vegetable oil
    1 ounce low fat cheddar cheese
    1/8 cup onion
    1/8 cup tomato
    1/4 cup lettuce
    2 teaspoons chili peppers
3/4 cup refried beans, made with vegetable oil
6 carrot sticks
6 celery sticks
1/2 cup skim milk

**Dinner**
Chicken Taco
    2 corn tortillas
    3 ounces chicken breast without the skin
    1/2 teaspoon vegetable oil
    1 ounce low-fat cheddar cheese
    2 tablespoons guacamole
    2 tablespoons salsa
1 cup corn
    1 teaspoon tub margarine
1 cup Spanish rice, made with tub margarine
1 medium banana
1 cup coffee
    2 tablespoons skim milk

**Snack**
1 cup popcorn
    1 tablespoon tub margarine

| | | |
|---|---|---|
| Calories | 2,557 | 2,574 |
| Percent calories from fat | 29 | 28 |
| Percent calories from saturated fat | 8 | 6 |
| Cholesterol (milligrams) | 185 | 136 |
| Sodium (milligrams) | 2,100 | 2,395 |

*continues*

continued

## STEP I—1,800 CALORIES

**Breakfast**
1/2 cup cantaloupe
3/4 cup farina, made with 1 percent milk
1 slice white bread
   1 teaspoon tub margarine
   1 teaspoon jelly
3/4 cup orange juice
3/4 cup hot cocoa, made with 1 percent milk

**Lunch**
Beef Enchilada
   2 corn tortillas
   3 ounces lean roast beef
   2/3 teaspoon vegetable oil
   1/2 ounce low-fat cheddar cheese
   1/8 cup onion
   1/8 cup tomato
   1/4 cup lettuce
   2 teaspoons chili peppers
1/2 cup refried beans, made with vegetable oil
4 carrot sticks
4 celery sticks
1/2 cup 1 percent milk

**Dinner**
Chicken Taco
   2 corn tortillas
   3 ounces chicken breast without the skin
   2/3 teaspoon vegetable oil
   1/2 ounce low-fat cheddar cheese
   1 tablespoon guacamole
   1 tablespoon salsa
1/2 cup corn
   1/2 teaspoon tub margarine
1/2 cup Spanish rice, made with tub margarine
1/2 medium banana
1 cup coffee
   2 tablespoons 1 percent milk

**Snack**
1/2 cup ice milk

*Note: No salt is used when making the food.*

## STEP II—1,800 CALORIES

**Breakfast**
1/2 cup cantaloupe
3/4 cup farina, made with skim milk
1 slice white bread
   1 teaspoon tub margarine
   1 teaspoon jelly
3/4 cup orange juice
3/4 cup hot cocoa, made with skim milk

**Lunch**
Beef Enchilada
   2 corn tortillas
   2 ounces lean roast beef
   2/3 teaspoon vegetable oil
   1/2 ounce low-fat cheddar cheese
   1/8 cup onion
   1/8 cup tomato
   1/4 cup lettuce
   2 teaspoons chili peppers
2/3 cup refried beans, made with vegetable oil
4 carrot sticks
4 celery sticks
1/2 cup skim milk

**Dinner**
Chicken Taco
   2 corn tortillas
   3 ounces chicken breast without the skin
   2/3 teaspoon vegetable oil
   1/2 ounce low-fat cheddar cheese
   1 tablespoon guacamole
   1 tablespoon salsa
1/2 cup corn
   1/2 teaspoon tub margarine
1/2 cup Spanish rice, made with tub margarine
1 medium banana
1 cup coffee
   2 tablespoons skim milk

**Snack**
1 cup popcorn
   1 tablespoon tub margarine

| | Step I | Step II |
|---|---|---|
| Calories | 1,852 | 1,860 |
| Percent calories from fat | 29 | 28 |
| Percent calories from saturated fat | 9 | 6 |
| Cholesterol (milligrams) | 169 | 127 |
| Sodium (milligrams) | 1,616 | 1,787 |

Source: "Step by Step: Eating to Lower Your High Blood Cholesterol," National Heart, Lung, and Blood Institute, NIH Publication No. 94–2920, August 1994.

# The Heart-Healthy Eating Plan

## INTRODUCTION

The foods you eat play a big part in keeping your heart healthy. But, what exactly is a heart-healthy eating plan? And is a heart-healthy eating plan important for everyone? All healthy Americans, 2 years of age or older, should eat in a way that is lower in total fat, saturated fat, cholesterol, sodium, and extra calories. Heart disease is still the number one killer of both men and women in the United States. High blood cholesterol, high blood pressure, smoking, being overweight, and physical inactivity increase your risk of getting heart disease. The good news is that you can change these risk factors and reduce your risk of heart disease.

## IN ORDER TO HELP YOUR FAMILY EAT IN A HEART-HEALTHY WAY, FOLLOW THESE RECOMMENDATIONS

1. **Choose foods low in saturated fat.** All foods that contain fat are made up of a mixture of saturated and unsaturated fats. Saturated fat raises your blood cholesterol level more than anything else you eat. The best way to reduce blood cholesterol is to choose foods lower in saturated fat. Less than 10 percent of the calories in your diet should come from saturated fat. One way to help your family do this is by choosing foods such as fruits, vegetables, and whole grains—foods naturally low in total fat and high in starch and fiber.

2. **Choose foods low in total fat.** Since many foods high in total fat are also high in saturated fat, eating foods low in total fat will help your family eat less saturated fat. Less than 30 percent of the calories in your diet should come from fat. When you do eat fat, substitute unsaturated fat—either polyunsaturated or monounsaturated—for saturated fat. But, watch the amount. Fat is a rich source of calories, so eating foods low in fat will also help you eat fewer calories. Eating fewer calories can help you lose weight and, if you are overweight, losing weight is an important part of lowering your blood cholesterol.

3. **Choose foods high in starch and fiber.** Foods high in starch and fiber are excellent substitutes for foods high in saturated fat. These foods—breads, cereals, pasta, grains, fruits, and vegetables—are low in saturated fat and cholesterol. They are also lower in calories than foods that are high in fat. But limit fatty toppings and spreads like butter and sauces made with cream and whole milk dairy products. Foods high in starch and fiber are also good sources of vitamins and minerals.

    When eaten as part of a diet low in saturated fat and cholesterol, foods with soluble fiber—like oat and barley bran and dry peas and beans—may help to lower blood cholesterol.

*continues*

continued

4. **Choose foods low in cholesterol.** Remember, dietary cholesterol can raise blood cholesterol, although usually not as much as saturated fat. So it's important for your family to choose foods low in dietary cholesterol. Strive for less than 300 milligrams of cholesterol a day. Dietary cholesterol is found only in foods that come from animals. And even if an animal food is low in saturated fat, it may be high in cholesterol; for instance, organ meats (like liver) and egg yolks are low in saturated fat but high in cholesterol. Egg whites and foods from plant sources do not have cholesterol.

5. **Choose foods lower in salt and sodium.** Americans eat more salt (sodium chloride) and other forms of sodium than they need. Often, when people with high blood pressure cut back on salt and sodium, their blood pressure falls. Cutting back on salt and sodium also prevents blood pressure from rising. Some people like African Americans and the elderly are more affected by sodium than others. Since there's really no practical way to predict exactly who will be affected by sodium, it makes sense to limit intake of salt and sodium to help prevent high blood pressure.

   Americans, especially people with high blood pressure, should eat no more than about 6 grams of salt a day, which equals about 2,400 milligrams of sodium (the daily reference value you see on the new food label.) That's about 1 teaspoon of table salt. But remember to keep track of ALL salt eaten—including that in processed foods and added during cooking or at the table.

6. **Maintain a healthy weight, and lose weight if you are overweight.** People who are overweight tend to have higher blood cholesterol levels. And, as body weight increases, blood pressure increases. Overweight adults with an "apple" shape—bigger (pot) belly— tend to have a higher risk for heart disease than those with a "pear" shape—bigger hips and thighs. Whatever your body shape, when you cut the fat in your diet, you cut down on the richest source of calories. So it is not only what you eat but how much you eat. An eating pattern of foods high in starch and fiber, instead of fat and calories, in moderation is a good way to help control weight.

7. **Be more physically active.** Being physically active helps improve blood cholesterol levels. Being more active also can help you lose weight, lower your blood pressure, improve the fitness of your heart and blood vessels, and reduce stress. And being active together is great for the entire family.

Source: "The Sports Guide: NHLBI Planning Guide for Cardiovascular Risk Reduction Projects at Sporting Events," Office of Prevention, Education, and Control, National Heart, Lung and Blood Institute, NIH Publication No. 95–3802, October 1995.

# Your Diet after Coronary Artery Bypass Graft

## NUTRITIONAL GOALS

The nutritional guidelines following coronary artery bypass graft are divided into two segments. During the initial eight to 10 weeks following surgery, the goal is to meet nutrient needs to promote normal wound healing, including adequate amounts of calories, protein, vitamins (A, C, and B complex), and zinc. The next phase incorporates a heart-healthy diet.

## A HEART-HEALTHY DIET

A heart-healthy diet is vital as part of your medical management. To improve your cardiovascular health, the main areas for special attention are cholesterol, saturated fat, sodium intake, and weight control. A diet high in cholesterol and saturated fat intake from high-fat meats, whole milk, egg yolks, and other high-fat dairy products will increase your serum cholesterol, which circulates in your blood and can clog your arteries. A diet low in fats (particularly animal fats), moderate in sodium, high in complex carbohydrates, and high in soluble fiber can be heart protective. In addition, your total calorie intake should allow you to maintain your best body weight. If you have not already received a detailed plan for your heart-healthy diet, please ask your nurse or home care dietitian.

## DIETARY GUIDELINES

- Do not add salt in cooking or to any foods once prepared.
- Limit high-fat products (less than 30 percent of your total calorie intake should come from fat).
- Avoid regular processed, high-sodium foods.
  - pickles
  - luncheon meats (e.g., salami, corned beef, pastrami) and cured meats (e.g., bacon, smoked ham)
  - processed cheeses
  - salted potato chips, pretzels, and other visibly salted snacks
  - canned soups, meats, and vegetables
  - condiments containing sodium (e.g., soy sauce and many others)
- Choose reduced-sodium, low-fat products (< 250 mg sodium/serving).
- Avoid or minimize caffeine and alcohol intake, as directed by your physician.
- There are many foods that can be included in your diet.
  - freshly prepared, skinless meats, poultry, or fish
  - fresh or canned fruits in their own juice
  - fresh, frozen, or low-sodium canned vegetables
  - reduced-sodium cheeses made with skimmed or partly skimmed milk
  - unsalted snack foods
- Consume small, frequent meals.

Source: Barbara Stover Gingerich and Deborah Anne Ondeck, *Clinical Pathways for the Multidisciplinary Home Care Team,* Aspen Publishers, Inc., © 1996.

# Congestive Heart Failure and Your Diet

## NUTRITIONAL GOALS

As part of your medical therapy, your physician has ordered a sodium-controlled diet to reduce cardiovascular stress and fluid retention. In addition, eating a variety of foods divided into small meals and snacks will help ensure adequate vitamin and mineral intake and minimize heartburn. This restricted-sodium diet is intended to prevent any increased fluid accumulation. Therefore, it is very important to follow your diet carefully. If you have not received an individualized, sodium-controlled diet, please request one from your nurse or home care dietitian.

## GUIDELINES

Sodium comes in many forms. Table salt is one of the more prevalent forms of sodium. It is important to read food labels carefully and avoid foods that list "salt" or "sodium compounds" as one of the first three ingredients. General guidelines to reduce sodium intake include the following:

- Do not add salt in cooking or to any foods once prepared.

- Avoid regular processed products (i.e., products with >250 mg sodium/serving).
  - luncheon meats (e.g., salami, corned beef, pastrami) and cured meats (e.g., bacon, smoked ham)
  - processed cheeses
  - salted potato chips, pretzels, and other visibly salted snacks
  - canned soups, meats, and vegetables
  - condiments containing sodium (e.g., soy sauce and many others)
- Choose reduced-sodium products (<250 mg sodium/serving).
- Avoid or minimize caffeine and alcohol intake as directed by your physician.
- There are many foods that can be included in your diet.
  - freshly prepared, skinless meats, poultry, or fish
  - fresh or canned fruits
  - fresh, frozen, or low-sodium canned vegetables
  - reduced-sodium cheeses
  - unsalted snack foods
- Be sure to check with your physician or nurse if you need to restrict your fluid intake.

Source: Barbara Stover Gingerich and Deborah Anne Ondeck, *Clinical Pathways for the Multidisciplinary Home Care Team,* Aspen Publishers, Inc., © 1996.

# Myocardial Infarction and Your Diet

## NUTRITIONAL GOALS

A heart-healthy diet is vital as part of your medical management. To improve your cardiovascular health, the main areas for special attention are cholesterol, saturated fat, sodium intake, and weight control. A diet that is high in cholesterol and saturated fat intake from high-fat meats, whole milk, egg yolks, and other high-fat dairy products will increase your serum cholesterol, which circulates in your blood and can clog your arteries. A diet that is low in fats, particularly animal fats; moderate in sodium; high in complex carbohydrates; and high in soluble fiber can be heart protective. In addition, your total calorie intake should allow you to maintain your best body weight. If you have not already received a detailed plan for your heart-healthy diet, please ask your nurse or home care dietitian.

## GUIDELINES

1. Do not add salt in cooking or to any foods once prepared.
2. Limit high-fat products (<30 percent of your total calorie intake should come from fat).
3. Avoid processed high-sodium foods, for example
   - pickles
   - luncheon meats (e.g., salami, corned beef, pastrami), cured meats (e.g., bacon, smoked ham)
   - processed cheeses
   - salted potato chips, pretzels, and other visibly salted snacks
   - canned soups, meats, and vegetables
   - sodium-containing condiments (e.g., soy sauce and many other condiments)
4. Choose reduced-sodium, low-fat products (<250 mg sodium/serving).
5. Avoid or minimize caffeine and alcohol as directed by your physician.
6. There are many foods that can be included in your diet.
   - freshly prepared skinless meats, poultry, fish
   - fresh or canned fruit in its own juice
   - fresh, frozen, or low-sodium canned vegetables
   - reduced-sodium cheeses made with skimmed or partly skimmed milk
   - unsalted snack foods
7. Eat small frequent meals.

Source: Barbara Stover Gingerich and Deborah Anne Ondeck, *Clinical Pathways for the Multidisciplinary Home Care Team,* Aspen Publishers, Inc., © 1996.

# Shop to Your Heart's Content

## INTRODUCTION

Use this handy guide to shop for a variety of heart-healthy foods. By eating a variety of foods each day, you will get the nutrients you need. Remember to use the new food labels. Look for the words low-fat, lean, and light. The federal government has defined these words to help consumers find heart-healthy foods that contain less saturated fat, cholesterol, and sodium.

| | CHOOSE MORE OFTEN | CHOOSE LESS OFTEN |
|---|---|---|
| **Meat, Poultry, Fish, and Shellfish** | Lean cuts of meat with fat trimmed before cooking: <br> *Beef*—round, top loin, sirloin, chuck, arm pot roast <br> *Lamb*—leg shank, fore shank, whole leg, loin, sirloin <br> *Pork*—tenderloin, sirloin, top loin <br> *Veal*—cutlets, ground, shoulder, sirloin, rib roast <br> Turkey and chicken, skinless <br> Most seafood* <br> Low-fat lunch meat and hot dogs† | Fatty cuts of meat: <br> *Beef*—ribs, brisket, chuck blade roast, ground (regular) <br> *Lamb*—chops and ribs <br> *Pork*—spareribs, blade, center loin <br> Goose, duck <br> Liver, kidney <br> Sausage, bacon <br> Turkey and chicken with skin <br> Eel, pompano, and mackerel <br> Regular lunchmeat and hot dogs |
| **Dairy Products** | Skim or 1 percent milk <br> Nonfat or low-fat yogurt <br> Cheese with 3 grams of fat or less per ounce† <br> Low-fat or nonfat sour cream | Whole or 2 percent milk <br> Cream, most nondairy creamers <br> Whipped cream or nondairy topping <br> Whole-milk yogurt <br> Cheese with more than 3 grams of fat per ounce <br> Sour cream |
| **Eggs** | Egg whites <br> Cholesterol-free or cholesterol-reduced egg substitutes† | Egg yolks |

*Shrimp, abalone, and squid are low in fat but high in cholesterol.
†Choices may be higher in sodium.

*continues*

continued

| | CHOOSE MORE OFTEN | CHOOSE LESS OFTEN |
|---|---|---|
| **Fats and oils** | Unsaturated vegetable oils: corn, olive, canola, sesame, soybean, sunflower, safflower | Lard, butter, palm kernel oil, palm oil, beef tallow, cocoa butter, coconut oil |
| | Soft margarine made with unsaturated fats listed above as first ingredient | Hydrogenated fats and oils |
| | Low-fat or nonfat salad dressings | Margarine or shortening made with fats listed above |
| | Reduced or nonfat mayonnaise | Dressing made with egg yolk |
| | | Fried foods |
| **Fruits** | Fresh, frozen, canned, dried fruit, and fruit in its own juice | Fried fruit such as fried apples |
| **Vegetables** | Fresh, frozen, or canned†† vegetables | Vegetables prepared in butter, cream, sauce, or fried |
| **Breads, cereals, pasta, rice and grains, dry peas and beans** | Breads, white or whole grain, such as pita, bagel, English muffin, sandwich buns, dinner rolls | Croissants, pastry, doughnuts, coffee cake, butter rolls |
| | Rice cake | Snack crackers like cheese and butter crackers |
| | Corn tortilla | Pasta, grain, and potato dishes made with cream, butter, or cheese |
| | Low-fat crackers like matzo, bread sticks, rye crackers, saltines | Egg noodles |
| | Pancakes, waffles | Chow mein noodles, canned |
| | Lower-fat biscuits, muffins, hot cereals, most cold cereals†† | Regular granola cereals |
| | Rice, barley, bulgur | |
| | Dry peas and beans | |
| | Pasta | |

††Choices may be higher in sodium.

*continues*

continued

|  | **CHOOSE MORE OFTEN** | **CHOOSE LESS OFTEN** |
|---|---|---|
| **Sweets and snacks** | Nonfat and low-fat frozen desserts like sherbert, sorbet, Italian ice, frozen yogurt, frozen fruit juice bars<br><br>Low-fat or nonfat baked goods like brownies, cakes, cupcakes pastries, fig and other fruit bars, vanilla or lemon wafers, graham crackers, gingersnaps<br><br>Jelly beans, hard candy, fruit leather<br><br>Plain popcorn, pretzels, no-oil baked chips[tt]<br><br>*(Remember that baked goods and frozen desserts are high in sugar and may be high in calories.)* | High-fat frozen desserts, like ice cream, frozen tofu, whole-milk frozen yogurt<br><br>High-fat baked goods, like most store-bought pound and frosted cakes, pies, cookies<br><br>Milk chocolate<br><br>Fried chips and buttered popcorn |

[tt]Choices may be high in sodium

*continues*

continued

---

### Do You Know How Much You Are Serving

Learning about portion sizes is an important part of being in control of what you eat. Here are some tips to help you know just how much you're getting.

- **Jar lid:** A piece of meat the size of a pint or quart mayonnaise jar lid is about 3 ounces.
- **Deck of cards:** A standard deck of cards is about the same size as 3 ounces of meat, poultry, or fish.
- **Measuring cups:** To find out how much you're serving your family at meals, try dishing it up with measuring cups. After a few tries, it should be easy to judge how big the portions are.

---

### How Much Sodium Is in Your Food?

- Most canned vegetables, vegetable juices, and frozen vegetables with sauce are higher in sodium than fresh or frozen ones cooked without added salt.
- Sodium content of milk and milk products varies. Lowest are milk and yogurt. Natural cheese contains a bit more, followed by cottage cheese, then processed cheeses, cheese foods, and cheese spreads.
- Most fresh meats, poultry, and fish are low in sodium. Most cured and processed meats such as hot dogs, sausage, and lunch meats are higher in sodium because sodium is used as a preservative.
- "Convenience" foods such as frozen dinners and combination dishes, canned soups, and dehydrated mixes for soups, sauces, and salad dressings often contain a lot of sodium.

---

Source: "The Sports Guide: NHLBI Planning Guide for Cardiovascular Risk Reduction Projects at Sporting Events," Office of Prevention, Education, and Control, National Heart, Lung, and Blood Institute, NIH Publication No. 95–3802, October 1995.

## Serving Sizes for Meat and Cheese

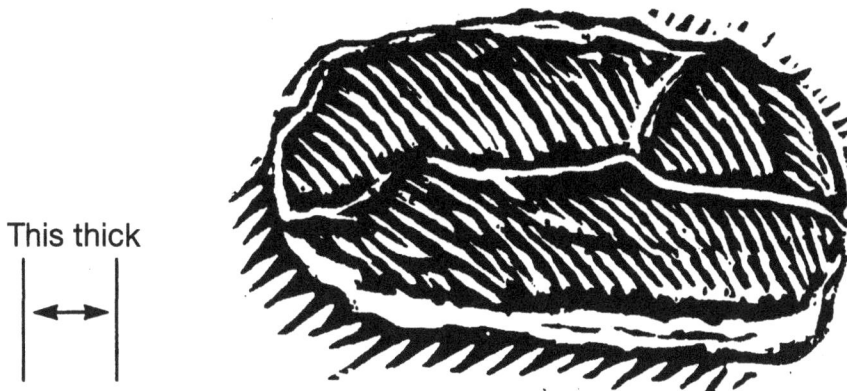

This thick

One piece of cooked roast beef or steak this size weighs 3 ounces.

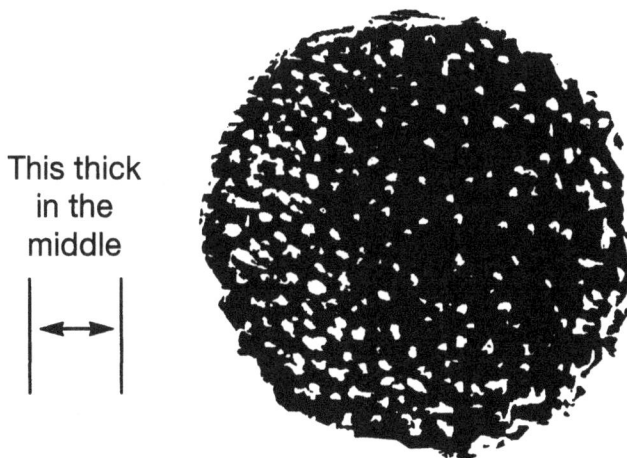

This thick
in the
middle

One cooked hamburger this size weighs 3 ounces.

*continues*

continued

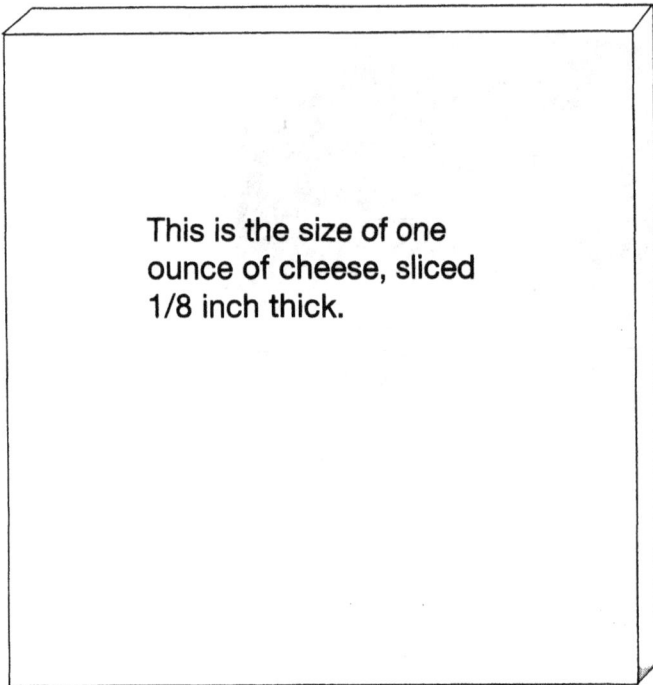

This is the size of one ounce of cheese, sliced 1/8 inch thick.

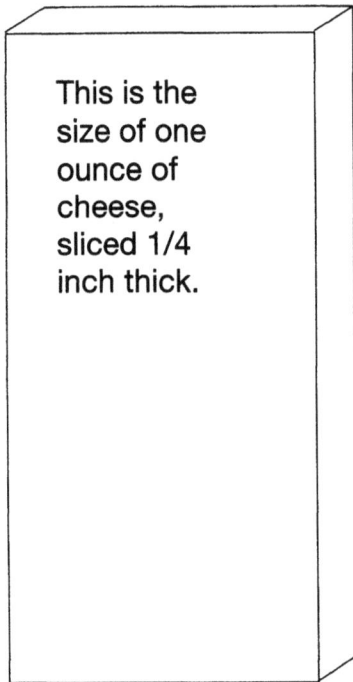

This is the size of one ounce of cheese, sliced 1/4 inch thick.

Source: "Step By Step Eating to Lower Your High Blood Cholesterol," NIH Publication No. 94–2920, U.S. Department of Health and Human Services, National Institutes of Health.

# ¡Reduzca la grasa—No el sabor!

## PROTEJA LA SALUD DE SU CORAZÓN Y EL DE SU FAMILIA SIRVIENDO ALIMENTOS BAJOS EN GRASA Y GRASA SATURADA

Las comidas latinas, tales como los frijoles (habichuelas), los vegetales, las frutas, el arroz y las tortillas de maíz, son parte de una alimentación saludable. Prepárelas de manera saludable para su corazón y el de su familia. Ayude a su familia a comer menos grasa y grasa saturada.

### COMPRE ALIMENTOS BAJOS EN GRASA

- Leche descremada o con 1% de grasa.
- Quesos, crema agria, aderezos para ensalada y mayonesa bajos en grasa o sin grasa.
- Pescado y pollo o pavo sin pellejo. Cortes de carne bajos en grasa en vez de carnes con alto contenido de grasa.
- Frutas, vegetales y granos como frijoles, arroz, tortillas de maíz y pastas.

### COCINE CON MENOS GRASA

- Hornee, ase o hierva en vez de freír.
- Use un sartén, que no pegue, humedecido con aceite en aerosol.
- Use sólo poca cantidad de aceite vegetal o margarina, en vez de manteca o mantequilla.
- Cocine los frijoles y el arroz sin manteca, tocino ni otras carnes con alto contenido de grasa. Déle sabor a los frijoles con chile verde, cebolla, ajo, orégano o cilantro.

### ELIMINE LA GRASA

- Antes de cocinar la carne de res y de cerdo, córteles la grasa.
- Antes de comer pollo y pavo, quíteles el pellejo.
- Escurra la grasa que sueltan las carnes al cocinarlas.
- Enfríe las sopas y los caldos, y quite la capa de grasa antes de recalentar.

### USTED PUEDE HACER CAMBIOS POCO A POCO.

### Marque los consejos que pondrá en práctica para comer menos grasa

- ☐ Comer frutas en vez de postres altos en grasa como flan, helado de leche, pan dulce o bizcochos.
- ☐ Tomar leche descremada o con 1% de grasa.
- ☐ Comprar quesos bajos en grasa o sin grasa.
- ☐ Hornear, asar o guisar el pollo en vez de freírlo.
- ☐ Quitar el pellejo al pollo.

Source: "Reduzca la Grasa—No el Sabor!" NIH Publication No. 96–4045, National Heart, Lung, and Blood Institute, National Institutes of Health, September 1996.

# Cooking the Heart-Healthy Way

Here are some easy cooking tips to cut down on saturated fat, cholesterol, and sodium.

## MEAT, POULTRY, AND FISH

**Before cooking meat, poultry, or fish:**

- Trim fat from meat; remove the skin and fat from poultry.
- If you buy tuna or other canned fish packed in oil, rinse it in a strainer before cooking. Better yet, buy canned fish packed in water. If you are watching your sodium to help lower blood pressure, be sure to rinse the fish whether it is packed in oil or water.

**Changes in your cooking style also can help to lower fat.**

- Bake, broil, microwave, poach, or roast instead of frying.
- When you do fry, use a nonstick pan and a nonstick cooking spray or a very small amount of oil or margarine.
- When you roast meat or make meatloaf, place the meat on a rack so the fat can drip away.
- When a recipe calls for ground meat, brown the meat and drain well before adding to other ingredients.
- If you baste meats and poultry, use fat-free ingredients like wine, tomato juice, lemon juice, or defatted beef or chicken broth instead of the fatty drippings.

## SAUCES, SOUPS, AND CASSEROLES

- After making sauces or soups, cool them in the refrigerator and skim the fat from the top. Treat canned broth-style soups the same way. Try low sodium or reduced sodium soups.
- When making casseroles with cheese, try lower-fat cheese. Or use less regular cheese than the recipe calls for. If you use a sharp-flavored cheese, you won't taste the difference.
- When you make creamed soup or white sauces, use skim, 1 percent, or evaporated skim milk instead of 2 percent milk, whole milk, or cream. To make a low-fat sauce, thicken it with cornstarch or flour.
- Make main dishes with pasta, rice, or dry peas and beans. If you add meat, use small pieces just for flavoring instead of as the main ingredient.

*continues*

continued

## SEASONING AND CONDIMENTS

- Use small amounts of lean meats instead of salt pork or fatback to flavor vegetables while cooking.
- Flavor cooked vegetables with herbs or butter flavored seasoning instead of butter or margarine.
- Use herbs, spices, and no-salt seasoning blends to bring out the flavor of foods. Try using garlic, garlic powder, onion, or onion powder instead of garlic salt and onion salt.
- Use salt sparingly in cooking, and use less salt at the table. Reduce the amount a little each day until no salt is used.
- Limit salty condiments like olives and pickles.

## CONVENIENCE FOODS

**And for those times when you don't feel like cooking:**

- Use your own convenience foods—low-fat casseroles and soups that you have cooked ahead and then frozen in small batches.
- Check the nutrition label to choose frozen dinners and pizzas that are lower in saturated fat, cholesterol, and sodium. Make sure the dinners have vegetables, fruits, and grains—or add them on the side.
- Use fewer sauces, mixes, and "instant" products, including flavored rices, pastas, and cereal, which usually have added salt.
- Use vegetables that are fresh, frozen without sauce, or canned with no salt added.

Source: "The Sports Guide: NHLBI Planning Guide for Cardiovascular Risk Reduction Projects at Sporting Events," Office of Prevention, Education, and Control, National Heart, Lung, and Blood Institute, NIH Publication No. 95–3802, October 1995.

# New Ways To Use Favorite Recipes

## INTRODUCTION

Lots of special cookbooks and recipe booklets can help you lower the fat, saturated fat, cholesterol, and sodium when you cook. But you don't have to throw out your favorite cookbook or recipes that you've been using for years. Just cut down on the high-fat, high-sodium ingredients, and substitute ingredients that are lower in saturated fat, cholesterol, and sodium as much as possible. Some recipes may change in texture and consistency when you use these substitutions.

## RECIPE SUBSTITUTIONS

| Instead of | Use |
|---|---|
| Whole milk | Skim or 1 percent milk |
| Evaporated milk | Evaporated skim milk |
| Light cream | Equal amounts of 1 percent milk and evaporated skim milk |
| Heavy cream | Evaporated skim milk |
| 1 cup butter | 1 cup soft margarine or 2/3 cup vegetable oil* |
| Shortening or lard | Soft margarine* |
| Mayonnaise or salad dressing | Nonfat or light mayonnaise or salad dressing; mustard in sandwiches |
| 1 whole egg | 1/4 cup egg substitute or 2 egg whites |
| Cheese | Lower-fat cheese† |
| Cream cheese | Nonfat or light cream cheese |
| Sour cream | Nonfat or low-fat sour cream or yogurt |
| Fat for greasing pan | Non stick cooking spray |
| 1 ounce baking chocolate | 3 tablespoons cocoa powder plus 1 tablespoon vegetable oil |
| Regular bouillon or broth | Low sodium bouillon and broth |
| Fatback, neck bones, or ham hocks | Skinless chicken thighs |
| Pork bacon | Turkey bacon, lean ham, or Canadian bacon (omit if on low sodium diet) |
| Pork sausage | Ground skinless turkey breast |
| Ground beef and pork | Ground skinless turkey breast |

*The texture of baked goods may be different when you use these substitutions. "Light" margarine is not recommended for baking. Experiment to find out what works best for you.

†Some salad dressings, processed cheeses, and cottage cheeses are very high in sodium. Omit if you are on a low-sodium diet or substitute a product that is low in sodium and fat.

If you or someone you know is on a low-cholesterol or low-sodium diet, you can contact the NHLBI Information Center at P.O. Box 30105, Bethesda, MD 20824-0105 for more information on how to follow these eating plans.

Source: "The Sports Guide: NHLBI Planning Guide for Cardiovascular Risk Reduction Projects at Sporting Events," Office of Prevention, Education, and Control, National Heart Lung, and Blood Institute, NIH Publication No. 95–3802, October 1995.

# Eat Right When Eating Out

*Eating out while following a heart-healthy diet is getting easier: Many restaurants have at least some menu items that are low in saturated fat and cholesterol. Here are some menu items to choose—and some to decrease:*

## BREAKFAST

*Choose:*

- egg substitute
- hot or cold cereal
- toast with margarine and jam
- English muffin or bagel with nonfat cream cheese
- fruit or juice

*Decrease:*

- egg yolks, any style
- fried potatoes
- bacon or sausage
- biscuit, croissant, or sweet roll

## LUNCH

*Choose:*

- salad (with dressing on the side)
- regular-sized hamburger (hold the mayo)
- turkey, chicken, or roast beef sandwich (hold the mayo)
- soup (other than cream-based)

*Decrease:*

- deluxe sandwiches
- hot dogs or sausage
- breaded and fried chicken or fish
- cream-based soups
- french fries, onion rings, or chips

## DINNER

*Choose:*

- pasta with low-fat sauce
- grilled or broiled fish or skinless chicken
- lean steak, trimmed of fat
- vegetarian entree (little or no cheese)
- baked potato with a little margarine or nonfat yogurt
- vegetables, plain or with a little oil
- low-fat desserts like fresh fruit, sorbet, sherbert, ice milk, or nonfat frozen yogurt

*Decrease:*

- prime rib or untrimmed steaks or chops
- fried chicken or fish
- cream sauces or gravies
- rich desserts, such as cake, cheesecake, tortes, etc.

*continues*

continued

Here are more tips for eating out:

- Choose restaurants that have low-fat, low-cholesterol menu choices. And don't be afraid to make special requests: it's your right as a paying customer.
- Control serving sizes by asking for a small serving, sharing a dish with a companion, or taking some home.
- Ask that gravy, butter, rich sauces, and salad dressing be served on the side. That way, you can control the amount you eat.
- Ask to substitute a salad or baked potato for chips, fries, or other extras—or just ask that the extras be left off your plate.
- When ordering pizza, order vegetable toppings like green pepper, onions, and mushrooms instead of meat toppings or extra cheese.
- At fast food restaurants, go for salads, grilled (not fried or breaded) chicken sandwiches, regular-sized hamburgers, or roast beef sandwiches. Go easy on the regular salad dressings and fatty sauces. Limit jumbo or deluxe burgers or sandwiches.
- At the salad bar, fill up on vegetables. Limit foods like eggs, bacon, and cheese, and prepared salads like potato or macaroni salad. Go easy on the salad dressing—and choose low-calorie dressing or oil and vinegar when it's offered.
- Try different ethnic cuisines. Many, such as Chinese and Middle Eastern, offer lots of low-fat choices.

---

### Quick Check

Eating Out—TRY IT!

Check off one of these things to try. Do it today!

- ☐ The next time I go out for lunch, I'll try a regular hamburger instead of the deluxe—and save on saturated fat and cholesterol.

- ☐ The next time I order pizza, I'll spice it up with vegetable toppings instead of fattier meat toppings like sausage or pepperoni.

- ☐ The next time I'm out for dinner, I'll ask that salad dressing and other sauces be served on the side. To cut down on fat, I'll use just a little bit.

---

continues

continued

## Tips for Eating at Social Events

Eating at social events like parties, receptions, family gatherings, and church socials can be a challenge to your heart-healthy eating style. Since you can't control what is served, you may feel pressured to eat foods high in saturated fat and cholesterol.

Here are some tips that will help you eat healthfully at social events:

- At a buffet, look ahead in line to see what low-fat foods are available. Fill up on low-fat items and take only small servings of high-fat foods.
- Bring a low-fat dish to a potluck dinner. That way, you'll have at least one low-fat item from which to choose.
- At parties, focus on activities other than eating. Sit away from the area where the food is being served so you won't be tempted to overeat.
- Ask for help from your family and friends who know you are following a cholesterol-lowering diet. See if they will include some low-fat dishes instead of the high-fat favorites.
- Have a few ready answers to politely say no to high-fat foods. For example, "Thank you, but I couldn't eat another bite—everything was delicious."
- If you do eat too many high-fat foods at a social event, don't feel guilty. Just eat lightly the next day and get back on track.

**NOTES:**

Source: "Step by Step: Eating to Lower Your High Blood Cholesterol," National Heart, Lung, and Blood Institute, NIH Publication No. 94–2920, August 1994.

# Saturated Fat, Total Fat, Cholesterol, Calories, and Sodium in Basic Foods

## INTRODUCTION

This table gives the saturated fat, total fat, cholesterol, calories, and sodium for some basic foods. Remember, there are 9 calories in each gram of fat. The foods within each group are ranked from low- to high-saturated fat. Choose most often the foods from the top part of each group; they are lower in saturated fat and cholesterol. The examples are meant to show the differences in fat and cholesterol in select foods.

### MEAT, POULTRY, FISH, AND SHELLFISH (3 oz. cooked)

### Beef (Fat trimmed to 1/8 in. unless otherwise noted)

|  | Saturated Fat (grams) | Cholesterol (mg) | Total Fat (grams) | Total Calories | Sodium (mg) |
|---|---|---|---|---|---|
| Liver, beef, braised* | 2 | 331 | 4 | 137 | 60 |
| Eye of round, roasted | 3 | 60 | 8 | 171 | 52 |
| Top round, broiled | 3 | 73 | 8 | 185 | 51 |
| Top sirloin, broiled | 5 | 77 | 13 | 204 | 52 |
| Ground, extra lean, broiled medium | 6 | 71 | 14 | 217 | 59 |
| Ground, lean, broiled medium | 7 | 74 | 16 | 231 | 65 |
| Salami, cooked | 7 | 51 | 17 | 216 | 984 |
| (3 oz. is about 4 slices, 4 in. around, 1/8 in. thick) | | | | | |
| Chuck, arm pot roast, braised | 8 | 86 | 19 | 277 | 52 |
| Short loin, T-bone steak, broiled (1/4 in. trim) | 9 | 70 | 18 | 253 | 52 |
| Chuck, blade roast, braised | 9 | 88 | 23 | 308 | 56 |

*Liver and most organ meats are low in fat but high in cholesterol

### Lamb (Fat trimmed to 1/8 in.)

|  | Saturated Fat (grams) | Cholesterol (mg) | Total Fat (grams) | Total Calories | Sodium (mg) |
|---|---|---|---|---|---|
| Leg, whole, roasted | 5 | 79 | 12 | 207 | 58 |
| Loin, broiled | 7 | 81 | 16 | 229 | 71 |
| Shoulder, arm braised | 8 | 103 | 19 | 289 | 62 |

*continues*

continued

## Pork (Fresh unless noted otherwise; fat trimmed to 1/4 in.)

| | Saturated Fat (grams) | Cholesterol (mg) | Total Fat (grams) | Total Calories | Sodium (mg) |
|---|---|---|---|---|---|
| Cured, ham steak, boneless, extra lean, cooked, served cold | 1 | 39 | 4 | 105 | 1,080 |
| Loin, tenderloin, roasted | 2 | 67 | 5 | 147 | 47 |
| Leg (ham), rump half, roasted | 5 | 81 | 12 | 214 | 52 |
| Cured, shoulder arm picnic, roasted | 7 | 49 | 18 | 238 | 912 |
| Ground pork, cooked | 7 | 80 | 18 | 252 | 62 |

## Chicken

| | Saturated Fat (grams) | Cholesterol (mg) | Total Fat (grams) | Total Calories | Sodium (mg) |
|---|---|---|---|---|---|
| Chicken, roasting, light meat without skin, roasted | 1 | 64 | 4 | 130 | 43 |
| Breast, without skin (3 oz. is about 1/2) | 1 | 72 | 3 | 140 | 63 |
| Chicken roll, light meat, about 2 slices or 2 oz. | 1 | 27 | 4 | 87 | 321 |
| Drumstick, without skin (3 oz. is about 2) | 2 | 79 | 5 | 146 | 81 |
| Breast, with skin (3 oz. is about 1/2) | 2 | 71 | 7 | 168 | 60 |
| Wing, without skin (3 oz. is about 4) | 2 | 72 | 7 | 173 | 78 |
| Chicken, roasting, dark meat without skin, roasted | 3 | 63 | 7 | 152 | 81 |
| Drumstick, with skin (3 oz. is about 1 1/2) | 3 | 77 | 10 | 184 | 77 |
| Thigh, without skin (3 oz. is about 1 1/2) | 3 | 81 | 9 | 178 | 75 |
| Chicken hot dog, about 1 | 3 | 55 | 11 | 142 | 754 |
| Thigh, with skin (3 oz. is about 1 1/2) | 4 | 79 | 13 | 210 | 71 |
| Wing, with skin (3 oz. is about 2 1/2) | 5 | 71 | 17 | 247 | 70 |

## Turkey

| | Saturated Fat (grams) | Cholesterol (mg) | Total Fat (grams) | Total Calories | Sodium (mg) |
|---|---|---|---|---|---|
| Breast, without skin | <1 | 71 | <1 | 115 | 44 |
| Breast, with skin | <1 | 77 | 3 | 130 | 45 |
| Wing, without skin | 1 | 87 | 3 | 139 | 66 |
| Leg, without skin | 1 | 101 | 3 | 135 | 69 |
| Turkey roll, light meat, about 2 slices or 2 oz. | 1 | 23 | 4 | 81 | 269 |
| Leg, with skin | 1 | 60 | 5 | 145 | 68 |
| Wing, with skin | 2 | 98 | 8 | 176 | 62 |
| Ground turkey, meat and skin, cooked | 3 | 87 | 11 | 200 | 90 |
| Turkey bologna, about 2 slices or 2 oz. | n/a | 54 | 8 | 110 | 483 |
| Turkey hot dog, about 1 | n/a | 59 | 10 | 125 | 785 |

*continues*

continued

## Fish (Baked, broiled, or microwaved)

|  | Saturated Fat (grams) | Cholesterol (mg) | Total Fat (grams) | Total Calories | Sodium (mg) |
|---|---|---|---|---|---|
| Haddock | <1 | 63 | <1 | 95 | 74 |
| Halibut | <1 | 35 | 3 | 119 | 59 |
| Bluefin tuna, fresh | 1 | 42 | 5 | 157 | 43 |
| Sockeye salmon | 2 | 74 | 9 | 183 | 56 |

## Shellfish (Steamed, poached, or broiled)

|  | Saturated Fat (grams) | Cholesterol (mg) | Total Fat (grams) | Total Calories | Sodium (mg) |
|---|---|---|---|---|---|
| Northern lobster | <1 | 61 | <1 | 83 | 323 |
| Clams | <1 | 57 | 2 | 126 | 95 |
| Clams, canned, drained solids | <1 | 57 | 2 | 126 | 95 |
| Shrimp | <1 | 167 | 1 | 85 | 192 |
| Oyster | 1 | 89 | 4 | 116 | 359 |

## DAIRY FOODS

### Milk (1 cup)

|  | Saturated Fat (grams) | Cholesterol (mg) | Total Fat (grams) | Total Calories | Sodium (mg) |
|---|---|---|---|---|---|
| Skim milk | <1 | 4 | <1 | 86 | 126 |
| Buttermilk | 1 | 9 | 2 | 99 | 257 |
| Low-fat milk, 1% fat | 2 | 10 | 3 | 102 | 123 |
| Low-fat milk, 2% fat | 3 | 18 | 5 | 121 | 122 |
| Whole milk, 3.3% fat | 5 | 33 | 8 | 150 | 120 |

### Yogurt (1 cup)

|  | Saturated Fat (grams) | Cholesterol (mg) | Total Fat (grams) | Total Calories | Sodium (mg) |
|---|---|---|---|---|---|
| Plain yogurt, nonfat | <1 | 4 | <1 | 127 | 174 |
| Plain yogurt, low-fat | 2 | 14 | 4 | 144 | 160 |
| Plain yogurt, whole milk | 5 | 29 | 7 | 139 | 105 |

*continues*

continued

## Soft cheeses (1 oz.)

| | Saturated Fat (grams) | Cholesterol (mg) | Total Fat (grams) | Total Calories | Sodium (mg) |
|---|---|---|---|---|---|
| Pot cheese or uncreamed dry curd cottage cheese, 1/3 cup | <1 | 3 | <1 | 41 | 189 |
| Cottage cheese, low-fat (1%), 1/2 cup | <1 | 5 | 1 | 82 | 459 |
| Ricotta, part-skim (1/4 cup) | 3 | 19 | 5 | 86 | 78 |
| Cottage cheese, creamed, 1/2 cup | 3 | 17 | 5 | 117 | 457 |
| Ricotta, whole milk, 1/4 cup | 5 | 32 | 8 | 108 | 52 |

## Hard cheeses (1 oz.)

| | Saturated Fat (grams) | Cholesterol (mg) | Total Fat (grams) | Total Calories | Sodium (mg) |
|---|---|---|---|---|---|
| Fat-free, low-cholesterol imitation cheese | <1 | 1 | <1 | 41 | 439 |
| Swiss cheese, reduced-fat | 3 | 9 | 4 | 70 | 35 |
| Reduced-fat and low-sodium cheese— American, cheddar, colby, monterey jack, muenster, or provolone[†] | 3 | 18 | 4 | 71 | 88 |
| Mozzarella, part-skim | 3 | 16 | 5 | 72 | 132 |
| Reduced-fat cheese—American, cheddar, colby, monterey jack, muenster, provolone, or string cheese[†] | 3 | 15 | 5 | 79 | 150 |
| Mozzarella | 4 | 22 | 6 | 80 | 106 |
| Swiss | 5 | 26 | 8 | 107 | 74 |
| American processed cheese | 6 | 27 | 9 | 106 | 406 |
| Cheddar | 6 | 30 | 9 | 114 | 176 |

[†]The nutrient values shown for these cheeses are averages of the different types and brands.

## EGGS

| | Saturated Fat (grams) | Cholesterol (mg) | Total Fat (grams) | Total Calories | Sodium (mg) |
|---|---|---|---|---|---|
| Egg white (1) | 0 | 0 | 0 | 17 | 55 |
| Egg yolk (1) | 2 | 213 | 5 | 59 | 7 |

*continues*

continued

## NUTS AND SEEDS (1 OUNCE—ABOUT 1/4 CUP—UNLESS NOTED OTHERWISE)
## (NOTE: ALL NUTS AND SEEDS ARE UNSALTED)

|  | Saturated Fat (grams) | Cholesterol (mg) | Total Fat (grams) | Total Calories | Sodium (mg) |
|---|---|---|---|---|---|
| Almonds | 1 | 0 | 15 | 167 | 3 |
| Sunflower seed kernels, roasted | 2 | 0 | 14 | 165 | 1 |
| Pecans | 2 | 0 | 19 | 190 | 0 |
| English walnuts | 2 | 0 | 17 | 182 | 3 |
| Pistachio nuts | 2 | 0 | 14 | 164 | 2 |
| Peanuts | 2 | 0 | 14 | 159 | 5 |
| Peanut butter, smooth, made with added salt, 2 Tbsp. | 3 | 0 | 16 | 190 | 149 |
| Brazil nuts | 5 | 0 | 19 | 186 | 0 |

## BREADS, CEREALS, PASTA, RICE, AND DRY PEAS AND BEANS

### Breads

|  | Saturated Fat (grams) | Cholesterol (mg) | Total Fat (grams) | Total Calories | Sodium (mg) |
|---|---|---|---|---|---|
| Corn tortilla, 1 (6–7 in. wide) | <1 | 0 | <1 | 56 | 40 |
| English muffin, 1 muffin | <1 | 0 | 1 | 134 | 265 |
| Bagel, plain 1 (3 1/2 in.) | <1 | 0 | 1 | 195 | 379 |
| Whole wheat bread, 1 slice | <1 | 0 | 1 | 70 | 149 |
| Hamburger or hot dog bun, plain, 1 | <1 | 0 | 2 | 123 | 241 |
| Croissant, butter, 1 medium (4 1/2 × 4 × 1 3/4 in.) | 7 | 0 | 12 | 232 | 424 |

### Cereals

|  | Saturated Fat (grams) | Cholesterol (mg) | Total Fat (grams) | Total Calories | Sodium (mg) |
|---|---|---|---|---|---|
| Oatmeal, instant (1 packet, 3/4 cup) | <1 | 0 | 2 | 108 | 180 |
| Oatmeal, quick, cooked without salt (1 cup) | <1 | 0 | 2 | 145 | 1 |
| Corn flakes, 1 cup | n/a | 0 | <1 | 98 | 240 |
| Granola, 1/2 cup | 3 | 0 | 17 | 298 | 6 |

*continues*

continued

## Pasta (1 cup cooked)

|  | Saturated Fat (grams) | Cholesterol (mg) | Total Fat (grams) | Total Calories | Sodium (mg) |
|---|---|---|---|---|---|
| Spaghetti or macaroni | <1 | 0 | 1 | 197 | 1** |
| Egg noodles | <1 | 53 | 2 | 212 | 11** |

## Grains (1 cup cooked)

|  | Saturated Fat (grams) | Cholesterol (mg) | Total Fat (grams) | Total Calories | Sodium (mg) |
|---|---|---|---|---|---|
| White rice | <1 | 0 | <1 | 205 | 1 |
| Brown rice | <1 | 0 | 2 | 216 | 9 |

## Dry Peas and Beans (1/2 cup cooked)

|  | Saturated Fat (grams) | Cholesterol (mg) | Total Fat (grams) | Total Calories | Sodium (mg) |
|---|---|---|---|---|---|
| Kidney beans, canned, solids, and liquid | <1 | 0 | <1 | 104 | 445†† |
| Kidney beans, dry | <1 | 0 | 1 | 112 | 2 |
| Garbanzo beans/chickpeas, canned, solids, and liquid | <1 | 0 | 1 | 143 | 359†† |
| Black-eyed peas, canned, solids, and liquid | <1 | 0 | <1 | 92 | 359†† |

†Pasta cooked without salt.
††Rinsing canned beans and peas with water will reduce the sodium content.

## FRUITS AND VEGETABLES

### Fruit, raw

|  | Saturated Fat (grams) | Cholesterol (mg) | Total Fat (grams) | Total Calories | Sodium (mg) |
|---|---|---|---|---|---|
| Peach, 1 | <1 | 0 | <1 | 37 | 0 |
| Orange, 1 | <1 | 0 | <1 | 62 | 0 |
| Apple, 1 | <1 | 0 | <1 | 81 | 1 |
| Banana, 1 | <1 | 0 | <1 | 105 | 1 |
| Avocado, 1/6 (or 2 Tbsp.) | <1 | 0 | 5 | 54 | 4 |

*continues*

*continued*

## Vegetable, cooked (1/2 cup)

|  | Saturated Fat (grams) | Cholesterol (mg) | Total Fat (grams) | Total Calories | Sodium (mg) |
|---|---|---|---|---|---|
| Potato | <1 | 0 | <1 | 68 | 3 |
| Corn | <1 | 0 | 1 | 89 | 14 |
| Carrot | <1 | 0 | <1 | 35 | 52 |
| Broccoli | <1 | 0 | <1 | 23 | 8 |

## SWEETS AND SNACKS

|  | Saturated Fat (grams) | Cholesterol (mg) | Total Fat (grams) | Total Calories | Sodium (mg) |
|---|---|---|---|---|---|
| Hard candy (1 oz). | 0 | 0 | 0 | 106 | 11 |
| Angel food cake, purchased, 1/12 of 9 in. cake | 0 | 0 | <1 | 73 | 212 |
| Ginger snap, 1 (about 1/4 oz.) | <1 | 0 | <1 | 29 | 46 |
| Frozen yogurt, fruit or vanilla, nonfat (1/2 cup) | <1 | 2 | <1 | 82 | 39 |
| Vanilla wafer, 1 | <1 | 2 | <1 | 18 | 12 |
| Fig bar, 1 (about 1/2 oz.) | <1 | 0 | 1 | 56 | 56 |
| Pretzels, salted (1 ounce, about 5 twists, 3 1/4 × 2 1/4 × 1/4 in.) | <1 | 0 | 1 | 108 | 486 |
| Popcorn, air popped without salt (1 oz. is about 3 1/2 cups) | <1 | 0 | 1 | 108 | 1 |
| Chocolate chip cookie, 1 (2 1/4 in. around) | <1 | 0 | 2 | 48 | 32 |
| Sherbet, orange, (1/2 cup) | 1 | 5 | 2 | 132 | 44 |
| Ice milk, vanilla, hard (1/2 cup) | 2 | 9 | 3 | 92 | 56 |
| Potato chips (1 oz.) | 3 | 0 | 10 | 152 | 168 |
| Pound cake, purchased, 1/10 of 10.75 oz. cake | 3 | 66 | 6 | 117 | 119 |
| Ice cream, vanilla, regular, (1/2 cup) | 5 | 29 | 7 | 132 | 53 |

## FAST FOODS

|  | Saturated Fat (grams) | Cholesterol (mg) | Total Fat (grams) | Total Calories | Sodium (mg) |
|---|---|---|---|---|---|
| Tossed salad, no dressing (1 1/2 cup) | 0 | 0 | <1 | 32 | 53 |
| Grilled chicken sandwich | 1 | 60 | 7 | 288 | 758 |
| Cheese pizza, 1/8 of 12 in. pizza | 2 | 9 | 3 | 140 | 336 |
| Roast beef sandwich, plain | 4 | 52 | 14 | 346 | 792 |
| French fries, regular order | 4 | 0 | 12 | 235 | 124 |
| Hamburger, plain | 4 | 36 | 12 | 275 | 387 |

*continues*

continued

| | Saturated Fat (grams) | Cholesterol (mg) | Total Fat (grams) | Total Calories | Sodium (mg) |
|---|---|---|---|---|---|
| Hot dog | 5 | 44 | 15 | 242 | 671 |
| Fish sandwich with tartar sauce | 5 | 55 | 23 | 431 | 615 |
| Chicken, breaded and fried, boneless pieces, 6 | 6 | 62 | 18 | 290 | 542 |
| Cheeseburger, plain, single patty | 7 | 50 | 15 | 320 | 500 |
| Chicken fillet sandwich, plain | 9 | 60 | 30 | 515 | 957 |
| Egg & bacon biscuit, 1 | 10 | 353 | 31 | 457 | 999 |
| Cheeseburger, large, double patty with condiments | 18 | 141 | 44 | 706 | 1,149 |

## FATS AND OILS (1 tbsp.)

| | Saturated Fat (grams) | Cholesterol (mg) | Polyunsaturated Fat (grams) | Monounsaturated Fat (grams) |
|---|---|---|---|---|
| Margarine, diet | 1 | 0 | 2 | 3 |
| Canola oil | 1 | 0 | 4 | 9 |
| Safflower oil | 1 | 0 | 11 | 2 |
| Corn oil | 2 | 0 | 8 | 4 |
| Olive oil | 2 | 0 | 1 | 10 |
| Margarine, soft tub | 2 | 0 | 5 | 4 |
| Margarine, liquid, bottled | 2 | 0 | 5 | 4 |
| Margarine, stick | 2 | 0 | 4 | 5 |
| Lard | 5 | 12 | 2 | 6 |
| Butter | 7 | 28 | <1 | 3 |

in. = inches
oz. = ounces
Tbsp. = tablespoon
< = less than
n/a = not available

## SOURCES

*Composition of Foods—Raw-Processed-Prepared, Agriculture Handbook 8. Series and Supplements.* United States Department of Agriculture, Human Nutrition Information Service.

*New beef and lamb nutrient data for cuts trimmed to 1/8 in. external fat.* United States Department of Agriculture, Human Nutrition Information Service, unpublished data, 1994.

*Minnesota Nutrition Data System (NDS)* software, developed by the Nutrition Coordinating Center, University of Minnesota, Minneapolis, MN. Food Database version 5A, Nutrient Database version 20.

*continues*

continued

# FOOD LABEL CLAIMS AND WHAT THEY MEAN

Here are the main label claims used on food packages—and what they mean:

## Saturated Fats

- **Saturated-fat-free\*:** Less than 1/2 gram saturated fat in a serving; levels of trans fatty acids must be not more than 1 percent of total fat.
- **Low saturated fat\*\*:** 1 gram saturated fat or less in a serving and 15 percent or less of calories from saturated fat. For a meal or main dish (like a frozen dinner): 1 gram saturated fat or less in 100 grams of food and less than 10 percent of calories from saturated fat.

## Cholesterol

- **Cholesterol-free\*:** Less than 2 milligrams (mg) cholesterol in a serving; saturated fat content must be 2 grams or less in a serving.
- **Low-cholesterol\*\*:** 20 mg cholesterol or less in a serving; saturated fat content must be 2 grams or less in a serving. For a meal or main dish: 20 mg cholesterol or less in 100 grams of food, with saturated fat content less than 2 grams in 100 grams of food.

## Fat

- **Fat-free\*:** Less than 1/2 gram fat in a serving.
- **Low-fat\*\*:** 3 grams total fat or less in a serving. For a meal or main dish: 3 grams total fat or less in 100 grams of food and not more than 30 percent calories from fat.

**Percent fat-free:** A food with this claim must also meet the low-fat claim.

## Calories

- **Calorie-free\*:** Less than 5 calories in a serving.
- **Low-calorie\*\*:** 40 calories or less in a serving.

## Sodium

- **Sodium-free\*:** Less than 5 mg sodium in a serving.
- **Low-sodium\*\*:** 140 mg sodium or less in a serving. For a meal or main dish: 140 mg sodium or less in 100 grams of food.
- **Very low sodium:** 35 mg sodium or less in a serving.

*continues*

continued

**Light**—A product has been changed to have half the fat or one-third fewer calories than the regular product; or the sodium in a low-calorie, low-fat food has been cut by 50 percent; or a meal or main dish is low-fat or low-calorie.

"Light" also may be used to describe things like the color or texture of a food, as long as the label explains this: for example, "light brown sugar" or "light and fluffy."

**Reduced/Less/Lower/Fewer**—A food (like a lower-fat hot dog or a lower-sodium cracker) has at least 25 percent less of something like calories, fat, saturated fat, cholesterol, or sodium than the regular food or a similar food to which it is compared.

**Lean and Extra Lean**—Two terms that are used to describe the fat content of meat, poultry, fish, and shellfish.

**Lean**—Less than 10 grams fat, 4.5 grams or less of saturated fat, and less than 95 mg cholesterol in a serving.

**Extra lean**—Less than 5 grams fat, less than 2 grams saturated fat, and less than 95 mg cholesterol in a serving.

*Words that mean the same thing as free: "no," "zero," "without," "trivial source of," "negligible source of," and "dietarily insignificant source of."
**Words that mean the same thing as low: "contains a small amount of" and "low source of."

## RECOMMENDED AMOUNTS OF SATURATED FAT AND TOTAL FAT

**If you eat this many calories a day . . .**

| Calories | 1,200 | 1,500 | 1,800 | 2,000 | 2,500 |
|---|---|---|---|---|---|

**. . . This is the recommended amount of fat for each day:**

| | 1,200 | 1,500 | 1,800 | 2,000 | 2,500 |
|---|---|---|---|---|---|
| Saturated Fat*, in grams | 12 | 15 | 18 | 20 | 25 |
| Total Fat**, in grams | 40 | 50 | 60 | 65 | 80 |

*Amounts are equal to 9 percent of total calories; the recommendation is to eat less than 10 percent of total calories as saturated fat. Remember, 1 gram of fat is equal to 9 calories.

**Amounts are equal to 30 percent of total calories (rounded down to the nearest 5); the recommendation is to eat this much or less.

Note: On average, women consume about 1,800 calories a day and men consume about 2,500 calories a day.

Source: "Facts about Blood Cholesterol," National Heart, Lung, and Blood Institute, NIH Publication No. 94–2696, August 1994.

# Index

www.ingramcontent.com/pod-product-compliance
Lightning Source LLC
Chambersburg PA
CBHW061338210326

41598CB00035B/5816